MEASUREMENT in PHYSICAL THERAPY

CLINICS IN PHYSICAL THERAPY
VOLUME 7

MEASUREMENT in PHYSICAL THERAPY

Edited by

Jules M. Rothstein, Ph.D., P.T.

Assistant Professor of Physical Therapy
School of Allied Health Professions
Medical College of Virginia
Virginia Commonwealth University
Richmond, Virginia

CHURCHILL LIVINGSTONE
NEW YORK, EDINBURGH, LONDON, MELBOURNE
1985

Acquisitions editor: Kim Loretucci
Copy editor: Margot Otway
Production designer: Michiko Davis
Production supervisor: Eileen Ziegman
Compositor: Maryland Composition Company, Inc.
Printer/Binder: The Maple-Vail Book Manufacturing Group

Distributed in the United Kingdom by Churchill Livingstone, Robert
Stevenson House, 1–3 Baxter's Place, Leith Walk, Edinburgh EH1
3AF and by associated companies, branches and representatives
throughout the world.

First published 1985

Printed in the U.S.A.

ISBN 0-443-08282-0

9 8 7 6 5 4 3 2 1

Library of Congress Cataloging-in-Publication Data
Main entry under title:

Measurement in physical therapy.

   (Clinics in physical therapy ; v. 7)
   Includes bibliographies and index.
   1. Physical therapy—Measurement. 2. Function
tests (Medicine) I. Rothstein, Jules M. II. Series.
[DNLM: 1. Biometry. 2. Diagnosis. 3. Physical
Therapy. W1 CL831CN v. 7 / WB 460 M484]
RM701.M39   1985   615.8′2′0287   85-17398
ISBN 0-443-08282-0

Manufactured in the United States of America

To those who ask questions,
to those who have the strength to seek answers,
and most of all to those who have the courage to learn, to change, and to
grow

Contributors

Suzann K. Campbell, Ph.D., P.T.
Professor of Physical Therapy, Department of Medical Allied Health Professions, University of North Carolina at Chapel Hill School of Medicine, Chapel Hill, North Carolina

Rebecca L. Craik, Ph.D., P.T.
Assistant Professor of Physical Therapy, Beaver College, Glenside, Pennsylvania

John L. Echternach, Ed.D., P.T.
Professor and Chairman, Department of Community Health Professions, and Director, Program in Physical Therapy, Old Dominion University, Norfolk, Virginia

Ali A. Ehsani, M.D.
Associate Director of Medicine and Preventive Medicine, and Director, Cardiac Rehabilitation Program, Irene Walter Johnson Institute of Rehabilitation, Washington University School of Medicine, St. Louis, Missouri

Alan M. Jette, Ph.D., P.T.
Associate Professor of Gerontology and Physical Therapy, Institute of Health Professions, Massachusetts General Hospital; Lecturer, Department of Social Medicine and Health Policy, Harvard Medical School, Boston, Massachusetts

Robert L. Lamb, Ph.D., P.T.
Associate Professor of Physical Therapy, and Director of Graduate Studies, School of Allied Health Professions, Medical College of Virginia, Virginia Commonwealth University, Richmond, Virginia

Thomas P. Mayhew, M.S., P.T.
Doctoral Student, Department of Physical Therapy, School of Allied Health Professions, and Department of Anatomy, School of Basic Sciences, Medical College of Virginia, Virginia Commonwealth University, Richmond, Virginia

Peter J. Miller, M.S., P.T.
Supervisor, Edwardsville Physical Therapy and Sports Medicine Clinic, Professional Physical Therapy, Inc., Edwardsville, Illinois

Carol A. Oatis, Ph.D., P.T.
Partner, Philadelphia Institute for Physical Therapy, Philadelphia, Pennsylvania

Elizabeth J. Protas, Ph.D., P.T.
Associate Professor and Coordinator of Graduate Programs, School of Physical Therapy, Texas Women's University, Houston, Texas

Jules M. Rothstein, Ph.D., P.T.
Assistant Professor of Physical Therapy, School of Allied Health Professions, Medical College of Virginia, Virginia Commonwealth University, Richmond, Virginia

David R. Sinacore, M.H.S., P.T.
Instructor, Program in Physical Therapy, and Staff Member, Cardiac Rehabilitation Program, Irene Walter Johnson Institute of Rehabilitation, Washington University School of Medicine, St. Louis, Missouri

Foreword

At the outset of this foreword, I wish to state that it is high time that a book such as this has become available in physical therapy and for physical therapists.

As an *aficionado* of the measurement literature in other fields for at least the last dozen years, and as a former practitioner—a long time ago—for fourteen years, I have often wished retrospectively that my wits in measurement had been challenged in my early years in the clinic, if not during my student days. Thanks to the remarkable endeavor by Jules Rothstein, the work of other contributors to this book, and the interest of the publisher, physical therapists who are engaged in practice, and others whose primary pursuit is teaching, research, or learning, will be able to use this book to challenge their wits in measurement.

Measurement is the *sine qua non* for effective practice in physical therapy. Without measurement, there can be no effective practice. This brief statement is not merely an article of faith, to be taken for granted and applied unquestioningly in practice. For practice to be effective, one must demonstrate and document its effectiveness. To demonstrate and document effectiveness, one must measure. If the reliability of the measurement has not been demonstrated, the measurement may not be valid. If the validity of the measurement has not been demonstrated, the *use* to which one puts the results of the measurement (for example, planning a treatment program, claiming improvement after treatment, or predicting performance of some other important activity) *may be flawed*.

The brief paragraph above is but a hint of what this book is all about, namely, that there is much more to measurement in physical therapy than methods or how to do measurements of various kinds. Knowing the methods of measurement is necessary for effective practice but it is not enough. This book is a major contribution to what else the physical therapist needs to know and think about.

One thing this book cannot be is the "final word" on what else the physical therapist needs to know and think about in measurement. I know the editor and the contributors well enough to be confident that they would agree with me on this point. The reader is urged to read the editor's preface, especially the last paragraph, and to think seriously about the invitation and challenge posed there.

This book is an excellent start on measurement as a serious, intellectual area in the practice of physical therapy. Taking up the editor's call, I urge all who take this book in hand to let it be a start of the dialogue, the constructive criticism, and the thinking he invites.

Even though I may disagree with a point here or there in a careful study of the full text, a foreword is not the proper place to join in intellectual debate. Do as I will do. Read the book. Think about it. Use it as a frequent reference. And track down the ideas you find in it—get to their base. Then think about how to improve the measurement done in physical therapy. That, finally, is what the book is all about.

Eugene Michels
Associate Executive Director
Research and Education
American Physical Therapy Association

Preface

First, I want to express my appreciation to anyone who reads this preface, let alone the rest of the volume. Physical therapists who use this volume are doing something their colleagues have never been able to do before—systematically examining the quality of the measurements that form the basis for our clinical judgments and the foundation of our science. This is not a "how-to" book, but rather a "why-to" book. The reader will not be shown how to take measurements; instead, the authors will discuss the purpose and value of measurements. Within this volume we raise fundamental questions about the nature of our practice. This book, as difficult as it was to produce, was in many ways a labor of love on the part of the contributors and the editor, because we share the belief that these fundamental questions must be asked.

The first outline for this book called for more chapters than appear here. For example, we wanted to include chapters on orthopedic assessment and on the evaluation of the neurological patient. The reason those chapters are missing is because we lack a body of scientific knowledge dealing with measurement in those areas. Many techniques have been described in the literature, but few of them have been examined scientifically. The problem is not an isolated one. The chapter on gait assessment is an interesting example. Although the emphasis of this book is primarily on the practical aspects of clinical measurement, that chapter is forced to discuss theoretical rather than practical considerations, because we have no systematic means of assessing gait clinically. As a result, the theoretical issues raised in the gait chapter are presented so that they can guide the clinicians in thinking about what they will choose to measure, and what we will need if we are to ever have a satisfactory means of evaluating gait clinically.

As readers will notice as they progress through this volume, the state of measurement is highly variable. We have some excellent tools, and some really questionable methods. In the past there has been no source that examines which tools and methods are better documented than others. More troublesome is our observation that there has been a tendency to use assessment procedures because they were available, not necessarily because they were reliable and valid.

Very few entry-level programs in physical therapy prepare students to critically analyze the measurements they will use in clinical practice. Measurement science is a rarity in entry-level curricula. The prerequisites for measurements—reliability and validity—are often described in the context of research and ignored in courses geared toward clinicians. We feel that this orientation is misguided. The heart of our profession is clinical practice; therefore, we have great concern for the quality of measurements used to guide clinical decision making.

The incredible work that went into compiling this volume was made bearable because we believe therapists must critically examine the way they assess patients. We believe therapists must be able to discuss the quality of the measurement tools they are using. That is one reason why the reader of this volume is to be congratulated, because although the topic is important, the material is not easily understood.

With the exception of the first chapter, the chapters review the literature that describes specific types of tests. Chapter 1 is provided for the reader who has had no training in measurement theory. Basic concepts, such as operational definitions, reliability, and validity, are explained. In addition, some of the statistics referred to throughout the book are described in Chapter 1. Readers who are unfamiliar with measurement theory and basic statistics are urged to read the first chapter before proceeding through the book.

Our profession has shown remarkable progress because therapists have been willing to face the need to change and to grow. We hope that this book will contribute to that growth.

As editor I want to express my heartfelt appreciation to the contributors. They were asked to do what no one else has ever done before. This meant that they had little precedent and had to rely on disorganized and fragmented bodies of literature in preparing their chapters. Their products were improved by a collection of reviewers who assisted the editor in making suggestions for the chapters. Some of these reviewers were also chapter authors, and I want to express special thanks to them, especially to Robert Lamb who was always willing to check one more thing out—until he had checked everything out. Despite their assistance, I am sure that a few errors still remain. I hope they are more random than systematic.

I also wish to thank all of those whose assistance made this book possible. The following people assisted in the review process; Robert Lamb, Neil Spielholz, Gary Soderberg, Leo Selker, Otto Payton, Jan Tecklin, Ann VanSant, Elizabeth Protas, Nora Donahue, and Alan Jette. Illustrations and photographs were contributed by Ann VanSant, Fred Langschultz, and Katie Hudson. Manuscripts were prepared by Valeria Norville, Madeline Bliley, Marilyn Rothstein, Jill Mayhew, Nancy Knowles, and Laura Spittle. Present and former students assisted by proofreading, searching for references, and performing assorted chores. These students are Barbara Vorwald, Sheryl Gilbertson, Patti Kohne, Denise Calvin, Barbara Lemmel, Daniel Riddle, Martha Walker, and Heidi Welti. I also want to thank all of the many students who have helped me by doing what students do best—asking questions. The questions helped me clarify my thinking.

Steven Wolf and Otto Payton deserve special commendation for appreciating the need for this volume and for encouraging its creation. Most of all

I want to thank my family for accepting this intrusion into their lives. My wife Marilyn not only tolerated the endless piles of papers and a man possessed, but she also managed to help edit. My children did more than put up with the distraction. Katherine proved that she was a superb typist who could conquer a computer and Jessica managed to keep her endless artwork off of the more important manuscript pages. This volume was made possible by the loving support of my family, for that and for so much more, I am forever indebted to them.

Lastly, I wish to thank someone who will not be able to read this foreword, my father. His illness introduced me to physical therapy. Although this book promotes the scientific approach to patient care, the memory of his courage reminds me to state my belief that science must be combined with caring if physical therapists are to properly serve their patients.

This volume is offered to the reader. I eagerly await your judgments on the many controversial topics discussed here. The contributors and I hope that this book will stimulate dialogue. If readers believe that we have erred, we hope they will let us know. No greater compliment can be paid to this volume than for therapists to become so concerned with measurement that they make this text obsolete. A future edition should be more complete and should reflect recent advances in our profession. I look forward to the day when this book may be revised, though I suspect the task will try the will and patience of the contributors and family members alike. I hope we get the chance to see if we can survive it.

Jules M. Rothstein, Ph.D., P.T.

Contents

MEASUREMENT in PHYSICAL THERAPY

1 | Measurement and Clinical Practice: Theory and Application

Jules M. Rothstein

The debate continues as to what is the rightful role of the physical therapist. Changing times and changing roles must lead to a reexamination of traditional patterns of practice and professional preparation. Central to this process must be a consideration of how we assess our patients, both in terms of their initial status and in terms of how patients are affected by treatment. Without a scientific basis for the assessment (and measurement) process, we face the future as independent practitioners unable to communicate with one another, unable to document treatment efficacy, and unable to claim scientific credibility for our profession. Physical therapy, like medicine and law, will always remain partially an art, but without measurement it can be nothing more than an art. However, not all clinicians need concern themselves with considerations of the quality of measurements. Older models of practice persist in which therapists apply various modalities (including exercise) because authorities, namely, physicians, have requested specific treatments. For therapists unable to break out of this antiquated technician's role, measurement and assessment is irrelevant, as is professional status. On the other hand, therapists who plan treatment must be able to justify their decisions and discuss the quality of measurements.

The first step toward knowing whether a treatment is appropriate is defining the patient's problems; this is primarily the task of the patient. However,

1

after the patient's problems have been identified, the therapist must then, through an interview and an examination, generate hypotheses as to why the problems exist. Why can't the patient walk without circumducting? Why can't the shoulder flex more than 40°? Only after hypotheses have been generated can therapists generate treatment plans. A treatment plan without hypotheses suggests that therapists may not be treating a specific patient who has a unique combination of signs, symptoms, and functional deficits, but rather a stereotypical condition they learned of in school or in some course. Therapists who engage in such a practice may not realize that they also need not consider the assessment process, because measurements have not really been used to formulate a treatment strategy. Therapists who engage in practice by unproven protocol are really not very different from the technicians who are guided by physician edict.

Unless a therapist uses assessment tools (i.e., measurement) to generate treatment plans, and unless a therapist controls the treatment, the consideration of the scientific value of measurements may be nothing more than an academic exercise. However, when therapists contend that they are practitioners who evaluate and then design treatments accordingly, they must consider the basis for that procedure. Similarly, if therapists want to claim efficacy for their practice, they are totally dependent on the quality of the measurements used to show change in their patients. As more and more therapists have adopted the role of assessors and treatment planners, as well as that of treatment givers, it is ironic that they have not been more concerned with the measurements that justify this role.[1]

The training of therapists often focuses on evaluation and treatment, two critically important elements in modern practice, but little consideration is given to the quality of measurements that are used in evaluative procedures.[1] Those who are proud of their ability to assess patients and to plan treatments must justify their methods. We must ask whether our measurement techniques really yield information, or whether they merely give the *illusion* of clinical data. If I can see or feel spasticity in a patient but a colleague cannot, have I really determined anything about a patient? If I feel a mobile left sacroiliac joint but a colleague cannot, can I justify a treatment based on what is real to me, but is illusion for my peer? These are issues of *reliability*. If I say that my patient is unable to walk because of a weak quadriceps and a colleague says that she has seen a thousand patients who have equal quadriceps "strength" walk, am I justified in a program of quadriceps strengthening? Or, are we justified in saying that weakness causes postural defects simply because a colleague says that weakness causes postural problems? This second group of issues deals with *validity*, or what we can legitimately infer from our measurements.

In the jargon of measurement theory, we say that unless measurements are shown to be valid and reliable they do not yield *information*, but rather numbers or categories that give a false impression of meaningfulness. Measurements can give the impression of science and precision, but unless someone has demonstrated that these measurements truly convey information (i.e., they have reliability and validity) they may actually mislead us.

The purpose of this chapter is to discuss measurement theory as it relates to clinical practice. Much of this chapter will focus on reliability and validity, their definitions, their various forms, and their importance to clinical practice. Another section reviews the classification schemes used to categorize various "levels of measurement." These classification schemes are clinically relevant because many clinicians, as well as clinical reports in our journals, ignore the fundamental limitations associated with the various levels of measurement and, as a result, have reached some rather dubious conclusions. Only by knowing the classification schemes and their limitations can clinicians avoid misuse of measurements.

Although it is beyond the scope of this chapter to serve as a statistics text, a third section will include a discussion of some of the statistical procedures used for the analysis of measurements (for the establishment of reliability, validity, and normative data). Concepts underlying the various statistical approaches rather than the mathematical principles will be emphasized.

TERMS AND CONCEPTS

Operational Definitions

Before something can be measured, it must be defined. A definition that guides one through the process of measurement is called an operational definition because it specifies the procedures (operations) used in taking measurements.[2] For an operational definition to have any utility for clinical practice, it must have two qualities: (1) universality—specifically the ability to be understood and used by all similarly trained people; and (2) sound theoretical assumptions.

The need for operational definitions is clear when we consider the measurement of such things as tone, strength, or sitting balance. In research papers, it is considered obligatory for the authors to identify the means they use to measure their variables. Therefore, at least theoretically, all papers dealing with strength or tone should contain operational definitions of the terms used. However, it should be remembered that such definitions are really the author's way of saying that the definition is applicable only in terms of that paper and the measurement systems available to that author. Because authors define terms and methods primarily in the context of their own studies, there can be limitations to their conclusions. For example, both Fowler and Gardner[3] and DeLateur and Giaconi[4] examined the "strength" of patients with muscular dystrophy. In the title of both articles, the word "strength" appeared, and measurement of strength was an essential feature of the studies. However, Fowler and Gardner measured strength with either a cable tensiometer or a hand-grip dynamometer, whereas DeLateur and Giaconi measured strength with an isokinetic dynamometer. Did both sets of investigators measure the same quality? That is a researchable question. The important issue is that unless there is an operational definition that is similar to the definition that we use clinically, we must be cautious in generalizing from the literature.

In clinical practice, we do not often ask each other to define terms operationally, although we should do so. If a colleague reports that a patient has increased "tone," can we really understand the term without knowing the operational definition that the colleague used? The therapist could have assessed resistance to passive movement,[5] the vigor of the deep tendon reflex,[6] or may have made a judgment based on the way in which the patient moved.[7] It is clear that we lack the first requirement for an operational definition: universality. A lack of universality exists because we, as a profession, and others interested in the issue of tone do not agree upon the theoretical assumptions that would lead to the development of one method of measurement.

A discussion of the two requirements for operational definitions naturally leads to a consideration of reliability and validity. Universality of use is really a reliability issue, whereas theoretical soundness is a validity issue. However, there is one other point that must be considered before these two topics can be considered. Measurement, especially in clinical practice, should be purposeful because therapists are attempting to assess some important or relevant characteristics in a patient. Some of these characteristics are global, such as the inability to locomote (see Ch. 6) and sometimes they are focal, such as the capability of muscle to contribute to the development of forces (see Ch. 2). In both of the above cases, the reason why the therapist might want to measure these qualities may be obvious, but that is not always the case.

A Brunnstrom-oriented[8] therapist may have an entirely different reason for assessing a patient's domination by primitive reflexes than does a Bobath-oriented therapist.[9,10] However, if they both claim to assess the same qualities, albeit for different reasons, they should share the same operational definitions. If they do not, communication is chaotic, and therefore meaningful assessment of clinical practice is impossible.

Therefore, without an operational definition, no measurement can be made. Stevens, one of the founders of modern measurement theory, put it most succinctly when he said, "In its broadest sense, measurement is the assignment of numerals to objects or events according to rules."[11] In this chapter, we will accept the expanded version of that concept, which also considers categorization (or classification) as a form of measurement.[11–13] Whether we assign numerals or categorical names to a performance or a characteristic, we are measuring. However, unless we do this according to rules governed by operational definitions we are *not* measuring.[2]

Clinically, we must assess many aspects of our patients, and ideally we should measure these characteristics (variables). In reality, however, we cannot always accomplish our aims. Clinicians are then faced with the task of knowing when they are obtaining measurements and when they are making decisions based only on "clinical impressions." To deny a role for clinical impressions at this stage of our profession's development would lead to a paralysis of practice, but to require a differentiation between impressions and *measurements* lays the ground work for the development of scientific practice.

Clinicians may find it useful to ask themselves whether they have operational definitions for the things they assess, e.g., gait, activities of daily living (ADL), or movement characteristics, or whether they are forming clinical impressions. Clinicians might also find it useful to ask colleagues if they share these operational definitions.

RELIABILITY

The two main prerequisites of a measurement, reliability and validity, are difficult to differentiate because they are conceptually interdependent. Therefore, any discussion of either requires some definitions and considerations that apply to both. It is most important that we review our purposes for measuring things. Although measurement is an attempt to place quantitative or qualitative labels on a variety of characteristics, in applied professions such as physical therapy, measurement is much more. In Galenic times, it might have seemed appropriate to develop measurement systems for the vital, natural, and animal spirits[14] because they were of central interest to the physicians of that day. Today, any health practitioner who proposed to measure the "spirits" would gain more infamy than recognition. Why can something be worth measuring (or attempting to measure) in one period of time, but be totally irrelevant in another? Physicists may want to measure anything and everything simply because, like Everest, it is there. The task of those scientists is to describe the world. In clinical practice, it is presumed that we measure because the information garnered helps us make decisions regarding treatment, prognostication, or referral.

Because clinical physical therapists are highly purposeful in the need to measure, we can agree that the element that is being assessed has great practical significance. For example, when we want to know if loss of motion is responsible for a patient's inability to perform a functional task, e.g., walking, we measure the motion of a relevant limb segment. If that measurement is to help us in our inquiry, we must be sure that the numbers obtained, in terms of degrees of motion, really reflect the item of interest, i.e., joint motion. In both research and in measurement theory, we call the item of interest, or the thing that we are measuring, a variable.[15] Measurement is actually the process of quantifying aspects of variables. Clinical assessment is the process of looking for changes in variables (i.e., do we change anything with our treatments or are we making our patients better?).

Reliability is basically the consistency of a measurement.[15–17] Implied in this rather simple definition is that consistency will be present when all conditions, to the best of the measurer's knowledge, are held constant. Because we attempt to quantify variables, we are hoping that all changes in obtained measurement reflect changes in the item of interest. When measurement systems do not yield reliable results, we say that measurements reflect not only true variability (true variance), but also some error (error variance).[15]

Reliability can only be fully appreciated when we keep in mind why we are measuring things and what the measurement will tell us. Consider the following examples.

A usually friendly patient once arrived for treatment in a rather gruff mood and told the following possibly apocryphal story. He had been out fishing the previous, cold September day, and after several hours of casting from his boat, he had many fish that he thought were of legal size. Much to his dismay and financial pain, he realized that he was mistaken when a game warden pulled alongside and proceeded to measure the fish. Most were indeed legal, but some were not. The patient was at a loss to explain his predicament. He had measured each and every fish as he caught it, using a metal yardstick affixed to the stern of the boat. The variable of interest, both to the fisherman and the game warden, was length, yet measurement error had somehow crept into the process, leading to a fine for violation of game laws. How did it happen? Most likely the metal yardstick had been a little shorter earlier in the day as a result of the cold; at day's end it was longer, after having been exposed to the sun's rays. The problem was not a wanton disregard of game laws by the patient, but a failure to appreciate how the coefficient of linear expansion could account for measurement error.[18] The same fish, measured at different times during that day, would have been assigned different length values, and different decisions might have been made regarding whether the fish could be kept.

A source of variability (variance) was present when the patient measured his fish, a source that was not known or accounted for by the process of measurement; therefore, it was a source of error variance. As a result of error variance, the measurement of length was not reliable. Had the patient appreciated the role of temperature on his measurement device (the yardstick), he could have made corrections for this element and eliminated this source of error variance. This fishing example also demonstrates how reliability relates to accuracy. Length has a rather precise operational definition attached to it. Standards for length are maintained by the International Bureau of Weights and Measures.[18] Had a nonvariable standard been available for comparison, the fisherman could have checked his measurements and determined inaccuracies.

When measurements are precisely defined and accuracy is obtained, only one value is possible; therefore, reliability is guaranteed. If a measurement is accurate, it must be reliable: however, consistent errors can lead to reliability (consistency) in measurement. Had the yardstick been inappropriately marked but resistant to temperature changes, the patient would have made reliable measurements (in that they all would have agreed when the variable was the same) but they would have been inaccurate. The patient still may have made the wrong judgment; that is, based on the measurements made, he would have kept illegal fish. That, however, is an issue of validity.

A second example demonstrates the complexity of the issue of reliability and the ways in which it can be threatened by inexplicable changes in the variable of interest. A therapist may see a patient who has undergone a total hip arthroplasty the day before, and need to know whether that patient will have sufficient upper extremity "strength" for ambulation. The therapist may use a manual muscle test to determine the strength of the triceps brachii muscles bilaterally. Based on the finding of grades below "fair," the therapist may decide to initiate a triceps exercise program. This judgment may seem vindicated if several days later the muscle test grades prove greater than "good" bilaterally. However, there are many problems with this judgment.

Can such patients be reliably assessed for "muscle strength" one day after surgery? Does such a measurement really reflect muscle performance or general health, the presence or absence of pain medications, or even the anemia that may exist after such surgery? And, therefore, is the change in the muscle grade really related to a change in *muscle* or does it reflect general health status, decreased pain, or the fact that the patient may have had a transfusion? Although these issues border closely on the subject of validity (was the inference about the triceps correct?), they are also relevant to reliability. Each of these elements, and many more, can vary independently of triceps capability and can, therefore, lead to changes in muscle test values that have nothing to do with the muscle. All of these elements can contribute to error variance in the measurement of "triceps strength" and are, therefore, threats to reliability.

There may be a temptation on the part of the functionally oriented clinician to consider the above concern irrelevant because the genuine issue is whether the patient can use the triceps. Had the muscle test been used in terms of some type of global assessment, all of the factors mentioned would have been part of the variable being measured and would have not contributed error to the measurement process. However, since the measurement presumed to *focus* only on the triceps, the factors did contribute to error. The problem occurs because the conclusions drawn lead to a treatment (focal exercise) that was not necessarily justified by the measurement.

A third example will reveal another source of error variance. Let us imagine that a therapist is attempting to assess whether a patient is independent in wheelchair use. The first time the therapist assesses this skill, he or she is rushed; there is a line of patients waiting for attention, and the therapist briskly asks the patient to lock his wheelchair brakes, waits 15 seconds and then concludes the patient cannot perform the task. The second time that the therapist assesses the same skill in the patient there is no rush; perhaps the department is fully staffed that day. The therapist carefully explains what the patient is to do and then waits 30 seconds. During that time the patient locks the wheelchair brakes. The patient's true skill or independence in wheelchair activities may have been the same on both occasions. Error was introduced to the measurement because of a lack of standardization in the testing procedure. Had an accepted measurement protocol (operational definition) been present and rigidly adhered to, the results of both testing sessions might have been the same.

The three examples described demonstrate the different factors that can threaten reliability. In the case of the fisherman, the measurement tool itself was flawed; it could not yield consistent results. In the second case, the inability to obtain consistent results reflecting the variable of interest had to do with the type of patient being tested. In the last example, the problem arose because of a failure on the part of the tester. What makes all these examples so clear-cut is the omniscience that our hypothetical examples permit us. In the real world, we can never be sure whether any or all of these three factors are contributing error to our measurements unless we conduct serial experiments designed to examine each element.

In summary, the three elements that may be the sources of error that make tests unreliable are:

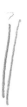

1.   Inherent flaws in instrumentation (this may even include bias in paper and pencil tests);
2.   An inherent lack of consistency in the variable of interest in the type of patient being examined; and
3.   Errors made by those persons taking the measurement.

Of these three factors, therapists may have the most difficulty understanding the second, which relates to the type of individual being tested. A biologist might want to know the length of some single-celled organism seen under a microscope; but who would attempt to measure the length of a living amoeba? Descriptions of posture are also frequently used by physical therapists. But who would attempt a postural assessment of a patient with athetosis? Some measurements as applied to some patients may reflect situations that are momentary events and are therefore useless for the purpose of making judgments because they are so labile that we don't know what they reflect. The lack of reliability inherent in such measurements is really the issue.

One reason to question the use of manual muscle testing (MMT) for the patient with damage to the central nervous system (CNS) is the lability of such measurements in this type of patient.[19] Many non-"muscular" factors, such as the release of primitive reflexes, can affect MMT measurements in such patients.[10,20] Therefore, the use of MMT for the CNS patient has been questioned from a standpoint of validity. Can such measurements really reflect muscle function? Because many of the factors that affect MMT grades in the CNS patient vary in ways that cannot be accounted for by the measurement process (e.g., autonomic excitation);[20] however, we must also question the use of MMT for CNS patients on the basis of whether such measurements can be reliably attained.

Population-Specific Reliability

Some measurements may be reliably obtained on some people but not on others. Population-specific reliability can only be demonstrated through research. We can imagine that there might be reliability of quadriceps torque measurements in healthy subjects when these measurements are made with an isokinetic dynamometer,[21] but can patients with knee pathologies be reliably measured? The presence of pain, which can vary independently of muscle "strength," can be a source of error in such measurements.

Fowler and Gardner[3] in a study describing measurement of the "strength" of muscular dystrophy patients by means of a cable tensiometer, reported reliability coefficients of 0.87 and 0.98 on normal subjects (from other studies). Then, however, they examined the reliability of their measurements on two different subcategories of patients with dystrophy. This reliability investigation may be contrasted to the approach of DeLateur and Giaconi, who also tested patients with muscular dystrophy.[4] These investigators never discussed the issue of the reliability of their measurement (isokinetic torque) as it was applied to their population.

We can also imagine how we can reliably measure the range of motion (ROM) on some patients and for some joints, because placement of the goniometer is relatively easy (see Ch. 4 for a full discussion). However, can we assume equal reliability when measuring deformed joints, when measuring patients who cannot be positioned correctly, or when measuring joints that allow for only small arcs of movement?

Reliability studies that demonstrate the consistency of a measurement must, therefore, describe the type of patients studied. For the clinician to be assured of reliability, the sample in the study must be clinically relevant. Often there is a failure on the part of researchers to consider the importance of population-specific reliability. Consider the report of Frost et al. dealing with the use of linear measurements to assess spinal range of motion.[22] To participate in the study, subjects had to have had no recent history of back pain. The authors apparently wanted to eliminate pain as a source of error variance. Although this is an admirable goal, the study essentially examined the reliability of a measurement as it was applied to a group that would almost never be measured in clinical practice. Had the authors reported the method to be generally reliable, which they did not, what would it have meant? From the study, we could not have concluded that the measurement was reliable for the patients in whom we most want to measure spinal motion.

Reliability studies cannot realistically be carried out on every imaginable patient population with every instrument used by therapists for measurement. We must consider how closely a sample mirrors a patient population before we can assume that a measurement will be reliable for that population.

Clinicians must know how reliable any given test is and on what types of patients its reliability was assessed. Clinicians, based on their knowledge of patients (e.g., pathologies, behavioral factors), must then judge whether the reliability demonstrated for one group of patients can be assumed to exist for another group of patients. Such assumptions can only be fully justified or invalidated through research.

Population-specific reliability, then, is the degree of reliability that a test has for a specific group being measured. There is a second form of population-specific reliability that must be considered, but in this case the "population" refers to the type of people taking measurements. We would not expect a random sample of people drawn from the general population to be able to measure reliably the ROM of the knee joint. We might expect a random sample of physical therapists to be able to measure ROM of the knee reliably (see Ch.

4). We assume that physical therapists by virtue of their training have the necessary skills either to replicate their own measurements (intra-tester reliability) or someone else's measurements (inter-tester reliability). We assume that all physical therapists are relatively equal in this ability.

The practice of physical therapy includes many different kinds of tests. Some do not seem to require vast amounts of experience or special training. Others may only be reliable with special training or repeated clinical practice. Many of the manual therapy tests that involve palpation skills are probably in the latter category. In seeking information about the reliability of such tests, clinicians must ask: Has reliability been established? Two more questions then become relevant. What types of patients have been examined? What was the level of training of the therapists who performed the evaluation?

Measurement tools, including questionnnaires (such as ADL instruments), are frequently developed in large clinical research centers. General reliability cannot reasonably be assessed in such settings. Therapists with special knowledge of a measurement device or system (e.g., they helped to develop it or are in communication with the developers) are different from the average therapist. When only specialized personnel are involved in establishing the reliability of an instrument, it can be assumed that only those expert users of the test can obtain reliable measurements. For us to make generalizations of reliability to the average user of a measurement device, appropriate studies that involve typical test users must be conducted.

Types of Reliability

We have previously defined reliability as the consistency of a measurement when all conditions are thought to be held constant. The argument was made that only when measurements do not randomly vary can obtained values or assigned categories possibly reflect the variable of interest. Non-random errors are also possible, but since they are systematic, correction factors can be applied to derive true measurements. Reliability must therefore be considered in terms of specific conditions. There are four types of reliability that can be described:[15-17]

1. Intra-tester reliability or stability over time;
2. Inter-tester reliability or stability between examiners;
3. Parallel forms of reliability, that is, whether different forms of the same test (or two different types of instruments) yield the same results; and
4. Internal consistency, that is, whether parts of a single test (or examination) that are designed to test the same element yield similar results.

Each of these forms has applicability to physical therapy and must be considered.

Intra-Tester Reliability.   Although intra-tester reliability appears simple to understand, some rather complex issues are associated with it. In essence, intra-tester reliability is assessed by having the same person measure the same thing on different occasions. The relationship between these multiple measures of the same thing is commonly assessed with a correlation coefficient. Statistical methods will be discussed later in this chapter. Because one person performs the multiple measurements, a period of time must elapse between test sessions, and this type of reliability, therefore, reflects stability over time.

Measurements that do not have intra-tester reliability can be considered so full of error as to be useless because the numbers obtained do not reflect the variable being measured.[15] Clinicians should remember that error means variability (changes) in obtained values that cannot be accounted for by the measurement protocol being used. Therefore, we do not know what the measurement really reflects. Threats to intra-tester reliability are caused by the same three factors previously described: the instrument, the person administering the test, and the characteristics of the subjects being tested.

A major concern in determining acceptable levels of intra-tester reliability deals with the time interval between the successive tests that are used to produce the measurements used for comparisons. For example, if we wished to know whether ROM measurements were reliable, how much time should elapse between the taking of the two measurements to be compared? There is no single answer and clinical judgments will have to be used. Let us imagine that in a clinic we find that we usually measure patients' hip motions over a two-month period. Because this is the standard clinical practice, it would be useful to establish whether ROM measurements vary meaningfully over that period of time. Let us also imagine that we have determined that normal subjects measured with a two-month inter-test interval have an average of 20° difference in the paired measurements. This information would tell us that under the best of circumstances (i.e., testing of normal subjects whose motion is not expected to change), we would see a variability of ± 20°. Therefore, in terms of patients, any changes less than that amount could be considered to be a function of error. Only changes in excess of 20° could be assumed to be actual changes.

Because intra-tester reliability studies should deal with patient groups, use of long inter-test intervals is problematic because disease can change the variable over time. Some reliability studies even have multiple measurements taken during the same patient visit.[23] Although this does establish some reliability for a measurement, it does not describe how stable the measured element is *over time*. Therefore, intra-tester reliability has two unique aspects: one deals with whether a single examiner can replicate results and the other with whether time can significantly change measurements. Both of these, however, can clearly be affected by the three common threats to reliability (that of the instrument, the tester, and the subject tested).

Sometimes intra-tester reliability is almost impossible to evaluate in a reasonable manner. In goniometric studies, we have "blinded the goniometer" so that a single therapist taking multiple measurements cannot know what values were obtained.[23] However, when sitting balance or accessory motions of patients is assessed or when a variety of other tests are performed, it is almost impossible for a therapist's second measurement not to be influenced by his first measurement. Another problem relates to whether the very process of measuring for the first time affects the element being measured. However, it is generally agreed that if all subjects change similarly between first and second measurements, a test should be considered reliable because the change is sytematic, i.e., free of random error.[16] Users of such tests should appreciate, however, that with serial (i.e., repeated) testing of the same patients, successive measurements may be too high or too low. The problem then is one of interpretation of measurement, not merely an issue of reliability.

In general, clinicians should consider reliability assessments, and especially intra-tester reliability estimates, as tools that can be used to understand a fundamental quality of any measurement. Measurements are used to make judgments (or valid inferences), and unless we know how much error is associated with a measurement, approporiate inferences are impossible. One-way reliability can be viewed is as an index of the fallibility of a measurement. There is no single or standard that states what levels of reliability are acceptable. Rather it is up to every person who uses measurements to interpret those measurements in view of the reliability associated with them. The more reliable a measurement, the more certain we can be in our judgments based upon it.

Inter-Tester Reliability.   When different people obtain measurements of the same thing, they should agree. The assessment of this level of agreement provides an index of inter-tester reliability. There are several reasons why this form of reliability is especially important in clinical practice. In some settings, different therapists may be called upon to measure the same patient at different times. If therapists do not routinely agree with each other when measuring the same thing, such procedures could lead to illusory results. Patients may be thought to be improving or regressing when in fact the differences in obtained values result in part from errors in measurement (i.e., a failure of therapists to agree).

Even when different therapists do not usually measure the same patient, inter-tester reliability becomes important. If clinical information is to be shared in a meaningful fashion, we must know whether the information (i.e., measurements) that we are sharing represents the same phenomenon. For example, a clinician reports that a procedure increases ROM 15° in a given type of patient. However, unless we can reasonably assume that we measure in the same way he did (i.e., we would expect the same numbers), we cannot really expect an equal treatment effect. Assessment of the quality of care often involves determining whether desired outcomes have been achieved. Such outcomes can only be quantified through measurement. For this process to be worthwhile, we must know whether therapists are actually measuring the same thing in the same way.

By knowing the amount of error associated with inter-tester reliability, measurements can be more appropriately used. Beekman and Hall demonstrated considerable variability in inter-tester agreement on the assessment of the degree of scoliosis as seen on a spinal roentgenograms.[24] Even though the two raters were trained physicians, they only agreed on the side of the curvature 80 percent of the time and on the location of the curve (± 2 levels) 70 percent of the time. A mean difference of 4.2° was observed between the two raters when they attempted to measure the curves. The conclusion drawn by Beekman and Hall[24] shows how useful it is to know the error associated with a measurement:

> Because of these findings, 4 degrees was chosen as the criterion for assessing whether lateral spinal curvature has changed in our study on the effects of an exercise program on the minimal idiopathic scoliosis curve. Changes of less than 4 degrees were considered to have resulted from measurement variability, while those of 4 degrees or greater were regarded as representing actual change.

There are many ways in which studies on inter-tester reliability can be performed. First one therapist and then a second therapist may measure the same patient. In order to eliminate the effect of time, and to consider only the effect of using multiple measures, the time interval between measurements should be kept to a minimum. However, the effect of taking the first measurement may alter the second, e.g., more motion may be measured the second time than the first time. This is similar to the problem noted with intra-tester reliability. Once again, as long as the change is similar among all patients being measured the second time, the test is usually considered reliable. When possible, the best way to assess inter-tester reliability is probably to have therapists take their measurements or make their judgments simultaneously. In evaluating the inter-tester reliability of visual assessment systems for gait, all of the therapists would have to evaluate the patient at the same time. Their judgments would have to be made without consultation. It is obvious that this approach cannot be used when measurements require the therapist to interact with the patient, as in manual muscle testing.

Parallel Forms.   Sometimes more than one version of a test may be used. All of us who have taken a state licensing exam (the one prepared by the Professional Examination Services) have taken a parallel form of a test. In the case of the PES, multiple forms exist because the test is offered so often. The use of multiple forms can only be justified when it can be shown that all forms lead to an approximately equal score when the test is taken by the same person. This may not appear to be terribly relevant to physical therapy because parallel forms reliability is most often associated with paper and pencil tests. However, we do have different tests within physical therapy that claim to test the same thing. The most obvious example is that of the two systems used for MMT (see Ch. 2 for a full discussion).[19,25] Will the grades obtained with the Kendall and Kendall system be the same as those obtained with the Daniels and Worthingham system? Clinicians usually favor one test over another. The arguments in favor of each may be academic if it can be shown that results are essentially interchangeable, i.e., they are parallel forms of the same test. No one, however, has ever examined this question, so the clinical debate continues.

Sometimes we use different instruments to measure the same thing, e.g., different goniometers. When we examine the interchangeability of obtained values we are really considering a type of parallel forms reliability. Clinicians should consider the different forms of tests used and the different instruments used clinically to measure the same thing. They must then ask if the results are the same. The choice of instruments is often a matter of opinion based on a variety of theoretical considerations. If we examine whether different approaches yield the same results we might lessen the need for debate or at least limit discussions to those situations in which the use of different instruments or systems really makes a difference (i.e., gives different results).

Internal Consistency.   Internal consistency is another form of reliability that is most commonly associated with paper and pencil tests. If a test asks what you know about a disease, it may have sections on pathology, epidemiology, medications, and management. If a question in any one section deals with the same body of knowledge as does another question, it is reasonable to assume that all persons taking the test should answer similarly to both questions. The assessment of internal consistency is performed with a variety of statistical techniques that are beyond the scope of this chapter.[17]

One potential application of the concepts inherent in internal consistency testing is relevant to physical therapy. If parts of a test battery agree with each other consistently, we might question whether all of the elements are needed. For example, in isokinetic testing, it has been suggested that slow-speed testing quantifies a different element of muscle performance than does high-speed testing.[26,27] A lack of internal consistency is implied because the two speeds are supposed to be testing unique elements. However, it has been shown that torques at both speeds are very highly correlated.[28] This finding implies a commonality or internal consistency that should lead to a reevaluation of whether the speeds actually measure different aspects of muscular performance.

Summary of Reliability

Reliability has been an overlooked issue in the development and use of physical therapy tests. As a result, many of our measurements are greeted with skepticism by others and at times are not taken seriously by members of our own profession. Yet, reliability in measurement is a hallmark of any scientific endeavor. Student physical therapists sometimes measure too much and develop bad habits as a result. More than once a student has suggested that every patient must be measured, regardless of the condition, so that "baseline information" may be obtained. Can a meaningful baseline really be obtained when threats to reliability exist, such as when the patient is uncooperative or confused? If we disregard such concerns, how can we justify our measurements and make legitimate inferences? How would we feel, if after arriving for a fasting glucose tolerance test, we admitted to having eaten breakfast only to have the physician say, "We will do it anyway to get a baseline." The very idea of analyzing nonfasting blood seems bizarre because no one would know how to interpret the results.

Kerlinger[15] has put the issue of reliability in appropriate context:

To be interpretable a test must be reliable. Unless one can depend upon the results of the measurement of one's variables, one cannot with any confidence determine relations between the variables. One goal of science, again, is to discover the relations among variables. Since unreliable measurement is measurement overloaded with error, the discovery of these relations becomes a difficult and tenuous business . . .

. . . High reliability is not a guarantee of good scientific results, but there can be no good scientific results without reliability.

Although Kerlinger discusses reliability in terms of scientific inquiry, the issues are even more important when clinical practice is considered. In the absence of reliable measurements, how can we know the initial or final status of any patient? How can we know whether a treatment has any effect? Studies of the reliability of existing clinical measurement systems is the single greatest need in physical therapy research. Such studies would not only provide usable tools (i.e., measurements) for clinical research, but they would go a long way toward establishing scientific credibility for clinical practice.

VALIDITY

Reliability, the first fundamental requirement for a measurement, can be defined and tested in a straightforward manner. This is in contrast to validity, which is neither easily defined nor *directly* testable. Evidence for the validity of a measurement may be hard to secure; this is not surprising because universal definitions for validity are not even readily available. Here, two definitions will be offered; one has been used in the physical therapy literature, while the other is a more complex description that has become almost universally accepted among behavioral scientists.

Validity has been defined as evidence that a test measures what it is supposed to measure. Therefore, in a widely cited article that introduced isokinetic testing, Moffroid and her associates demonstrated "validity" by showing that the obtained values from the machine agreed with those that would be expected when weights were applied to the machine's lever arm.[29] Because the values agreed, it was concluded that the machine was "valid" i.e., it measured the physical quantities it was supposed to measure within an acceptable level of error.

An alternative view of validity is offered in *Standards for Educational and Psychological Tests and Manuals*.[16] This manual was developed by a joint committee of the American Psychological Association, the American Educational Research Association, and the National Council on Measurement in Education, and is considered to be the standard reference on tests. The global definition put forth in the manual states:

Questions of validity are questions of what may properly be inferred from a test score; validity refers to the appropriateness of inferences from test scores or other forms of assessment. The many questions surrounding validity can, for convenience, be reduced to two: a) What can be inferred about what is being measured by the test? b) What can be inferred about other behavior?

The definition in the manual focuses validity not only on whether a test measures the element it is supposed to measure but also on *whether the measurements obtained can be legitimately used to make judgments (inferences)*. In line with this definition, we can characterize both fundamental qualities of a measurement thus: reliability deals with whether a measurement consistently reflects something whereas validity deals with how the measurement is used. Reliability is essential for a measurement. However, if a measurement has reliability but no validity, it has no justifiable use or application.[29]

The issue of use makes the first and simpler definition of validity impractical.

Kerlinger[15] has suggested that:

> When measuring certain physical properties and relatively simple attributes of persons, validity is no great problem. There is often rather direct and close congruence between the nature of the object measured and the measuring instrument. . . . With some physical attributes, then, there is little doubt of what is being measured.

In an attempt to differentiate behavioral properties from physical, Kerlinger may have oversimplified. For instance, a thermometer may be used in different ways: measurements of temperature and the volume of a container may be combined with a constant to *derive* a value to indicate the pressure of a gas within the container (through use of Charles' Law).[18] Here, two measurements are used to derive (infer) a third. The legitimacy of the procedure is based on experimental evidence confirming Charles' Law—experimental evidence confirming the validity of the inference.

In applied fields, inferences are more obvious and are *always* present, even when we do not realize it. A patient's temperature is taken not because we want to infer something about the kinetic energy of molecules (which in itself is an inference), but rather because it has been established that an elevated temperature can be used to infer a variety of phenomena, e.g., the presence of postoperative pyrogens, infection, CNS dysfunction, etc. The knowledge that a person has an elevated temperature has only limited value unless we do something with that knowledge. The justification we bring to this use is directly associated with validity. Why can we infer the presence of a dysfunction or a disease from an elevated temperature? We can make the inference because over a long period of time such phenomena have been associated with such findings. Unless data on the relationship of an elevated temperature with clinical findings in patients had been obtained, we would have little inferential capacity with regard to the febrile state.

Now, consider the "validation" of isokinetic testing with weights. What does it tell us about how we can use the measurements obtained from that machine? We can say that the machine accurately reflects forces (actually torques), work, and power when weights are applied. But isn't the clinical function of the machine to allow therapists to assess a patient's muscular performance? Does the machine reflect a patient's performance? What do variations in that performance mean? What is good performance? What is bad performance? Is there a relationship between function and the measurements? What can we really infer? These questions remain unanswered, possibly because people assume any machine-derived measurement to be valid. See Chapter 3 for a discussion of these issues in reference to instruments used for muscle testing.

This section will use the definitions of validity that have been presented in *Standards for Educational and Psychological Tests*[16] because they are widely accepted and because they are the most logical. My premise here is that *all* measurements are used to make inferences and, therefore, *all* devices or tests, especially those used clinically, must be examined for validity. When there is no evidence for the validity of measurements, such measurements may contribute to the data that therapists can use to form "clinical impressions" or judgments. There is nothing inherently wrong with this, especially in view of how little we know about the validity of most of our tests. However, clinicians are urged to remember that the judgment is then their own, and somewhat objective. What is more important is that anyone who writes in professional journals or who presents material in courses must present evidence of validity when discussing measurements. If speakers do not present such evidence, it should be noted that they are presenting their *opinions* as to what measurements reflect and that their opinions have not been scientifically tested. Evidence demonstrating the legitimacy of an inference is evidence for validity.

Types of Validity

Face validity is sometimes called the lowest form of validity because it reflects only whether a test *appears* to do what it is supposed to do.[30] Face validity is really based on the personal opinions of those either taking or giving a test. No evidence is presented in discussions of the topic.

Professionals are obligated to understand the measurements they make, and, therefore, they should know when data exist to support the usefulness of a measurement. For the clinician, face validity appears to be the last resort for justification of measurement use, and such use is then based on nothing more than the clinician's opinions. Measurements with only face validity are those that each of us must use in our own way. In other words, when we use data obtained from a test that has no more than face validity, we are taking a number and using it to make a conclusion without evidence to support that conclusion. We may have to do this in clinical practice; however, we should be cognizant of our actions and use more caution in making clinical judgments.

At the risk of overstating the need for face validity, we might want to consider face validity as it applies to those being measured. If patients do not believe that what we are asking them to do is meaningful (i.e., *if it does not have some face validity for them*), they may not make a maximal effort. This element may be important in performance testing. Brunnstrom's tests to determine whether a patient is not in synergy clearly require effort on the part of the hemiplegic patient.[8] If patients do not appreciate the reason for the test or cannot simply trust the therapist's judgment, they may not make the effort. Varying degrees of effort by various patients could then introduce a significant amount of error into the measurement process; i.e., some patients who are in reality less dominated by synergies during functional activities may appear to have greater problems with synergies than other patients. It is possible that a test without face validity will not be taken seriously.

Although face validity itself cannot be tested, it can be argued that if patients do not fully participate in testing because they do not perceive face validity, measurements of reliability will be affected. However, consistent minimal efforts on the part of subjects could lead to consistent, and therefore potentially reliable, results. It is clear that the best way to rule out errors caused by a lack of the appreciation of face validity on the part of test takers is to base the use of tests on the far more rigorous forms of validity (see below) especially the criterion-related validities. When such forms of validity are less than ideal, developers of tests and measurement systems may want to consider whether this lack was caused by variations in motivation that can be traced to whether or not the patients were fully motivated to perform.

Construct validity is based on a logical argument that supports the idea that a measurement reflects what we want it to measure. The manual on tests[16] describes this process thusly:

> Evidence of construct validity is not found in a single study: rather, judgments of construct validity are based upon an accumulation of research results. . . . Taken together, such hypotheses form at least a tentative theory about the nature of the construct the test is believed to be measuring. Since a construct cannot be tested directly, this form of validity is classified as a "theoretical form."

Most of the literature on tests and measurements has been generated by psychologists and educational researchers, and it is not surprising that they recognize construct validity as one of the most important concepts ever developed in the field.[15] Such researchers attempt to measure what we may consider vague concepts such as intelligence, anxiety, emotional state, etc. They must first define their variables (develop a construct). Although behavioral scientists necessarily must deal with construct validity, this necessity is less obvious in some of the basic sciences. However, it can be argued that the need is still present. Newton's First Law ($F = mA$) is a good example of a basic construct that is expressed in the form of a formula.[18] Physicists routinely measure forces with incredible accuracy; when gravitational forces are at issue, however, we may still ask why one body attracts another. The question transcends physics and approaches theology. The fact that masses attract one another is "explained" by a concept of gravitational force based on acceptance of a construct inherent in Newtonian laws.

The construct behind most physical therapy tests is at best implied; at times it has been lost during the historical evolution of the test. MMT is a good example. Although the original literature describing the test never specifically mentioned construct validity, we can infer that the construct was based on the purpose the test developers had in mind. MMT was first described by Lovett[31] during the era of polio epidemics and was used to characterize patterns of weakness associated with anterior horn cell lesions. The construct was: destruction or injury to the anterior horn cell will be reflected in weakness of the muscle innervated by that cell. This early use of the test is different from attempts to infer functional performance from MMT grades, and it can be seen that this latter use is not based on the original construct (see Ch. 2 for a discussion of the relationship of MMT grades and function).

The term "strength" has a variety of operational definitions and each should be based on a construct if we want to infer something from strength measurements. Similarly, we may talk about "endurance" and attempt to measure it, but what is the construct? A common endurance test used in isokinetic testing is the counting of the number of contractions that are necessary before a subject dips below 50 percent of the peak torque previously achieved at the same speed of movement.[27] What does this reflect? What does it allow us to infer? On what theoretical considerations was this test developed? Do variations in this measurement relate to functional performance (e.g., running or walking)? These issues should have been considered when the test was developed; they are issues of construct validity.

Content validity is the second form of "theoretical validity" and cannot exist without construct validity. In establishing construct validity, we go through the process of defining what we are measuring and for what purpose. Having defined the element or domain of interest, we must ask whether the measurements we will obtain can adequately reflect the domain. Content validity concerns the issue of whether a test reflects the variable as we have defined it.

When therapists attempt to make patients more functional, they may want to measure whether a patient's ability to carry out activities of daily living (ADL) has improved. To test ADL, there must be a definition of what constitutes activities for daily living (see Ch. 5 for examples of this). The arguments used in developing our definition are our case for construct validity. Having made a case for what we believe constitutes ADL, we must demonstrate that our test examines all relevant elements. If we have defined ADL as the ability to dress, groom, ambulate, work, and play, any test we use would have to include elements that reflect abilities in these areas. For content validity, we would have to make a case that each of these elements (e.g., groom) is fully examined by the test. Would an ADL test be content-valid if it examined only whether patients were capable of brushing their teeth? We might wonder whether patients could wash themselves or carry out toilet functions.

Because we can never test all aspects of the global elements described in the ADL example, how can content validity ever be examined? Let us say for the sake of argument that a body of research exists which shows that if patients can brush their teeth, they almost always can perform other grooming activities such as washing or toilet functions. Content validity does not require that every imaginable skill or element be examined, but only that the test contain a *sample of elements that are representative of the domain of interest.*

The ADL example is reasonably straightforward. Now we will consider more complex questions. Muscle "strength" is a concern of physical therapists. However, because a single uniform construct of "strength" is lacking, a variety of operational definitions have been used in the literature. Again, solely for the sake of illustration, let us use a simple construct and see how we could examine content validity. Based on our knowledge of anatomy, physiology, biomechanics, and kinesiology, we could argue that so-called strength of a muscle should reflect its capability of being used to generate tension and thus create forces that move limbs during functional activities. Although this construct is still somewhat vague, we can begin to list some of the elements needed before we can measure strength in a manner that has content validity.[32] We might, for example, want to know the following:

1. What forces can the muscle develop under static and dynamic conditions?

2. What forces can be generated during eccentric and concentric contractions (because both are used during functional activities)?

3. At various points in the ROM, what kinds of forces can be generated statically and dynamically, since we use isometrics to hold various positions and to generate different forces at different points in a motion (for example, when a subject is kicking a ball, does the quadriceps-generated force need to be greatest at a different point in the motion than when the subject is walking)?

The above list in only an initial attempt at defining some of the elements necessary for content validity. The task may seem staggering, but unless there is content validity, it is unlikely that the nontheoretical forms of validity, i.e., the criterion-related validities, can ever be demonstrated. As will be shown later, these criterion-related forms are developed through the use of evidence to show that inferences are justifiable. If we want to infer functional capacity from a "strength test," how can we expect to do this unless the test is content-valid? For example, because we use muscle isometrically, as well as dynamically and eccentrically and concentrically, how can we hope to reflect these elements unless our tests measure them? If some of these elements are so closely related that one can be used to predict the other, tests of each are not necessary for a test to be content-valid. Basic research tells us about the relationships of variables and helps to guide test makers in knowing how many elements must be measured for a test to be content-valid. Citations from such research are a primary mechanism used to make claims for content validity.

Although content validity has never been discussed in the MMT literature, it may be argued that the essential differences between two forms of MMT are based on content. The break test suggested by Kendall and Kendall[25] assesses muscular strength at one point in the ROM. Some clinicians think that testing through the ROM is a more functional test. In arguing for testing "through the range," clinicians are really saying that the break test, as far as they are concerned, does not adequately sample muscular performance. The concern may be admirable, but we must ask whether there is evidence for this assumption. Do the grades from both systems give meaningfully different results? If they do not, it can be argued that they are both testing the same thing and that neither has a greater claim to content validity. The choice of tests then could be based on personal choice, ease of administration, or upon relative reliability. *Content validity is not merely an academic exercise, but rather a statement of the minimal scope a measurement must have in order to allow inferences.* Clinicians may want to contemplate whether there is content validity present for the various assessment tools they use. First, however, they must consider what the constructs really are and—most important—they must ask: Why am I measuring?

Criterion-Related Validities. Construct and content validity were both demonstrated through the use of logical arguments or expert opinions, although these may rely heavily on research literature. These two forms of "theoretical validity" may be contrasted to the criterion-related validities that are demonstrated through direct research. Therefore, the criterion-related validities, concurrent and predictive, represent the greatest possible justification one can offer in defense of the validity of a measurement.

The term "criterion-related validity," is derived from the concept that validity for an inference can be justified by comparing an obtained measurement with some other observed standard (criterion).[16] If we think that Standard Achievement Test (SAT) scores can be used to infer college success or failure, we test this hypothesis by examining the relationship between SAT and college performance. The criteria to judge SAT scores would probably be grade point average (GPA). If we think that increased deep tendon reflexes (DTR) indicate hypertonicity, which in turn means that a patient will be less functional, we are inferring something. We can test this inference by examining the relationship between DTR testing and some form of ADL testing. It is clear that the criteria used (in this last case an ADL test score) should be derived from a test that is reliable and valid. When claims for criterion-related validity are made, the criteria must be critically examined. Do the criteria really relate to the inference? Can the criteria score be believed (i.e., does it meet minimal standards)?

The need to choose the criteria critically can be illustrated by an ongoing concern among physical therapy educators who want to know the best way to choose students for educational programs. In other words, how can they best infer which students will complete their programs and go on to be good therapists? There are many variables that can be examined during the admissions process, such as GPA, math and science GPA, letters of recommendation, interviews, history of professional involvement, and performance on admission tests. We do not lack measurements, although certainly they need better definition and reliability, but we do lack a criterion against which to test them.

Should we use GPA in physical therapy classes? GPAs may not predict who will be a good therapist. We can use grades from clinical affiliations, but will they predict who will be a good clinician? We are actually asking whether we can infer from either physical therapy GPAs or clinical education grades whether someone will be a good therapist. Unless we can be sure that either or both of these can be used to predict professional success, we certainly cannot use these in turn to validate admissions criteria.

Critical selection of the criteria used in validation guides the inferential process. If, for example, someone did justify a school's admission process based either on GPAs or clinical education grades, we must ask what inferences are warranted. Because neither of these two measures has been shown to predict whether a person may be a good clinician, we can say that use of these criteria has limited value. If the admissions criteria predict GPA in a program, we can say that variables used to make the admissions decision can be used to infer academic success. That is a reasonable goal but a limited one. Both goals are reasonable because unless a student completes academic and clinical requirements, he or she cannot become a therapist, let alone a good one. If we are concerned not only with whether students will get through the process but with whether they will make meaningful contributions to the profession, we need other criteria with which to compare admissions data. These criteria somehow would have to measure whether one was contributing to the profession, either as a clinician, researcher, academician, or administrator.

Other examples may further clarify the role criterion-related validities play in justifying inferences. Two examples are drawn from clinical medicine. The ultimate way in which one knows that the myocardium has suffered an infarct is through examination of heart tissue. Therefore, it can be argued that the only direct way in which one can be sure that a myocardial infarction has taken place is to examine the tissue grossly and under the microscope. It is fortunate that this is rendered necessary by the availability of a variety of indirect measurements (see Ch. 9).

Einthoven et al, using knowledge of the electrical properties of the heart and the body, developed the electrocardiogram (ECG).[33] Based on the properties of the heart and its conduction system, a *construct* was developed about how the ECG signal should change when various conditions exist (death of part of the myocardium, blocks, etc.). In addition, parts of the ECG wave were associated with contractions of different parts of the heart, i.e., the atria *v* the ventricles. The conceptual basis (the construct) for this relationship did not ensure that the inferences drawn from the ECG were valid. Criterion-related validity was established through the comparison of pathological findings with previously recorded ECGs. Did the defect inferred from the ECG actually exist? Animal models were used in this process, as were necropsy data from human subjects. For the physician, autopsy can be the ultimate form of criterion-related validation for the collective inferences called a diagnosis.

The ECG is an example of a construct leading to the development of a measurement system used to make inferences. Along the way, criterion validation was obtained through research. Some tests, albeit very few, are developed serendipitously and may never have a construct. Joseph Babinski was working in Charcot's clinic in Saltpetrier when he observed the clinical sign that bears his name. He was testing CNS-damaged patients for flexion-with-drawal reflexes when he noticed that if he stroked the lateral surface of the foot, the toes fanned.[34] This movement was only present in patients with CNS lesions. The Babinski sign has become pathognomonic for CNS disturbances not because we understand why it exists (we do not), but rather because re-peated examinations have shown that it is only present when a lesion is present (it has criterion-related validity).

Criterion-related validity is usually not easy to demonstrate because all too often there are no simple criteria available to test an inference. ADL tests exemplify this problem. If we developed an instrument to test ADL, how would we achieve criterion-related validity? To what would we compare our test scores? As Jette discusses in Chapter 5, the development of criterion-related validity is difficult and may involve complex statistical approaches. Sometimes, in the absence of previously established criteria, indirect evidence must be used. For example, if an ADL test leads us to conclude that a patient is in-dependent, we may conclude that the inference is correct if a large series of patients who are judged to be independent report on a questionnaire that they are able to function fully.

Malone et al suggested that when patients achieved 75 percent of the quad-riceps peak torque in an involved extremity (after knee surgery), they were ready to return to athletic activities.[35] What is implied is that these patients were no longer at risk. The inference that they were ready to return to athletics was never justified with any data. Would it not be useful to know how many patients are reinjured when they return to activity after meeting this criterion? Are the number of injuries different than would be expected if a lower or higher percentage was used? At best, Malone and his associates were offering a clinical opinion. Although that opinion may appear valid because it was rendered by experts, the clinician must remember that opinions are supported by obser-vations and interpretations, whereas validity is supported by data. When opin-ion is offered because data are not available, a minimum requirement clinicians should insist upon from experts is a description of the method used by the experts in reaching their conclusions. For example, how did Malone and his associates come to the conclusion that 75 percent was an acceptable figure? Did they look at various percentages and find that there were in some cases unacceptable risks (with too low a criterion) or unacceptable delays in returning to activity (with too high a criterion)? Opinion is no substitute for validity. Inferences made in the absence of criterion-related validity must be used cau-tiously. Inferences based on opinions should at least be supported by logical arguments and a record of observations.

Criterion-related validity, the presence of evidence to justify inference, is lacking for many physical therapy tests and measurements. How hard would it be to obtain? That question must be answered differently for almost every test and measurement. However, until there is an adequate appreciation for the need to demonstrate criterion-related validity, it is unlikely that the time and effort to do so will be expended. As long as we are willing to accept that certain manual therapy tests reveal ligamentous laxity, who will feel the imperative to use radiography to test this hypothesis? As long as we accept the idea that hypertonicity impairs the ability to move, who will test this inference? Unless we begin to examine our measurements critically, especially for reliability and the criterion-related validities, we may expect others to challenge us to justify the very existence of physical therapy. The questioning will not necessarily come from the manufacturers of new tests and new machines or from colleagues who believe that they have developed new measurement tools. The questioning must come from the user of these tools, the clinician whose task it is to best serve the patient. A case has been made for the importance of criterion-related validities. The two types are defined below.

Concurrent validity deals with whether an inference is justifiable at the *present time*. The use of an ECG to state whether someone has a conduction block is an example of an inference that relates to the criteria at the same point in time when the measurement is made. When MMT is used to infer the level of a spinal cord lesion the inference concerns what exists at the time of the test. One must demonstrate, through the use of a criterion, that the inference is justifiable. The presence of concurrent validity means that we can say something about what *is* at the time of the test: it does not allow us to predict what will be. MMT testing showing a lesion does not tell us to what extent recovery will occur. The ECG, by itself, does not permit us to predict the future course of cardiac disease.

Predictive validity allows us to measure something and infer something about the future. When Malone and his colleagues[35] stated that a minimum quadriceps torque was needed for the return to athletic activity, they were claiming predictive validity. Most screening programs have inherent claims of predictive validity for the measurements they use. Infant screening programs for developmental disabilities are predicated on the notion that results can be used to predict what will happen to that child in the future—*unless* intervention occurs. We can only justify intervention based on screening when we can make a case that our measurements have predictive validity. Unless one can be sure that something will occur without intervention, how can one justify the intervention? Or, for that matter, how can we ever be sure the intervention is accomplishing something?

Ghiselli et al[17] have given a rather clear-cut description of how to test predictive validity:

> Simply put, a predictive validity study involves 1) obtaining an appropriate sample of people, 2) measuring them on a predictor, 3) waiting for the necessary weeks, months, or years to pass, 4) obtaining the criterion scores for the same sample of people, and 5) computing the correlation between predictor scores and the criterion score.

Waiting the necessary time may seem like an impossible task, but the time interval should be specific to the inference or the prediction being made. Some of the most significant studies in medicine have actually been predictive validity studies. The Framingham study, which examined what factors contributed to the development of cardiovascular disease,[36] was an investigation into what measurements (factors) could be used to predict the future occurrence of disease. It is obvious that a major reason for the study was the assumption that if these predictors could be altered, the likelihood of the prediction (i.e., the development of disease) coming true would be lessened. Although we frequently assume that if we change the measurement used to make a prediction we may then change future events, it is not always true. This chapter is not meant to serve as a primer on research, and the reader is urged to examine some texts in the area to understand why it is inappropriate to assume that changes in predictive measurements can automatically change future occurrences. However, we must reiterate that predictive validity and concurrent validity deal with the relationships between our measurement and some other criteria. The presence of a relationship does not mean that one variable causes changes in the other. Causality can ultimately be demonstrated only through experimentation if variables are manipulated.[37]

General Issues in Validity

The standards for tests and measurements[16] has identified two essentials for valid tests. They are:

1. Whoever suggests the use of a test should present evidence for validity for each type of inference for which the test is recommended. If there is no evidence for the validity of some inferences (e.g., they are opinions) this should be made clear.

2. Test users are responsible for describing the evidence (i.e., in terms of reliability and validity) that justifies the use of their measurements.

An additional requirement not previously discussed must also be considered. Validity, like reliability, has a population-specific quality. An intelligence test written in English is unlikely to validly measure the intelligence of a non–English-speaking person. Clinicians must consider the circumstances in which they use tests and ask whether results can be valid. Can we validly test the receptive aphasic patient's ability to perform complex motor tasks when we do not know if the patient understands our instructions? The frequency of perceptual deficits found in hemiplegic patients should cause one to wonder whether tests of such deficits are valid. Perhaps the problem is not a perceptual deficit, but rather an inability to take the test because of cognitive, motivational, or attention problems.

Population-specific validity problems threaten much of the inferential potential of our tests. In the presence of pain, can we expect a person to generate much muscle tension? It does not matter whether we are muscle-testing such a patient with a machine or manually. Often such tests cannot be used to infer something about isolated muscle function. These tests, in theory, may be used to reflect a collection of variables, such as muscle performance, pain, and comfort. However, we have no way of knowing which factor (or factors) is causing a change in the measurement, and therefore, where we should focus treatment.

Tests whose validity is threatened by variables other than those being measured can lead to inappropriate treatments. The inappropriateness may not be noted if the success of the intervention is examined solely with the same test we first used. For example, if we muscle-test a patient in pain and find that the grade is too low, we might exercise the patient. We then claim success if we have improved the grade. Actually, the improvement may reflect decreased pain, not increased ability to generate muscle tension. The focus of testing should always relate to the reason we are testing the patient—which is to infer something. Perhaps we wish to infer why the patient cannot walk or perform some other meaningful activity.

Few patients care about their muscle test scores or seek treatment because they have poor muscle test grades. Patients seek treatment because they are having trouble with something that is meaningful to them, either because they cannot perform a task or because they have pain during an activity. How well do our measurements reflect these problems? If we wish to discover what factor is causing the problem, knowledge of why we are testing is essential. Therefore, when we observe change in the measured variable (such as a muscle test grade) we need to consider whether this has changed the problem we believe was caused by that poor grade, i.e., the function. Repeated checking of the grade misses the essence of the process, which is to infer, judge, make decisions, and effect treatments that change the problem, not just the measurement.

There is little evidence available to support the validity of most physical therapy measurements. Research is obviously needed. Clinicians must also become more critical consumers. We must question those who suggest they can measure things. We should assert ourselves. If there is no evidence of reliability, and if we believe a test is not valid, we must—as the standards[16] suggest—assume a sense of responsibility.

In the past, I have often asked questions of those who have developed tests for clinical practice only to hear, "You have to give the clinician something." Such an argument denigrates clinical practice and shows a wanton disrespect for clinicians and reality. The quality of clinical practice is not served when it is based on measurements that do not contain meaningful information. Convenience may be served when we uncritically accept measurements, but at what cost to our profession and our patients? We may say that an illusion of a measurement may give clinical practice face validity, but that is no substitute for more rigorous forms of validity. In the absence of more rigorous information supporting the use of tests, clinical practice need not be paralyzed, but rather practice can be elevated to the point at which individual clinicians assume the responsibility for their decision-making process based on *their own arguments and observations*.

Use of Standards for Inferences

The validity of a test was defined as the inferential capacity of a measurement. Essentially, there are three ways in which these inferences may be derived.[16] They deal with whether a test (and therefore a measurement) has been (1) criterion-referenced, (2) content-referenced or (3) norm-referenced. The definitions used here are those from *Standards for Educational Tests and Measurements*.[16]

Criterion-Referenced Tests. The term criterion-reference is closely related to the previous discussions on criterion-related validity and is defined thus: "Criterion-referenced interpretations are those where the score is directly interpreted in terms of performance at any given point on the continuum of an *external* variable."[16] In other words, a test has been criterion-referenced when we can *assume* performance on one variable by measuring another, or when we measure one thing to infer the value of another. Criterion-referencing is an argument for criterion-related validity.

Content-Referenced Tests. Content-referencing of a test introduces a new concept. The definition states: "Content-referenced interpretations are those where the score is directly interpreted in terms of performance at each point in the achievement continuum."[16] Here an inference is made based on how well a person scores. When teachers say that a 70 percent grade is a passing grade, they are content-referencing their exam since they are setting a level of achievement as a standard for what is good and necessary. However, we may ask where the teacher got the idea that 70 percent was a magic threshold?

Establishing an appropriate framework for content-referencing is difficult. In Chapter 4 of this volume, Miller has questioned the various means we use to judge a goniometric measurement as "good" or "acceptable." He argues persuasively that we should determine the ROM each patient needs and use that as a standard of what is good and necessary. He specifically discusses how clinicians might generate such criteria by examining the patient's functional deficits. Miller is arguing for evaluation of goniometric measurements on the basis of content-referencing. In order to content-reference, we must have basic knowledge of the ways in which the variables we are measuring relate to things we care about. To content-reference muscle performance adequately, we would need to know how force relates to the functional activities that the patient must perform. To content-reference a variable such as stride length in terms of gait, we would have to know how stride length relates to optimal locomotor proficiency.

Content-referencing provides a real challenge in physical therapy. It would be ideal for researchers to generate information regarding what levels are acceptable—much as physicians, for example, have shown that a blood glucose level of 100 mM is desirable.[38] Until information such as this is created in physical therapy, clinicians essentially are using their own criteria. Such criteria, like those suggested by others, are neither good or bad, just in need of logical justification. For example, if a clinician states that a patient needs quadriceps torque that is equal to body weight (actually the units of the two are different) for gait, we must ask where this criterion-reference originated. Content-referencing is a process that requires considerable thought and use of the literature.

Norm-Referenced Tests.   Norm-referencing uses a representative sample of people who are measured relative to the variable of interest. This sample is then thought to reflect the population of interest. Use of norm-referencing permits comparison of a single individual's measurement with those expected from the rest of the population. The most obvious comparison is whether a subject's measurement is above or below the mean, or what is considered "normal." However, use of means alone for comparison can be less than illuminating and can even lead to some rather questionable conclusions. In order to use norm-referencing meaningfully, some basic statistical concepts must be understood.

During the second half of the 19th century, several researchers began to observe a similar phenomenon.[39,40] After measuring various properties of humans, e.g., chest girths of soldiers, heights of peasants, etc., these founders of statistical science noted that there was a characteristic distribution for these measurements. When the frequency of observations (the number of observations) was plotted along the ordinate (*y*-axis) and the magnitude of the measurements along the abscissa (*x*-axis), the distribution took on a "bell shape" (see Figs. 1-1 and 1-2). The center of the bell (its highest point) where the most measurements were observed was the mean. This bell-shaped distribution has been called a "normal distribution" (or a Gaussian distribution, after one of the mathematicians who described it). A key element of this type of curve is that the mean, the median (the score that separates a top and bottom 50 percent), and the mode (the most commonly obtained score) are all the same.

When measurements are normally distributed, most observations are relatively close to the mean. Measurements that are greatly above or below the mean become less common in this type of distribution. In other words, any measurement that is close to the mean has a greater likelihood of having been taken on a subject from the population than would any measurement that greatly deviates from the mean. The further a measurement is from the mean, the more likely it is that the subject measured was not really part of the originally defined sample used to estimate the distribution of the population.

Galton, who was amongst the first to describe the "normal distribution," measured the chest girths of soldiers (see Fig. 1-2). The mean for this measurement was approximately 39.5 inches. The most commonly observed chest girths were 39, 40, and 41 inches. Therefore, these data show that any soldier who was measured at that same time and had a girth of 40 inches was very much like the rest of the army. However, if we measured a soldier and found that his chest girth was 30 inches we would have to say that that soldier was very different.

Let us assume now that Galton's data represented not a sample of soldiers, but rather a sample of adult men who did not have a disease. We could say that anyone with a girth of 40 inches was certainly within "normal limits."

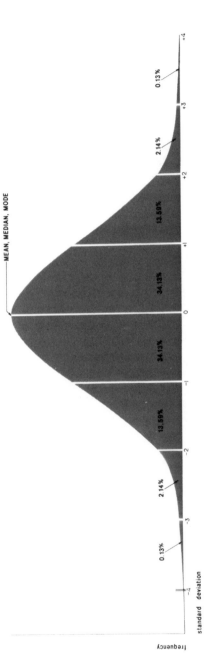

STANDARD DEVIATIONS

Fig. 1-1. When data are "normally" distributed (i.e., they fit a normal curve) the mean, the median, and the mode are all the same. The symmetry of the curve permits prediction of percentages (of observations) below or above a single observation when the SD is known. For example, 34.13 percent of the scores will fall within 1 S.D. and 50 percent of all scores will be above or below the mean.

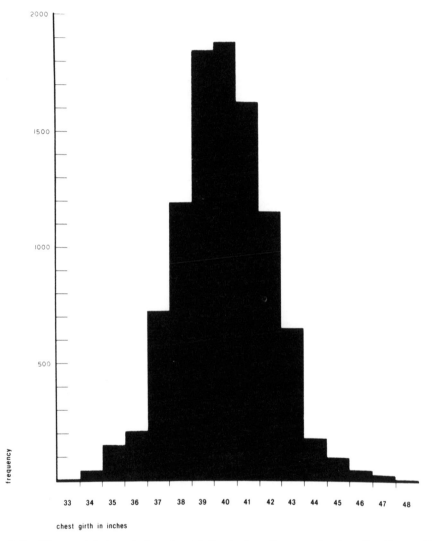

Fig. 1-2. The graph is loosely based on Galton's data. Because the data fit a "normal" distribution, they can be used to determine when a value (i.e., a measurement of chest girth) is so deviant from the mean that it represents an observation that was probably not made on a member of the original population (i.e., healthy soldiers).

Even someone with a girth of 37 inches would (Fig. 1-1) have a good chance of being part of the population sampled (i.e., normal adult men). However, what would we say about someone with a girth of 30 or 50 inches? The possibility exists that they *could* be part of the population (i.e., normal) but it is more *likely* that they are part of another group. That other group may be composed of persons with growth disturbances or lung disease. The use of the "normal curve" permits statements about the probability of any one person belonging to the population measured to generate the curve.

From the above example (and from analysis of Fig. 1-1), it should be clear that the mean tells only part of the story. To judge what is "within normal limits," you must also consider how a given measurement varies in a defined population. It is fortunate that a method exists that permits reasonably precise estimations of the probability of various measurements coming from a given population—if the variable being measured is normally distributed. The mean (and the median and the mode) are measures of *central tendencies*.[15] A measurement of variability is also needed. One very useful measurement of variability is the standard deviation (SD).[15]

The first step in obtaining the SD (at least conceptually), is to take each score and find how much it deviates from the mean. These values are called the deviation scores. Because the sum of these scores will always equal zero (which is the definition of the mean) they cannot be averaged to assess variability. However, if these deviation scores are squared, they can then be averaged to derive a statistic called the variance. The SD is the square root of the variance and is, therefore, expressed in the same units used for the measurements. In practice, deviation scores need not be obtained to calculate the variance because computational formulas exist. In addition, when estimating the variance and SD of a population from a sample, a "correction factor" is used; that is not of great importance relative to the theoretical application of the SD discussed here.[15]

Use of the SD permits judgments as to the probability of whether a given score was obtained from members of a defined population. At least 68 percent of all scores will be found when a variable is normally distributed. Within ±2 SDs, 96 percent of all scores will be found, and with ±3 SDs, 99 percent of all the scores will be found (Fig.1-2).

If 68 percent of all scores fall within 1 SD from the mean, we can also say that a score 1 SD higher than the mean is higher than 84 percent of the other scores. A score above the mean for a normally distributed value will be higher than 50 percent of the scores since the mean is not only the average for such a distribution but also the median (the score that divides the distribution in half). Because plus *or* minus 1 SD encompasses 68 percent of the scores, +1 SD would include 34 percent (68/2 = 34). We add the 34 percent to the 50 percent (since we know that half the scores are below the mean). Therefore, we can say that any score 1 SD above the mean is higher than 84 percent of the scores. Another way of saying this is to state that such a score is in the top 16 percent of all scores.

We can see the utility of norm-referenced scores. If we know the distribution for a given variable, we can then make judgments about how likely it is that our patient's measurement belongs to that group. Let us imagine that we know the mean score found for shoulder flexion ROM in a described population. We see a patient who has a value that is 4 SD below the mean. We can see from Figure 1-1 that there is less than a 1 percent chance that our measurement was made on a subject who belonged to the measured (described) population. A much more reasonable conclusion is that this person is not part of the population (based on the use of the shoulder flexion criteria) and is not "within normal limits." The same process is used to determine *abnormal* values for many laboratory tests.

In order to use normal values (such as those offered in many texts on goniometry) one must know the SD of the measurement. Unfortunately, this has not been presented (see Ch. 4). Normal values, which are really a loose form of norm-referencing, are almost useless unless we know how much variability is associated with a "normal value." Only through the use of a normal value (a mean), and a measurement of variability (i.e., SD), can one meaningfully, judge measurements.

Norm-referencing permits interpretation of how a subject performs relative to members of the same group (or population). If we consider that Americans, on average, tend to be overweight, we can see that someone who is "normal" is not necessarily healthy (i.e., when weight is judged on the basis of content-referencing). In the latter case, we are basing a judgment on what is desirable. Norm-referencing does not deal with desirability but with the probability that someone is relatively on a par with the rest of the population.

There are logical requirements for normative data. As has been noted, norms have no inferential use without descriptions of the variability associated with the measurement. For the rest of the requirements, we will paraphrase what *Standards for Educational Psychological Tests*[16] considers essential:

1. Norms should be presented whenever a test is first described.

2. Norms reported should refer to specifically defined and clearly described populations, and these populations should be the same as those for whom the test was designed.

3. In reporting norms, percentiles should be reported (i.e., what percentage will a given score be above), and measures of central tendency and variability should *always* be reported.

The second essential raises an important point. Norms must be population-specific. We know that ROM changes over a lifetime.[41] Therefore, one normal value cannot possibly be used to judge measurements taken on patients of varying ages.

We have emphasized the need to be age-specific. Imagine a sample of young subjects measured to obtain norms for hip ROM. For that sample to reflect the population meaningfully, it would have to be sufficiently large to minimize sampling error. The norms would be too high, if for example, the sample contained a large number of ballerinas. The sample must be *representative*. If men are significantly different from women, norms must be generated for each. If height or weight affects a variable, norms for different heights and weights are required.

Consider clinical reports that describe the quadriceps peak torque of a small group of football players.[42] There is nothing representative here that permits generalization to other players; these are not normative data. Perhaps, if the torque were from the world's greatest football players, a case could be made for the use of these values to establish a criterion-referenced standard; under no circumstance, however, can convenient small samples be used to generate meaningful "norms."

Ghiselli and his colleagues,[17] give a good example of how one defines the population used for norms:

> Various types of populations are used as a basis for establishing norms. In actual practice, of course, we ordinarily do not have all members of a population but only a sample. The selection of groups is a function of the purpose for which the measurements are being made. Thus, the norms for a typing achievement test might be based on the scores earned by trained typists in general or by tenth-graders who have completed a one semester course in typing, depending on the type of person in whom we are interested.

Which population is sampled to generate norms, therefore, depends on the use intended for the normative data.

MEASUREMENT

Levels of Measurement

What is a measurement? In this chapter, the term describes the assignment of a numeral or a name to a characteristic being examined. Therefore, classification is considered to be a type of measurement. Assignment of a number, such as is done when measuring motion or forces, is also a type of measurement. The term "test" describes the process used in obtaining a measurement. Although there is less than universal agreement on these definitions, they have support in the literature[11] and are highly useful. Because measurement has multiple meanings, further clarification of the term is in order. Traditionally this consists of describing the four levels of measurement, *nominal, ordinal, interval,* and *ratio.* Each level describes a different type of measurement and, what is more important, each defines the type of mathematical operations that can be used with that level.

Nominal measurement is nothing more than classification or categorization based on a variable.[11] Some authors do not even consider it a form of measurement.[43] Using an operational definition, we measure nominally when we assign individuals or things to previously named and defined, unranked categories. When we classify patients according to their diagnoses, we are nominally measuring. The characteristics of each group must be predetermined so that rules for assignment to groups are clear, and so that assignment can be made to one group and one group only. To classify stroke patients based on the side of involvement, we would nominally categorize patients into groups with left or right hemiplegia. Note that no subject could belong to both groups, but all hemiplegics must belong to one group or the other. This means that our *categories must be mutually exclusive (i.e., not overlapping)* and exhaustive *(i.e., have a place for everyone being measured)*. If our patient group contained subjects who have had multiple strokes, then we would need to add a third category called "both." The third category would be needed in order to be mutually exclusive and exhaustive.

Nominal measurement does not allow us to make statements about the relative merits of belonging to one group or another. We can only say that people or objects belong to a group.

Nominal measurement has great value in clinical practice. We know that not all patients with a given diagnosis are equal. By developing clinically useful categories to measure patients nominally, we may be able to determine which types of patients best respond to various treatments. McKenzie's system for treating low back disorders provides an example.[44] He classifies patients based on a series of tests into groups with dysfunctions, postural problems, and derangements.[44] He further subdivides the derangement group, and it is this classification that guides treatment. To date, the reliability of the categorizations has not been tested. The reliability of the nominal measurement will obviously depend on the reliability of the tests used to make the assignment to the various groups.

Better differentiation of the populations treated by physical therapists can only lead to better understanding of how treatment works. Only by developing meaningful classification schemes can we expect to test the effectiveness of treatments, because only then can treatments be selectively and effectively applied to the most appropriate patient populations. Although such classification is an obvious requirement for the advancement of physical therapy science, classification schemes as a form of measurement must be examined for reliability before they are used. The validity of the classification will support or limit the inference. If, as in the case of McKenzie's approach, classification is used to guide treatment, validity will be demonstrated by whether or not use of the classification scheme leads to more effective treatments.

In terms of analysis, the only mathematical operations that can be performed on nominal data deal with frequency counts, i.e., enumerating how many units or members are in a given category.

Ordinal measurement is very similar to nominal measurement in that categorization is made based on operational definitions that allow for assignments that are mutually exclusive and exhaustive. The major difference lies in the relationship between or among the categories. Ordinal scales have a logical hierarchy between categories. McKenzie categorized patients with low back problems in such a way that each belonged to a different group that presumably related to the etiology of the pain. One group was not higher or lower than the other; they were just differerent. If we want to categorize patients with low back disorders based on the severity of their complaints, we could assign them, using operational definitions, to a mild, moderate, or severe group. There is clearly a continuum depicted in the above example. Members of the mild group have less of the quantity of interest (back pain) than do those in the severe group. The name ordinal is derived from the fact that the groups are ordered along a continuum. A limitation of ordinal measurement is that we cannot assume equal intervals between categories. The difference in pain between those in the mild and the moderate pain groups need not be the same as the difference between those in the moderate and severe pain groups.

Ordinal measurements are used for MMT grades. We assign performance to a category (absent, trace, poor, fair, good, or normal).[19] The difference between the muscle tension needed to go from a trace grade to a poor grade is not necessarily the same as that needed to go from a poor to a fair grade. Because the limitations of ordinal measurements are the same as those of nominal measurements, we can note some misuse of MMT data in the literature.

There is a temptation to assume that if we assign numbers to ordinal or nominal groups we can then treat those numbers in any way we please. The way in which we name a group—with a word or number—does not change the way in which we can use the various levels of measurement. Because the only permissible operation for nominal and ordinal data is the analysis of frequencies (i.e., counting members of the groups) it is impossible to average MMT grades legitimately. Therefore, we cannot say that "an average MMT improvement of one grade was noted." How can you average numbers that do not really represent quantities equally spaced? How can you interpret such observations? The change between trace and poor would be entirely different in magnitude than the change between good and normal.

It is unfortunate that the Kendall and Kendall text on MMT encourages the misuse of MMT data by presenting a table that gives grades in percentages.[25] Percentages should only be calculated on ratio-scaled data, as will be seen later. When the Kendall approach is used, the labels that use the term "percentage" are really terms used for ordinal classification and offer no more information than if words had been used (see Ch. 2).

Interval-scale measurement involves subsesquent units with numerically equal distances between them. The difference between 1° C and 2° C is the same as the difference between 236° C and 237° C. The mathematical operations permissible with interval-scaled data are addition, subtraction, and limited forms of multiplication and division. An interval-scaled measurement cannot be divided by an interval-scaled measurement or, in other words, *ratios cannot be formed from interval-scaled data.* To use normal distributions and norm-referenced concepts, data must be at *least* interval scaled (i.e., they can also be ratio scaled).

Ratio Scale of Measurement. A ratio scale is essentially an interval scale with one noticeable difference: the zero point on the measurement scale represents *a total* absence of the quantity being measured. In interval scales, the zero, if present, is somewhat arbitrary. The classic example used to differentiate interval and ratio scales involves temperatures. Both the Fahrenheit and Celsius scales have zero points that are somewhat arbitrary, although the use of the freezing point of water in the Celsius system has some utility. Heat energy is present when the temperature is zero in either Fahrenheit or Celsius. Only when an absolute temperature scale is used can we really say that zero represents an absence of the quantity being measured. Use of a ratio scale of measurement is a requirement for the calculation of ratios (including percentages). If we attempt to use non-ratio–scaled data, the resultant numbers describe relationships erroneously.

Generation of inappropriate ratios with interval-scaled data is shown in the following example. When the temperature rises from 10° C to 20° C, we could conclude mistakenly that it is twice as hot as it was before (20/10 = 2). However, the real ratio can only be calculated after we change the data into degrees Kelvin. The first temperature would then be 283° K and the second 293° K. The real change in heat was 293/283 = 1.035. Instead of becoming twice as hot, it actually became 1.035 times as hot.

Sometimes measurements may appear to be ratio scaled when they are actually interval scaled. Torque, for example, is thought of as being ratio scaled because the zero normally represents a total absence of the quantity being measured. However, when measured with an isokinetic device, torque is no longer ratio scaled. Isokinetic devices measure only the torque needed to keep a limb segment from accelerating beyond the machine's present speed. A limb moving at less than the machine's speed is moving because muscular tension is resulting in a torque, but the isokinetic device still records zero. Thus, there is a varying amount of unaccounted-for torque when isokinetic devices are used.[45] If the muscle is working against gravity, torque is missing and the zero point is falsely high. If the muscle is moving with gravity, some of the machine's measured torque represents gravitationally generated forces rather than torque of muscular origin; the zero is then falsely low (i.e., torque can be measured even when the muscle may not be generating tension). For a more complete discussion of this issue, see Chapter 3 in this volume. The meaning of ratios generated from isokinetic measures are questionable. Future research that does not violate the basic rules applied to levels of measurement will be necessary before we can discover if the previously reported ratios of isokinetic torque values represent *real phenomena* rather than *artifacts* of the misuse of interval-scaled data.

Statistical Concepts Used in Measurement Theory

We have already briefly reviewed the importance of measures of central tendency (i.e., the mean) and measures of variability (i.e., SD) in interpreting scores. Review of all the relevant statistics and the theory one must know in order to evaluate reliability and validity fully is beyond the scope of this chapter. Readers desirous of more information in this area and on measurement theory in general are urged to examine the references carefully. A brief overview of some of the statistical techniques commonly applied to the analysis of measurements follows.

Correlation coefficients may be generated with many different types of data, although the level of measurement dictates the correlation coefficient that must be used. The term "correlation" was originated by Galton, who made some of the earliest observations on distributions. Galton observed that some paired observations tended to have a relationship. For example, the sons of tall fathers, he noted, tended to be taller than the sons of shorter fathers. In other words, the variability in one measurement, the father's height, seemed to predict (relate to) the variability in the other measurement, the son's height. The term correlation is used to describe the relationship between two sets of paired measures; it is an index of how these paired numbers covary (or *correlate*).

Correlation coefficients are an index of how well an equation can predict one variable from another. If there is a perfect rule of correspondence, based on the equation, the coefficient will be high (1 is the upper limit). When the relationship is less than perfect (i.e., there is some error in the prediction of one variable from the other), the correlation is less than one. A negative correlation occurs when an increase in one variable is accompanied by a decrease in the second variable. In this circumstance, a perfect inverse relationship is indicated by a -1 and a less than perfect inverse relationship by any number between -1 and zero.

Ghiselli, Campbell, and Zedeck[17] offer a succinct definition:

> *Correlation Coefficient:* An index of the degree of association between two variables or the extent to which the order of individuals on one variable is similar to the order of individuals on a second variable. This quantitative description of the relationship between two variables indicates the accuracy with which scores on one variable can be predicted from scores on another as to the extent to which individual differences on two variables can be attributed to the same determining factor.

The correlation coefficient is the most commonly used statistic in the analysis of measurements. Reliability is often assessed through the use of correlations, the assumption being that if paired measurements correlate highly, reliability is present. Intra-tester reliability is analyzed by correlating the measurements taken on one occasion with those taken on a second occasion by the same measurer. Inter-tester reliability is analyzed by correlating the measurements taken by two different measurers of the same person.

A perfect correlation (of 1) does not mean that the paired variables are identical, but rather that they are perfectly related. When correlation is used to describe reliability, a false impression may be given if only the correlation coefficient is reported. If we were testing the intra-tester reliability of a new kind of dynamometer and a single therapist measured ten patients' triceps force on one day and the same ten patients on the second day, a correlation of 1 may have been calculated. What does this mean, however? Any one of the three sets of paired scores in Table 1-1 would yield a coefficient of 1.

Table 1-1. Triceps Force (in Arbitrary Units)

Measurement	Set 1		Set 2		Set 3	
Patient	1	2	1	2	1	2
1	50	55	50	60	50	50
2	59	64	59	70.8	59	59
3	45	50	45	54	45	45
4	70	75	70	84	75	75
5	80	85	80	96	80	80
6	20	25	20	24	20	20
7	90	95	90	108	90	90
8	100	105	100	120	100	100
9	50	55	50	60	50	50
10	80	85	80	96	80	80

The reason why all three sets have a perfect correlation coefficient is that each has a perfect rule of correspondence. All the second numbers in Set 1 are five units higher than the first numbers. All the second numbers in Set 2 are 20 percent higher than the first. Only in Set 3 are both first and second numbers identical. If these three sets of numbers were obtained in different reliability studies, we would be able to say that there was minimum error, because *we can account for the variability* in one measure from another. However, in terms of clinical practice we would want to know, and account for, whether the process of taking a second measurement led to an increase in the measurement (as would be the case for Sets 1 and 2). This is why reliability reported solely on the basis of correlation coefficients does not tell the whole story. The formula that most often is used to describe the relationship between correlated variables is the linear regression equation.[17] The equation takes the following form: $Y = a + bX$, where Y is one variable, X is the second variable, a is the intercept and b is the slope. The intercept is an additive factor that must be added to one variable (i.e., X) to make that variable equal to Y. The slope is a multiplicative factor that must be multiplied by one variable (i.e., X) to make it equal to Y. The two may be considered corrections that must be used together to predict one variable from the other. For the three sets of triceps force, the equations would be (if X is the first number in each set):

$$\text{Set 1} \quad Y = 5 + 1X$$

$$\text{Set 2} \quad Y = 0 + 1.20X$$

$$\text{Set 3} \quad Y = 0 + 1X$$

The above example illustrates how reliability may be understood when both the correlation (an index of the strength of relationships) is reported along with a regression equation (the mathematical representation of the nature of the relationship). Careful examination of the linear regression equations reported with reliability data permits clinicians to determine how much change is simply a function of testing more than once, and how much is caused by *meaningful* change in the variable of interest.

Regression equations can only be calculated for interval- and ratio-scaled data. With such data, the correlation coefficient most commonly used is the Pearson product moment (*r*).[15] There has been an unfortunate tendency to rename this statistic when it is used to measure reliability. Calling it the "coefficient of objectivity," or the "reliability coefficient" may cause some confusion. The use of multiple names sometimes makes it difficult to know what statistic was used. There is no inherent property of this statistic that makes it a coefficient of reliability. Correlation coefficients are indices used to represent reliability only when a study is properly designed. Other correlation coefficients may be also used in reliability studies.

To avoid the necessity of interpreting both a correlation coefficient and an associated linear regression equation, a statistic that is sometimes used for reliability assessments is the intra-class correlation coefficient (ICC).[46–49,52] This statistic is derived from an analysis of variance model for repeated measures.[49] Users of the statistic (which takes the form of any number from 0 to 1) argue that since it measures the extent to which multiple measures *agree* (i.e., are equal) rather than are associated (i.e., covary) it is more appropriate for certain types of reliability assessment. In addition to being a means of assessing agreement rather than association, the ICC has the further advantage of permitting comparisons between any number of multiple measurements taken of the same person. The most commonly used forms of correlation coefficients are limited to comparing only two sets of paired scores at a time.

Correlation coefficients also play a critical role in validity studies, especially in investigations of criterion-related validities. In such studies, the measurement being validated is correlated with the criterion measurement. Because these paired measurements (made on the same subject) frequently have different units, we are less concerned with the nature of the relationship than we are with the strength of the relationship as indicated by the magnitude of the correlation coefficient or the coefficient of determination (r^2).

A statistical procedure, factor analysis, is sometimes used in the development and validation of tests.[15] Factor analysis is a special type of multivariate analysis that allows for the examination of many variables in order to determine relationships among these variables. Often the purpose of this analysis is to reduce the number of variables to a smaller number of clusters that reflect an underlying "factor" or "factors" of interest. As can be seen in the review of gait measurements by Craik and Oatis in Chapter 6, a plethora of gait variables may be measured. Some of these may contain redundant information. For example, a basic application of factor analysis could be the determination of whether measurements of stride and step length and associated variables may actually be a function of an underlying factor that could be labeled "ambulation speed." If stride and step length vary as a function of "ambulation speed," we do not really need to measure all of these variables. Measurement of "ambulation speed" would suffice. Factor analysis has been used to define those items that should be included in ADL tests (see Ch. 5). Factor analysis could be a useful tool for reducing variables in the future. Use of factor analysis may permit a reduction in the number of measurements needed to make inferences about important behaviors which physical therapists may want to measure clinically.

Two other statistics commonly appear in discussions of measurement and should be defined, the coefficient of variation (CV)[50] and the standard error of the measurement (SEM).[51] These are quite different from correlations since they, at least theoretically, relate to single sets of measurements that must meet certain requirements.

The concept of the normal distribution and the SD has been previously introduced. When a group of people are measured for a variable, the obtained measurements will be distributed along the classic bell-shaped curve. The assumption is that although people are different, their measurements tend to be relatively close to the mean for any given characteristic. When we measure a sample that is representative of a population, the SD is an estimate of the variability of that measurement in the population. The variability represented by the SD in this case represents the variability of the characteristic (e.g., height, weight, or whatever is being measured). To a lesser extent, the variability also reflects measurement errors, but we have no way of knowing how much variabilty results from error; this is one reason why reliability is essential.

If we measured the same characteristic on one subject many times, we would expect no variation in the measurement, except that caused by measurement error. Whenever we measure the same characteristic many times on the same subject or different subjects who should score equally on a variable, the obtained SD reflects only measurement error (here sampling error will be considered a form of measurement error).

The coefficient of variation (CV) is the SD as expressed as a percentage of the mean (CV = SD/mean × 100). This can be used to estimate the percentage of variation that can be expected in a measurement solely because of measurement error. As can be seen from review of pulmonary function measurements by Protas in Chapter 8, this is a useful way to analyze the reliability of instrument-based measurements.

The conceptual basis for the standard error of the measurement (SEM) and the underlying statistical principles are beyond the scope of this chapter (for a more complete discussion of this statistic, see Ghiselli et al).[17] The purpose of the statistic is to provide a number that represents the way in which a single score will vary if a test is administered more than once. Because a basic assumption for all reliability testing is that scores should remain stable between uniform conditions (because we have controlled for this), variations between tests are not caused by *true* changes in the variable of interest. Variability between test sessions is, therefore, solely caused by error and can be assessed by the SEM. Because the mathematics underlying SEM measurement are tied to the SD and associated assumptions, this statistic has some remarkable properties.

Let us assume that we know that the SEM for hip flexion ROM is 3°. Note that the SEM is expressed in the same units used for the measurement. If we then measure a patient and find that his hip flexion ROM is 90°, we would have to conclude, using the SEM, that the *true* measurement was somewhere between 87° and 93°. The SEM is really a special case of a SD, and since we have stated that our *true* measurement was between ±1 SD, we must note that this range will encompass the *true* measurement 68 percent of the time. The probability statement of 68 percent is derived from the observation that measurements tend (even error measurements), to be normally distributed, and therefore 68 percent of all scores are within ±1 SD. The SEM is practical because it provides a direct way in which reliability can be used in clinical practice.

When correlation coefficients (*r* values) are reported, they may be squared to derive a statistic called the coefficient of determination (r^2).[15] This statistic represents the average variability that can be accounted for when predicting one measurement from another. An *r* of .80 as an index of reliability would, therefore, mean that 64 percent of the variability in one measurement (i.e., a first measurement or a measurement by a first observer) could be accounted for by a second measurement (i.e., a second measurement or a measurement by a second observer). Although the use of the coefficient of determination gives a perspective on the degree of error associated with a measurement, it is less useful than the SEM, which allows each individual score to be considered with an error term. With r^2, we know the average error, but not the expected error for any single measurement. When we use the SEM, every single obtained measurement is associated with a degree of error (or uncertainty) that has a known probability. The SEM provides a more precise index for deciding how the measurement is to be interpreted. In the example previously presented, when the measurement of hip flexion ROM was 90° and the SEM was 3°, we would have to question whether a real change in motion occurred if subsequent measurements showed only a gain of 3°. However, if a gain of 6° was made, we could be reasonably assured that a real improvement in ROM had occurred (there would actually be less than a 2 percent chance that no change had occurred).

The SEM is probably the most desired index of reliability. The CV is really only useful in the rare circumstance where many measurements can be taken on the same subject. Correlation coefficients are the most commonly reported indices of reliability, but unless they are accompanied by either the data used or the associated regression questions, they have a more limited usefulness than the SEM. However, the requirements in terms of experimental design needed to generate correlation coefficients are easier to meet than those needed to calculate the SEM.

Objectivity and Subjectivity

The terms ''objective'' measurement and ''subjective'' measurement are sometimes used loosely. A subjective measurement may be defined as one that is affected by the measurer. An objective measurement is not affected by the person taking the measurement. A test is not *subjective* if it shows inter-tester reliability, since the hallmark of inter-tester reliability is the ability of different examiners to obtain the same test score from the same subject. It is obvious that if multiple examiners consistently obtain the same measurement, they are not bringing a unique part of themselves (biases, skill, etc.) to the measurement process. Inter-tester reliability demonstrates the fact that if biases are brought to taking measurements, they are at least shared by those who were testers in the reliability study. If there *are* biases, but those biases are shared or are nearly universal, the validity of a test *may* be threatened, but the reliability is not.

Objectivity: A Question of Reliabilty, Not Validity

MMT is sometimes called an "objective test." But is it? As Lamb notes in Chapter 2 of this volume, reliability is rather poor for measurements above fair. Apparently testers do bring a part of themselves into this part of the measurement process. As Lamb observes, MMT up to the grade of fair is objective, but above that, it is subjective. Some clinicians might even argue that in view of this we might abandon the terms good and normal and report grades only as absent, trace, poor, fair, and greater than fair. A case could be made that this grading system provides a more objective test, whereas existing MMT combines subjective and objective elements.

Some physical therapy evaluations have been denigrated as being "too subjective," and they usually involve the therapist's observational assessments—as when therapists evaluate gait or sitting balance. Need such measurements be called subjective? Yes—until reliability of the visual assessment is shown. Well-developed operational definitions have the potential to change the observational process so that there may be reliability. The clinician should remember that the human observer can be quite reliable if the task is reasonable.[52,53] What is most important is that subjectivity of a test is not a moot issue, but rather one that can be dealt with directly through reliability studies. Any well-thought-out measurement scheme, regardless of the apparatus used to take the measurement, can therefore be tested for objectivity (i.e., reliability).

SUMMARY AND CONCLUSIONS

S. S. Wilks has noted three major requirements for scientific measurements: (1) there must be an operational definition to guide the process; (2) measurements must be reproducible; and (3) measurements must be valid in that they must yield "true" measurements of the object being measured. Wilks adds that for a measurement process to be satisfactory, there must be a high degree of reliability and a high degree of validity.[3]

Much of this volume considers whether measurements used by physical therapists fulfill these requirements. In Chapter 7 on the assessment of the pediatric CNS patient, Campbell alludes to what she perceives as an antiquantitative bias on the part of some practitioners. That bias may be more widespread than we are willing to admit, but clearly such a bias is not unique to our profession. Shryock, in reviewing the history of quantification in medical science, describes centuries of resistance to quantification (i.e., measurement).[54] He cites an 18th century French physician as saying that "nearly everything depends on what is seen and on a certain instinct for interpretation; the outcome depends more on the artist's sensations than on any principle in the art."[54] Shryock observes that, "For the many practical men who held such views, to turn from patients to experiments and measurement was a flight from reality."[54] Antiquantification sentiment was so strong in the 18th century that the use of the thermometer was resisted and use of a watch to take a pulse was considered a waste of time.

Quantification can be discussed in purely scientific terms, but the issue of measurement in clinical sciences seems to evoke a visceral response from many practitioners. Apparently those who are proud of their clinical skills may perceive their art threatened by scientific quantification. Consider the French medical authority, Auber, who declared in 1839 that others were "arrogant" in claiming that quantification alone permitted judicious reasoning."[54] He went on to support his antiquantitative notions by arguing that many physiologic and pathologic phenomena were unmeasurable. This last argument has appeared throughout the history of science. Stevens even recounts how much resistance existed earlier in this century to the idea that sound energy (in terms of decibels) could be measured.[11] The resistance was so fierce that a commission of English scientists said the concept was foolish.[11] Yet, today we accept the value of such measurements, just as health professionals accept the value of taking temperatures and timing pulses with watches.

One of the great ironies of science lies in the argument that quantification has an arrogance attached to it and that measurement is somehow antihumanistic. Such arguments are untenable when one considers what measurement is all about and when measurement theory is fully comprehended. The empiricist sees through eyes that are potentially biased and makes judgments. Without measurement these judgments are never tested. Empiricism—basing decisions solely on personal observation—has a role when measurement is impossible, but when quantification is feasible, empiricism can be the arrogant approach if the observer assumes infallibility. That observer is suggesting that his opinions are more valid than information gained through scientific inquiry.

Measurement science is concerned with the quality of measurements. We desire to make our measurements perfect, or error-free, but we know that is impossible. By knowing the limitations of our measurements, we free ourselves from following false guidelines and from acting with unwarranted certainty. Measurement theory tells us what we can legitimately achieve with our measurements. Jacob Bronowski in his classic television production, "The Ascent of Man," put the issue in perspective when he said: "All knowledge, all information between human beings can only be exchanged within a play of tolerance. And that is true whether the exchange is in science, or in literature, or in religion, or in politics, or even in any form of thought that aspires to dogma."[55]

Our profession is burdened with untested dogma, untested not only by research, but also by the careful scrutiny of clinical practice that uses meaningful measurements. Bronowski argues that dogmatists open the door to tragedy and "betray the human spirit" because they close minds and turn followers into obedient ghosts. For Bronowski, a Polish scientist who lost much of his family in the Holocaust, the issue of how we know and how we act on our knowledge was central to his understanding of that great tragedy. Reflecting on the crimes at Auschwitz, he said, "When people believe that they have absolute knowledge, with no test in reality, this is how they behave. This is what men do when they aspire to the knowledge of gods."[59]

The critical phrase in his analysis is "no test in reality." Physical therapy is an inherently humanistic profession. As part of the dedication we share to our profession and our patients, we must consider the need to *test* what we do and the need to quantify. Our art has served patients well, but the same argument could have been made by physicians in the 18th century. The real issue is how we might best fulfill our professional mandate. Scientific practice offers the best hope for that fulfillment and the greatest promise that we may serve our patients. A science is only as good as the measurements on which it is based.

The state of measurement in physical therapy is not good. The issues that must be addressed have been discussed in this chapter and elsewhere in this volume. Whether clinicians use this knowledge to develop better methods and to become more critical consumers is a question that only time can answer. However, the present state and the dire need should not cause a frustration that leads to acceptance of the status quo. Ours is a young profession and the possibilities for future growth are great. The opportunities for the development of meaningful measurement systems are vast. Let us consider the challenge in perspective. Clinical medicine took nearly 100 years to accept the value of taking a patient's temperature. If we as a profession can begin to face the challenge of quantification after a little more than half a century of existence, we will have little explaining to do to future generations of therapists and patients. If we do not face the challenge, we may forfeit the right to professional status. Use of meaningful measurements for quantification by therapists can be thought of as a means of serving science, patient care, and the continued growth of physical therapy.

REFERENCES

1. Campbell SK: Measurement and technical skills—neglected aspects of research education. Phys Ther 61:523, 1981
2. Wilks SS: Some aspects of quantification in science, p. 5. In (Woolf H (ed): Quantification. Bobbs Merrill, New York, 1961
3. Fowler WM Jr, Gardner GW: Quantitative strength measurements in muscular dystrophy. Arch Phys Med Rehab 48:629, 1967

4. DeLateur BJ, Giaconi RM: Effect on maximal strength of submaximal exercise in Duchenne Muscular Dystrophy. Am J Phys Med 58:26, 1979

5. Chusid JG: Correlative Neuroanatomy and Functional Neurology. Lange, Los Altos, California 1982

6. Carr JH, Shephard R: Physiotherapy in Disorders of the Brain. Heinemann, London, 1980

7. Shephard RB: Physiotherapy in Pediatrics, 2nd Ed. Heinemann, London, 1974

8. Brunnstrom S: Movement Therapy in Hemiplegia, Harper & Row, New York, 1970

9. Bobath B: Abnormal Postural Reflex Activity Caused by Brain Lesions, 2nd Ed. Heinemann, London, 1971

10. Bobath K, Bobath B: Cerebral Palsy, p. 31. In Pearson PH, Williams CE (eds): Physical Therapy Services in the Developmental Disabilities. Charles C Thomas, Springfield, Illinois, 1972

11. Stevens SS: Measurement, psychophysics and utility. In Churchman CW, Ratoosh P (eds): Measurement: Definitions and Themes. Wiley, New York, 1959

12. Hays WL: Quantification in Psychology. Brooks Cole, Belmont, California, 1967

13. Lyle VJ: The Nature of Measurement in Educational Measurement, p. 8, 2nd Ed. American Council of Education, Washington D.C., 1971

14. Singer C: The Discovery of the Circulation of the Blood. Dawson, London, 1956

15. Kerlinger FN: Foundations of Behavioral Research, 2nd Ed. Holt, Rinehart, and Winston, New York, 1973

16. Standards for Educational and Psychological Tests: American Psychological Association, Washington, D.C., 1974

17. Ghiselli EE, Campbell JP, Zedeck S: Measurement Theory for the Behavioral Sciences, W. H. Freeman, San Francisco, 1981

18. Halliday D, Resnick R: Fundamentals of Physics. Wiley, New York, 1970

19. Daniels L, Worthington C: Muscle Testing: Technique of Manual Examination, 4th Ed. Saunders, Philadelphia, 1980

20. Farber SD: Neurorehabilitation: A Multisensory Approach, Saunders, Philadelphia, 1982

21. Johnson J, Siegel D: Reliability of an isokinetic movement of the knee extensors. Res Q 49:88, 1978

22. Frost M, Struckey S, Smalley LA, Darman G: Reliability of measuring motions in centimeters. Phys Ther 62:1431, 1982

23. Rothstein, JM, Miller, PJ, Roettger RF: Goniometric reliability in a clinical setting: elbow and knee measurements. Phys Ther 63:1611, 1983

24. Beekman CE, Hall V: Variability of scoliosis measurement from spinal roentgenograms. Phys Ther 59:764, 1979

25. Kendall H, Kendall F, Wadsworth G: Muscle Testing and Function, 2nd Ed. Williams and Wilkins, Baltimore, 1971

26. Thorstensson A: Muscle strength, fibre types and enzyme activities in man. Acta Physiol Scand 443 suppl.:1, 1976

27. Isolated Joint Testing and Exercise: A Handbook for Using Cybex II and the U.B.X.T. Cybex, Div Lumex, Ronkonkoma, New York, 1982

28. Rothstein JM, Delitto A, Sinacore DR, Rose SJ: Muscle function in rheumatic disease patients treated with corticosteroids. Muscle Nerve 6:128, 1983

29. Moffroid M, Whipple R, Hofkosh J, Lowman E, Thistle H: A study of isokinetic exercise. Phys Ther 49:735, 1969

30. Payton OP: Research: The Validation of Clinical Prctice. Davis, Philadelphia, 1979

31. Lovett RW, Masten EG: Certain aspects of infantile paralysis and a description of a method of muscle testing. JAMA 66:729, 1916

32. Rothstein JM: Muscle biology: clinical considerations. Phys Ther 62:1823, 1982
33. Einthoven W, Fahr G, deWaart A: Uber die Richtung und die manifeste Grosse der Potentialschwankungen im menschlichan Herzen und uber den Einfluss der Herzlage auf die Form des Electrokardiogramms. Arch Ges Physiol 150:275, 1913 (English translation, Hoff HH, Sekelj P, Am Heart J 40:163, 1950)
34. McHenry LC: Garrison's History of Neurology, Charles C Thomas, Springfield, Illinois, 1969
35. Malone T, Blackburn TA, Wallace LA: Knee rehabilitation. Phys Ther 60:1602, 1980
36. Shurtleff D: Some characteristics related to the incidence of cardiovascular disease and death: Framingham Study; 18-year follow-up U.S. Government Printing Office, Department of Health, Education and Welfare, Washington, D.C., NIH Publ #74:599, 1974
37. Campbell DT, Stanley JC: Experimental and Quasi-Experimental Designs for Research, Rand McNally, Chicago, 1963
38. Wallach J: Interpretation of Diagnostic Tests, 2nd Ed. Little, Brown, Boston, 1978
39. Galton F: Hereditary Genius: An Inquiry Into Its Laws. Horizon Press, New York, 1952
40. Tyler LE: Tests and Measurements, Prentice-Hall, Englewood Cliffs, New Jersey, 1963
41. Bell BD, Hoshizak TB: Relationship of age and sex with range of motion of seventeen joint actions in humans. Can J Appl Sports Sci 6:202, 1981
42. Gilliam TP, Sandy SP, Freedson, PS, Villanaci J: Isokinetic torque levels for high school football players. Arch Phys Med Rehab 60:110, 1979
43. Campbell NR: An Account of the Principles of Measurement and Calculations, Longmans, Green, London, 1928
44. McKenzie RA: The Lumbar Spine—Mechanical Diagnosis and Therapy. Spinal Pub, Worikanae, New Zealand, 1981
45. Winter DA, Wells RF, Orr GW: Errors in the use of isokinetic dynomometers. Eur J Appl Physiol 46:387, 1981
46. Bartko JJ, Carpenter WT: On the methods and theory of reliability. J Nerv Ment Dis 163:307, 1976
47. Ebel RL: Estimation of the reliability of ratings. Psychometrika 16:407, 1951
48. Lahey, MA, Downey RG, Saal FE: Intraclass correlation: there's more than meets the eye. Psychol Bull 93:586, 1983
49. Winer BJ: Statistical Principles in Experimental Design, 2nd Ed. McGraw-Hill, New York, 1971
50. Snedecor GW, Cochran WG: Statistical Methods, 7th Ed. Iowa State University Press, Ames, Iowa, 1980
51. Cronbach LJ: Essentials for Psychological Testing. Harper and Row, New York, 1949
52. Taplin PS, Reid J: Effects of instructional set and experimenter influence on observer reliability. Child Dev 44:547, 1973
53. Mitchell SK: Interobserver agreement, reliability, and generalizability of data collected in observational studies. Psychol Bull 86:376, 1979
54. Shryock RH: The history of quantification in medical science. In Woold H (ed): Medical Science, p. 85. Bobbs Merrill, New York, 1961
55. Bronowski J: The Ascent of Man. Little Brown, Boston, 1973

2 | Manual Muscle Testing

Robert L. Lamb

The word ''strength'' has multiple meanings within the profession of physical therapy. These multiple meanings have caused difficulty in communication, and occasionally have led to opposing conclusions among clinicians concerning a patient's functional ability. Therefore, it is essential that the term ''strength'' be clarified by specifying the method by which the strength is measured. The manual muscle test is one method by which muscle strength is operationally defined and measured.

The earliest description of manual muscle testing (MMT), as devised by Dr. Robert W. Lovett, was published by Wright in 1912.[1] Dr. Lovett's approach has been revised over the years, resulting in the appearance of several variations of the original test in the literature.[2-10] It is unfortunate that information is not available for determining which method is more appropriate as a clinical tool. Neither is it known to what extent each of the various methods is used in clinical practice. However, most physical therapists practicing in the United States today are probably familiar with the methods of testing and grading described by Daniels and Worthingham[10] and by Kendall et al.[9] Therefore, in the following text, these two sources have been used when needed for specific examples.

The manual muscle test uses the principles of gravity and applied external load to determine the ability of a patient to develop muscle tension voluntarily. Because muscle is the effector of body movement and a prime stabilizer, measurement of muscle performance must accurately reflect the function of the neuromuscular system as well as the integrity of other soft tissue. Thus, in conjunction with other tests and observations, MMT has been and still is considered a useful diagnostic and prognostic tool that can also be used to judge the effectiveness of therapeutic programs.

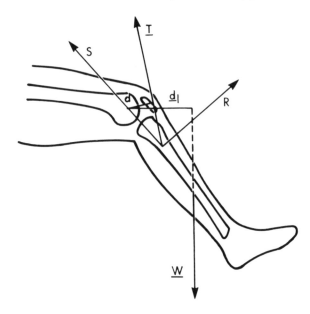

Fig. 2-1. Resolution of forces related to manual muscle testing principles. T = muscle force vector; S = stabilizing muscle force component; R = rotating muscle force component; d = muscle moment arm vector; W = segment weight vector; d_1 = weight moment arm vector.

PRINCIPLES

Muscle strength is a function of the ability of muscles to develop tension through its long axis. A direct measurement of muscle tension is not clinically practical. In its simplest situation, however, muscle tension (T) can be resolved into two forces: one acting along the long axis of the bone upon which the muscle functionally inserts, and the other perpendicular to that axis[11,12] (Fig. 2-1). The force along the axis of the bone has been termed the stabilizing component (S), and the perpendicular force (R) acting to rotate the body segment around a joint axis is called the rotating component. The rotational effect can be expressed as a moment or torque, which is defined as T multiplied by the perpendicular distance d from the joint axis to the line of muscle action. Both gravitational force (W) on the body segment and muscle tension can be resolved in the same manner. The effect of the rotational component of the segment weight is expressed as the product of its weight (W) and the perpendicular distance (d_1) from the joint axis to its line of action. The gravitational torque acts in the direction opposite to the muscle torque. The muscle torque must overcome the torque created by the weight of the extremity and any applied force in order to move or maintain the position of the body segment. MMT techniques make use of identified criteria that the practitioner can use to grade a patient's ability to voluntarily generate muscle torque. It is obvious that these grades are relative indices of muscle tension and not absolute measures of force production.

Most methods of MMT that I have reviewed use the same factors to define the criteria for grading strength. These factors are: (1) the extent of the arc of movement, (2) gravity, and (3) the amount of force applied by the examiner in

Table 2-1. A Comparison between the Criteria for Two Methods of Grading Muscles

Daniels and Worthingham[10]	Kendall et al.[9]
Normal—motion through full range against gravity and maximum applied force	100%—move into a test position against gravity and hold against maximum applied force, or hold in test position against gravity and maximum applied force
Good—motion through full range against gravity and less than maximum applied force	80%—move into a test position against gravity and hold against less than maximum applied force, or hold in test position against gravity and less than maximum force
Fair—motion through full range against gravity and hold	50%—move into test position against gravity and hold against gravity or hold test position against gravity
Poor—motion through full range with gravity diminished	20%—move through a small arc of motion with gravity diminished
Trace—palpable contraction but no movement	5%—palpable contraction but no movement
Zero—no palpable contraction	0%—no palpable contraction

a direction opposite to the torque exerted by the muscle group being tested. Occasionally, with some muscles, there is no consideration given to the effects of gravity. This occurs when the weight of the body segment is considered insignificant, when the full effect of gravity on a segment cannot be obtained with any reasonable body position, or when a patient's condition is severe enough to cause the examiner to make mental allowances for abnormal gravitational relationships.

The specific criteria for grading muscle groups are relatively simple and self-explanatory. Table 2-1 presents an abbreviated summary of the criteria used by two familiar methods. The presentation is abbreviated because each method uses additional grading increments in their system. For example, Daniels and Worthingham[10] describe a poor plus (P+) grade as the grade indicating the capability of the muscle group to move the segment through a full range of motion (ROM) in the gravity-diminished postion or in a partial range against gravity. Kendall et al.,[9] consider a muscle group with a grade of P+ (30 percent) as one that would be capable of moving the extremity through a larger arc of motion in the gravity-diminished position than that designated by the criteria for 20 percent grade. As noted in Table 2-1, the criteria for grading is relatively specific for fair grades and below. However, normal and good grades and the increments in between require a great deal of subjective judgment on the part of the examiner.

Although the grading criteria seem simple, the examiner must work from an in-depth knowledge of anatomy and kinesiology. The examiner must also be aware of the variables that affect measurement of strength. In general, these variables apply to all methods of strength measurement and have been discussed in detail in Chapter 3 and in several recent review articles.[13-16] However, there are variables important to MMT that warrant a brief discussion if the procedure is to be of any value clinically.

MMT requires attention to positioning, stabilization, and the method of applying external force to the body segment.[9,10] Standardization of these factors from one patient to another is important because the examiner must develop an experiential model with which the results of each muscle group tested will be compared. In addition, standardization is obviously important if the examiner expects to produce results that are meaningful during serial testing of a patient.

There are differences between testing methods in positioning, stabilization, and the way in which manual forces are applied. Daniels and Worthingham[10] recommend that testing of the elbow flexors be done with the patient in a sitting position with the arm stabilized at the side and, if the biceps brachii is of main concern, the forearm supinated. The patient, if possible, should move through the full arc of motion with the examiner applying force at the end of the arc of motion. The application of force against the extremity at the end of the arc of movement is my interpretation of the test procedures suggested by Daniels and Worthingham. It is not clear whether these authors advocate applying manual force to the extremity continuously through the arc of movement or at the end of the arc of motion (break test).

In contrast, for the same muscle group, Kendall et al.[9] have the patient either sitting or supine, moving the supinated forearm to a test position of 90° of elbow flexion or slightly less, or holding the test position against the applied force. The examiner's force is applied to the forearm in the test position of 90° of elbow flexion. Stabilization is maintained by the examiner, who places one hand under the patient's elbow. Although the two methods are clearly different, there is no direct evidence suggesting that the two approaches would yield significantly different results. However, there is some indirect evidence that a practitioner should be cognizant of both methods when using MMT as a clinical assessment tool.

Data suggest that variations in stabilization yield different strength measures.[13] The supine position, in the previous example, seemingly would provide more constraint to the patient than the sitting position and therefore provide more consistent results. The more constraint placed on the patient's posture, the more the test grade will represent the torque generated by the muscle group that is being considered.

Muscle torque is known to vary according to muscle length and moment arm or perpendicular distance from the joint axis of rotation to the line of action of the muscle.[13,16,17] In the example of elbow flexion, Daniels and Worthingham[10] apply external force at the end of the range of motion, where the flexors are mechanically and physiologically disadvantaged. Kendall et al.[9] apply force near midrange, where the mechanical and physiological properties of the muscles apparently are more appropriately congruent for maximum torque generation.[18] Kendall et al.[9] also place the forearm in a position that seems functionally more appropriate, and therefore the results might be a better indication of the functional capacity of the muscle. This hypothesis has not been tested, however.

The skill and consistency with which the examiner applies the external force to the body segment is important. The force should be applied gradually in the correct direction and at a consistent location on the extremity.[9,10] For example, differentiating between a normal (100 percent) and a fair plus (60 percent) grade depends on the ability of the examiner to apply the force and to judge the amount of force he or she thinks a patient should be able to generate against the applied force. The external force should be applied in the opposite direction to that of the muscle's rotational component (R) (Fig. 2-1). Because the patient is asked to hold the mobile or potentially mobile segment against this external force, one should consider the type of muscular contraction being graded, particularly if a break test is used. The muscle's ability to develop tension varies according to the type of muscle contraction.[17,19,20] Eccentric contractions generate the greatest amount of tension, followed by isometric and then concentric contractions. At what point, when applying external force, is the examiner grading the torque that is developed by an eccentric contraction? Is it of importance relative to the interpretation and functional significance of test results? These questions have not yet been answered, and further research is needed.

The effect of the external force in resisting muscle torque is a function of the distance of its application from the joint axis. If the examiner changes the distance at different times with the same patient and among patients, appropriate measurements and the development of the necessary experiential model of muscle strength related to sex, age, body type, and life style cannot be obtained. Because the patient is responding to the level of force deemed appropriate by the examiner, and because that force probably does vary with individual physical therapists, there is a possibility that judgments regarding a patient's clinical strength may be in error.

It should also be noted that the two different techniques of muscle testing use different grading systems (Table 2-1). Whether a practitioner uses a percent or letter grading system or even a numerical one is unimportant as long as there is consistency. However, it is important to remember that MMT techniques use an ordinal scale of measurement[21,22]; therefore, the practitioner cannot determine the amount of difference between two grades. A grade of 50 percent or fair is not indicative of the absolute amount of muscle tension developed; that is, a muscle grade of 50 percent is not equivalent to half the strength represented by a grade of 100 percent.

RELIABILITY

MMT seems to be a universally accepted clinical tool. One need only visit a physical therapy department, accompany a physician on rounds, or visit an amputee clinic, where musculoskeletal problems are common, to see MMT being performed in some form. One important criteria for any measurement tool is reliability.[23] If the manual muscle test is to be used in evaluating patients and the effectiveness of therapeutic intervention, one must be able to depend on the test. Thus, it would seem likely that a physical therapist would be concerned with whether MMT grades can be repeated on patients (intra-rater reliability) and if peers, using identical methods, can duplicate such grades (inter-rater reliability).

There was some genuine concern for the reproducibility of grades and the factors that influence these grades when poliomyelitis was a national health problem. Most concern was displayed in review articles identifying factors influencing grading from an empirical standpoint.[24,25] One study addressed the issue of intrarater reliability.[26] Two physical therapists performed the manual muscle test on a technically difficult post-poliomyelitis patient at 6-week intervals. Intra-examiner agreement occurred on 65 percent and 54 percent of the grades. Agreement occurred within a plus or minus grade on 82 percent and 84 percent of the muscles tested and within a full grade in 98 percent and 96 percent of the instances.

Most of the studies on inter-rater reliability were made while the effectiveness of gamma globulin and Salk vaccine on poliomyelitis were being investigated. In one study, physical therapists, nurses, and physicians were instructed in standardized methods of muscle testing.[27] They reported that the average difference between examiners was 7.1 percent. When two physical therapists were compared, the difference in grading was 3.0 percent. The comparison of two physical therapy instructors gives some credibility to the reproducibility of muscle testing grades. However, the data used to make the comparison are rather deceiving. The numerical scores used were the average grades of tested muscles weighted by a muscle bulk factor. Mathematically, this method of grading minimizes the actual differences between examiners. In addition, the grading method probably does not represent current clinical practice. The authors, recognizing that actual differences may be cancelled out of the muscle bulk factor, compared the examiners again, using only muscle grades. The two physical therapists were in agreement in 60 percent of the instances. In 95 percent of the cases, they were consistent within plus or minus one grade.

Iddings et al.,[26] had 10 physical therapists complete a manual muscle test on a poliomyelitis patient within a 2-week period. A training period was not provided; each examiner performed the test in his or her customary manner. Nine of the examiner's muscle grades were compared with the tenth. The nine physical therapists on the average agreed completely with the tenth in 45.3 percent of the cases. On the average, they agreed within a plus or minus grade in 63.8 percent of the cases and within one full grade in 90.6 percent of the cases. In order to compare results with the previously described study, they selected three pairs of examiners and compared their agreement on grading. The average agreement between the pairs of the examiners on the muscles tested was 44.5 percent. Agreement within plus or minus one full grade was 91.1 percent.

Silver et al.[28] standardized testing methods relative to positioning, stabilization, and grading of criteria. Therapists were trained to use the method on subjects with no known pathology. These same therapists then muscle-tested patients whose grades on 12 muscles or muscle groups ranged from zero to normal. The three therapists agreed completely with each other in 67 percent of the cases and within plus or minus a half grade in 97 percent of the muscles tested.

Given the results reported above, one might question the amount of variation in strength that a manual muscle test can detect. In all cases, exact agreement between examiners is relatively low. Agreement improves considerably as the scale of consensus is expanded as much as plus or minus one full grade. Apparently, one should not be concerned clinically with small changes in test grades (e.g., plus or minus one grade). These grade changes may be result from random error inherent in the MMT procedures rather than representative of true losses or gains in strength.

The studies that have attempted to address the issue of reliability are descriptive in nature and, in most cases, do not represent the use of MMT in the present clinical environment. Except for one study in 1978 that investigated the factors influencing the reliability of MMT,[29] recent literature demonstrates little interest on the part of physical therapists in establishing the reliability—or the validity—of the test as an assessment tool.

VALIDITY

For MMT to be valid, the test must measure what it was intended to measure, thus permitting an examiner to make some decision.[23,30] If an examiner obtains a grade of fair when testing the tibialis anterior, it is logical that the muscle will appear to have less strength than is expected. Thus, MMT has face validity, which is defined as the extent to which the test appears to measure what it was intended to measure.[23,30]

A judgment relative to face validity is based partially on content validity. Content validity reflects the adequacy with which the test construction in this case represents known physiologic, anatomic, and kinesiologic principles.[23,30] Referring to the previous example, these principles indicate that the tibialis anterior is a prime mover in inversion and dorsiflexion of the foot. The muscle, innervated by the deep peroneal nerve, should be able to move the foot through a full arc of motion against gravity. To some extent based on the experiential model of the examiner, the muscle should, be able to resist some degree of applied external force. It is rational that MMT has content validity because it seems to measure directly the torque-generating capability of the muscles being tested. However, does the MMT test all the types of contractions the muscle will need to make, and does it encompass important variables such as rate of tension development? Muscle testing appears to be of value as an aid to diagnosis because it has some content validity.

Agreement of knowledgeable persons that test construction is sound is an indication of a high degree of content validity of a test. There is certainly evidence that MMT is conceptually valid for some uses. However, there are evident differences between the two testing methods used as examples earlier in this chapter that should at least generate some questions. What methods have a higher degree of content validity? Will an examiner arrive at different conclusions by using one method rather than another? Does it really make a difference which method is used?

Another type of validity, particularly important to physical therapists, is construct validity. Construct validity, as related to MMT, represents the degree to which one can generalize the results of the test to relevant behaviors.[23,30] The "fair" grade obtained on the tibialis anterior indicates to the examiner that the muscle inverts and dorsiflexes the foot through a full ROM while the patient is sitting with legs over the edge of the table and with the leg in question stabilized.[10] Given the grade of fair, can the examiner answer questions relative to functional activities? How will the muscle perform in the non–weight-bearing flexor pattern of gait? How will it perform as a stabilizer or in the coordinate patterns of push-off and heel strike in the weight-bearing portion of gait? Because MMT procedures do not examine muscles during meaningful functional activities, their use may be limited, particularly for the neurological patient. Neither is there published evidence to which the examiner can relate the muscle torque-generating capabilities indicated by MMT to the functional capabilities of the patient.

Construct validity relates closely to predictive validity.[23,30] I believe that one of the major differences between the two is time. Predictive validity refers to the scientific generalizations one can make to the future. For example, given MMT grades representing a characteristic pattern of weakness, can the examiner make a decision as to the future behavior of the patient? Again, there is no published evidence that MMT has predictive validity.

CONCLUSIONS

Manual muscle testing is hypothesized as a valuable measurement tool for the clinical assessment of patients with neuromuscular problems. Information relevant to its reliability is sparse. More research must be done in today's clinical environment, using appropriate research design. MMT appears to have face and content validity. However, there is no published evidence that gives credence to the degree to which an examiner can generalize the results of MMT to immediate and future functional behaviors of patients.

REFERENCES

1. Wright W: Muscle training in the treatment of infantile paralysis. Boston Med Surg J 167:567, 1912
2. Lowman CL: A method of recording muscle tests. Am J Surg 3:588, 1927

3. Legg A, Merrill J: Physical therapy in infantile paralysis. In Mock HE, Pemberton R, Coulter J (eds): Principles and Practices of Physical Therapy. Vol. 2. W.F. Prior, Maryland, 1932

4. Kendall H, Kendall F: Care during the recovery period in paralytic poliomyelitis. U.S. Publ Health Bull No. 242, U.S. Government Printing Office, Washington, D.C., Rev. 1939

5. Brunstromm S: Muscle group testing. Physiotherapy Rev 21:3, 1941

6. Zausmer E: Evaluation of strength and motor development in infants. Part I. Phys Ther Rev 33:575, 1953

7. Zausmer E: Evaluation of strength and motor development in infants. Part II. Phys Ther Rev 33:621, 1953

8. Hines TF: Manual muscle examination. In: Therapeutic Exercise, p. 163. Lecht (ed) Waverly, Baltimore, 1965

9. Kendall H, Kendall F, Wadsworth G: Muscle Testing and Function, 2nd Ed., Williams and Wilkins, Baltimore, 1971

10. Daniels L, Worthingham C: Muscle Testing: Technique of Manual Examination, 4th Ed. W. B. Saunders, Philadelphia, 1980

11. MacConaill MA, Basmajian JV: Muscles and Movements: A Basis for Human Kinesiology, p. 85. Williams and Wilkins, Baltimore, 1969

12. Le Veau B: Biomechanics of Human Motion, p. 23. W. B. Saunders, Philadelphia, 1977

13. Smidt G, Roger M: Factors contributing to the regulation and clinical assessment of muscular strength. Phys Ther 62:1283, 1982

14. Rothstein J: Muscle biology: Clinical considerations. Phys Ther 62:1823, 1982

15. Westers BM: Factors influencing strength testing and exercise prescription. Physiotherapy 68:42, 1982

16. Soderberg GL: Muscle mechanics and pathomechanics. Phys Ther 63:216, 1983

17. Poland J, Hobart D, Payton O: The Musculoskeletal System, 2nd Ed. p. 8. Medical Examination, Garden City, New York, 1981

18. Clark H, Elkins E, Martin G, Wakins K: Relationship between body position and the application of muscle power to movements of the joint. Arch Phys Med 31:81, 1950

19. Komi PV, Buskirk ER: Effect of eccentric and concentric muscle conditioning or tension and electrical activity of human muscle. Ergonomics 15:417, 1972

20. Singh M, Kaspovich PV: Isotonic and isometric forces of forearm flexors and extensions. J Appl Physiol 21:1435, 1966

21. Michels E: Evaluation and research in physical therapy. Phys Ther 62:828, 1982

22. Michels E: Measurement in physical therapy. Phys Ther 63:209, 1983

23. Payton O: Research: The Validation of Clinical Practice, p. 111. F. A. David, Philadelphia, 1979

24. Williams M: Manual muscle testing, development and current use. Phys Ther Rev 36:797, 1956

25. Wintz M: Variations in current manual muscle testing. Phys Ther Rev 39:466, 1959

26. Iddings D, Smith L, Spencer W: Muscle testing: part 2, reliability in clinical use. Phys Ther Rev 41:249, 1961

27. Libenfeld A, Jacobs M, Willis M: Phys Ther Rev 34:279, 1954

28. Silver M, McElroy A, Morrow L, Heafner K: Further standardization of manual muscle test for clinical study. Applied in chronic renal disease. Phys Ther 50:1456, 1970

29. Nicholas J, Sapega A, Kraus H, Webb J: Factors influencing manual muscle tests in physical therapy. J Bone Joint Surg 60:186, 1978

30. Nunnally JC: Psychometric Theory, 2nd ed., p. 86. McGraw-Hill, New York, 1978

3 | Measurement of Muscle Performance with Instruments

Thomas P. Mayhew
Jules M. Rothstein

A discussion of all the methods used to assess muscle performance could fill a volume all by itself. This chapter represents a selective review of the literature with an emphasis on clinical practice. Devices and procedures that have been primarily used for research will not be discussed. Certain assumptions underlie the approach taken in this chapter. Physical therapists spend much of their time exercising patients or teaching their patients how to exercise. Frequently, although not always, this is done to improve the ability of muscles to generate tension. We are not suggesting that disability or pain is caused only by isolated muscle weakness. However, we do contend that individual muscle performance must be measured in order to determine whether focal weakness or patterns of weakness are contributing to pain or dysfunction.

MUSCLE PERFORMANCE

Presumably, we test muscles because we want information that will help us make decisions. The most common decision is whether or not we want to exercise specific muscles. We also determine patient restrictions and alternate movement strategies based on muscle evaluations. For such evaluations to be meaningful, they must reflect muscle performance and not other variables. In reviewing instruments in this chapter, we will therefore judge them in part on whether they can be used to reflect a muscle's capabilities. We believe that tests of coordination, neuromuscular timing, motivation, etc., should reflect those variables, and that muscle tests should be equally specific. We are not suggesting that any one type of test is more important than any other, but rather that each is useful only if it is specific, i.e., it measures the variable of interest.

Throughout this chapter, we have attempted to use terms as they are most commonly defined or as they are used in most scientific disciplines. We have avoided creating our own operational definitions because all too often they can be misinterpreted and lead to inappropriate generalizations, as can be seen from the first term defined.

Strength and Weakness

The terms used most often to describe muscle performance are "strength" and "weakness." Yet there are no units of measurement associated with either. A dictionary defines strength as "a physical force" and "a source of power," whereas weakness is a "lack of strength."[1] It is clear that a concept is conveyed with the definitions, but does that help us in the process of measurement? We think not. Strength is a nonscientific descriptor when applied to muscle. If we attempt to assess strength we must define it operationally, i.e., describe it through delineating a procedure used to measure it.

There is no one operational definition of strength currently in use. One definition suggests that it is the maximal force that can be exerted during a single isometric contraction.[2] That definition implies that all other forms of measurement, such as the use of isokinetics or even manual muscle testing through the range of motion (ROM), do not assess strength. What value is there in a term that has no inherent scientific meaning, but rather only a vague concept attached to it?

We believe that the use of the term "strength" has encouraged a chaotic approach to measurement. If someone tells you they have measured strength, you do not know what they did or what units they obtained. Did they measure force, torque, or power, and under what conditions and with what type of device did they measure it? However, when the term "strength" is used, we receive the false impression that the same thing is being measured in the same way. A fundamental question in muscle assessment concerns the best approach to measurement. Are force measurements better than torque, or does use of one type of device or one type of contraction tell us more than use of another? In a review of five years of publications in six journals that physical therapists might consult, we found more than a dozen ways in which authors said they were measuring strength. The authors were not measuring the same thing, yet they all described what they were measuring by using the same term. We have avoided using the term, "strength," in this chapter because it has the twofold deficit of being inherently ambiguous while appearing to be specific. Instead we will talk of "muscle performance." We prefer this term for the rather ironic reason that it gives an impression that is suitably vague so that it forces the user to operationally define how they measure performance. We can measure muscle performance isokinetically, isometrically, etc. Coincidentally, we have never had trouble communicating with colleagues in the clinic because we avoid using the term "strength."

"Weakness" obviously depends on a definition of strength; on that basis alone we might avoid using the term. However, the term also raises other questions. One of the major problems in the area of muscle assessment is the lack of data that can be used to make judgments. Without data, such as population-specific norms, statements about weakness are clinical opinions. As such, they have great value; nonetheless, we should use terms which indicate that we are expressing opinions rather than terms that imply documented levels of performance.

Units of Measurement

One of the advantages of using instruments to measure muscle performance is that they yield units that have universal meaning. If you are measuring force, although you may use English or metric units, it is always: force = mass × acceleration. Similarly, when you are measuring work, power, or torque, you know that:

For linear motions: work = force × distance.
For rotational motions: work = torque × arc of movement.
Power = work/time.
Torque = force × perpendicular distance from the axis of rotation.

It is apparent that there has been a temptation to redefine some of these terms, especially as they relate to isokinetic measurement. Such redefinition adds nothing to our understanding of muscle performance and frequently assumes relationships that are nonexistent or at best unproven. High-speed isokinetic testing does not assess power any more than does low-speed testing. As can be seen from the equations above, power can be measured at high or low isokinetic speeds.

Which of the units (i.e. force, torque, power, or work) best describes muscle performance? That will depend on the reason muscle performance is being measured. A full discussion of this issue is not possible within this chapter. Therapists must ask what aspect of muscle performance needs assessment. To do this properly requires a thorough understanding of muscle biology and kinesiology. However, some types of measurements have associated limitations that are worth noting.

Muscle has been described as a physiological transducer of chemical to mechanical energy. The chemical energy exists in the form of adenosine triphosphate (ATP) bonds, whereas the mechanical energy is manifested by the creation of tension. Muscle capabilities are best reflected by measuring tension, which is the common practice of physiologists. Tension is actually a type of force, and therefore the units are useful. However, in order to measure muscle tension, some type of measurement device (usually a strain gauge) must be attached to the muscle or the tendon. Unless we have the unique opportunity to test patients who are cineplastic amputees whose tendons are accessible,[3] we cannot measure muscle tension in humans. We must measure the forces created when muscle tension acts through the skeletal leverage system.[4] Although we may measure forces or torques in this way, only a part of these measurements actually reflect variations in muscle tension. Forces and torques will vary because of biomechanical factors (e.g., changes in the angle of insertion and changes in rotational and compressive components).[4] In a very real sense, even though forces and tension are both vectors (they both have magnitude, direction, a line of application, and an angle of application), *when we assess muscle, we are measuring forces of which only the magnitude element varies when the tension that a muscle can generate varies*. For example, when biomechanical factors are advantageous, we might measure more force with the biceps brachii flexing the elbow at 90° than we would at 120° degrees of flexion—even though there could be more tension developed at 120° of flexion.[4]

Having differentiated tension and force measurements, we can see why the two terms cannot be used interchangeably. The time-to-peak-torque during isokinetic contractions has been referred to as time-to-peak-tension.[5] It is not. We do not know when peak tension was achieved; we do know when peak torque was achieved. Peak torque occurs when it does because muscle tension and optimal biomechanical factors combine. Time-rate-of-tension is another measurement that cannot be made during any type of dynamic contraction. Forces or torques are measured during isometric contractions; therefore, these values can consistently reflect tension because the limb's position is held constant and the mechanics do not change; only the tension varies.

If we use the terms tension and force interchangeably, there may be a tendency to describe phenomena inappropriately. For example, if we think "time-to-peak-torque" is the same as time-to-peak-tension, we could try to explain measurement variations purely in terms of muscle (or neurological factors such as recruitment) when the measurement predominantly reflects mechanical factors.

Speed of Movement and Speed of Contraction

When a limb moves, we can measure its speed or, with isokinetic devices, we can control the angular speed. How fast the limb moves depends only in part on how fast a muscle generates tension. The rate of tension development is *speed of contraction*. Two legs may be moving through an arc with the same *speed of movement*, but if one has a greater mass, its quadriceps must develop more tension per unit time to move the heavier leg at the same speed as the lighter leg. Once again, we see that tension cannot be reflected with more conveniently obtained measurements.

Torque and Force

Is it better to measure force, which is a linear quantity, or to use the rotational measurement, which is torque? If we apply some type of measurement device, or even perform manual muscle testing (MMT), with resistance applied closer to the axis of rotation, the muscle we are assessing has a mechanical advantage over the resistance (i.e., the resistance will have a smaller level arm) as compared to when the resistance is applied more distally. When forces are measured, as with a cable tensiometer or a hand-held dynamometer, unless the devices are applied at the same anatomical position for each test, the force measurements could vary—even though muscle tension was identical. Torque can be difficult to derive, unless a device is used that has an axis of rotation aligned with the subject's anatomical axis of rotation. When this is not the case, torque for the resistive moment may be calculated (force × distance between resistance and axis of rotation). However, muscle torque can only be estimated by calculating from anatomical studies the distance from the muscle's insertion to the axis.

Although it would appear to be beneficial to measure torque, it is not always possible. When torque cannot be directly measured, great care must be taken to standardize the site at which resistance is applied to limbs when force measurements are made.

Issues

Muscle contractions have been described as eccentric, isometric, or concentric.[6] Physiologists have demonstrated that, per unit of muscle, the greatest tension can be generated eccentrically, less can be generated isometrically, and the least can be generated concentrically.[6] The force–velocity relationship is inverse for concentric contractions, although it is direct, up to a point, for eccentric contractions.[7,8] Eccentric contractions use less metabolic energy (ATP) per unit of tension than do other contractions.[6] The differences between contraction types are profound. Therefore, when we assess muscles, we must be aware of the type of contraction we are measuring.

A major clinical concern is whether the performance in any one mode reflects the others and whether training in one mode increases performance in the other. Because we do not yet know the answer to these questions, we must be aware of the types of contractions tested by different procedures. We must also be aware that a "break test," in which the examiner pushes against a limb until the subject can no longer hold the position, appears to be different than an isometric contraction. The extent and significance of this difference has not been documented, but given our present knowledge we should differentiate between the two.

Assessment Criteria

It is presumed that we measure patients to guide clinical practice. Therefore, we need a context to use when we judge obtained measurements. Normative values for various populations have not been established for clinically relevant populations. Comparisons between "affected" and "nonaffected" limbs may be useful, but there are no data that tell us how much inter-limb variation is normal. Such comparisons are also confounded by the alternate patterns of use that patients demonstrate as a result of their disease or disability. Walking with a limp is very likely to lead to selective hypertrophy of some muscles and atrophy of others.

This chapter offers no simple solutions for finding criteria to judge muscle performance measurements. We advocate good clinical sense—that is, we urge clinicians to use all available data and not to be tempted to rely on questionable criteria. Some of these questionable criteria are discussed in this chapter; however, we will illustrate the concept here. Some forms of "fatigue" tests measure the number of contractions it takes before a subject reaches a percentage of their maximal force or torque. Although such an index may reflect on a relative basis the biological properties of muscle that relate to "endurance," we wonder whether such tests are clinically relevant.

The problem arises because "fatigue" and "endurance" lack clinically applicable operational definitions. Using the criteria of the test described above, we would have to say that a weight lifter who could develop only 50 percent of his maximal force after five repetitions had less endurance than an elderly subject who could generate a very weak torque level ten or 20 times. In terms of functional capacity, the weight lifter could do a lot more with even 10% of his peak levels than the elderly subject could with 50 percent of his. We are not suggesting that the existing test is useless. We are asking: "What is the clinical relevance of this test?"

The best way to judge force or torque levels would be to know the amount of force or torque needed in a given subject for that subject to function. These values, which would have to be normalized for anthropomorphic factors (e.g., height and weight), could then be used as guidelines. It is clear that we need research in this area.

Organization of the Chapter

Whenever possible, we have tried to follow a consistent outline when we describe measurement devices. We first describe the device or technique; then we review the history before considering reliability and validity. There is almost no literature discussing the nature of the inferences that can be made from use of most of the devices. Therefore, there is little discussion of this type of validity. Most of the validity sections discuss ways in which measurements taken with various devices compare with each other, rather than what a given measurement tells us. Although a case can be made that this is not validity but rather a form of inter-device (or equivalence of forms) reliability,[9] we have placed these discussions in the validity section. That placement is in line with the claims made for most of the devices. Authors frequently contend that their methods are valid because their measurements relate to those taken with other devices.

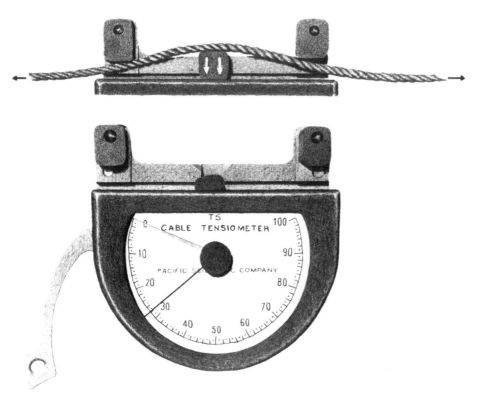

Fig. 3-1.   Standard cable tensiometer: note how the cable, when pulled, presses down on the riser.

CABLE TENSIOMETERS

The Device

Cable tensiometers were developed to measure the tension of airplane control cables.[10] To test muscle performance, one end of a cable is attached to some fixed (stable) object and the other end is attached to a limb segment. The tensiometer is placed at some point between the two sites of fixation. As the cable is pulled, it presses on the tensiometer's riser (a bar) which is connected to a gauge that measures in relative units (Fig. 3-1). However, the device can be calibrated so that the relative values can be converted into units, e.g., pounds or kilograms.

Although there is some variation in the way cable tensiometers are used, the essential features are common to all methods. The cable must be fixed to an immovable object (e.g., a wall, column, or floor). The other end of the cable must be attached to whatever body segment is being tested. The devices used for these attachments vary,[11–13] but in order for the measurement to reflect muscle performance, the cable must be in the plane of the movement (i.e., the cable must resist the movement). Therefore, the cable must make a 90° angle at its point of attachment to the body. The tensiometer situated along the length of the cable meaures cable tension when a subject attempts to move the body segment away from the cable. Because the subject is attempting to move but cannot, cable tensiometers measure isometric performance.

History

The cable tensiometer has been widely used for research,[11-13] primarily because of Clarke, who in 1948 reported how tensiometers could be used for the measurement of 28 muscles (movements).[14] Clarke has since revised testing procedures, eliminated some tests, and added others[10,11,15] A 1953 manual that describes 38 tests was his most comprehensive work;[15] it includes a description of the tensiometer and the attachment devices he developed. Instructions for fabricating the straps are included, as are directions for all aspects of testing, including positions and stabilization. Clarke also reported "objectivity coefficients" for each test. These coefficients were correlation coefficients for intertester reliability that had been, for the most part, previously published by Clarke.[10,11] Alderman and Banfield[13] and Currier[12] have also contributed to the literature on the reliability of tensiometers. Currier investigated the positions that would be most appropriate for testing elbow extension.[12] These studies will be discussed in the review of reliability.

Clarke compared the measurement characteristics of the tensiometer with those of a strain-gauge device, a spring scale, and a hydraulic myometer.[10] He concluded that the tensiometer was the best instrument. However, Wakim et al, found the strain gauge to be superior to the tensiometer.[16] A third opinion was offered by Kennedy, who concluded that the devices were essentially equivalent.[17] The reasons for these diverse opinions will be discussed later.

Reliability

No other device designed to measure muscular performance has been studied for reliability as extensively as the cable tensiometer, Clarke's systematic investigations using cable tensiometers represent the only series of studies that examine the reliability of a muscle-testing device in all its possible applications. After examining almost every feasible use of the cable tensiometer, Clarke concluded that acceptable reliability could be obtained for 38 different muscles (movements).[15] All of the reliability data is based on tests of nondisabled college students.

Usually, 64 subjects were tested twice within a single session by two different examiners. The number of examiners using the tensiometer and their level of training or professional background was not specified. The paired measures (the values obtained by each examiner) were correlated. Although the statistical methods were not described by Clarke, it appears that a Pearson product moment correlation was used. Clarke considered this a means of assessing the "precision" of the instrument and called the product moments

Table 3-1. Coefficients of Objectivity for 38 Motions Tested with the Cable Tensiometer

Motion	Coefficient of Objectivity	Motion	Coefficient of Objectivity
Finger flexion	.90	Neck flexion	.93
Finger extension	.93, .76, .81[a]	Neck extension	.92
Thumb adduction	.91	Neck lateral flexion	.97
Thumb abduction	.84, .75[a]	Trunk flexion	.90
Wrist dorsal flexion	.95	Trunk extension	.99
Wrist palmar flexion	.93	Trunk lateral flexion	.90
Wrist abduction	.84, .74[a]	Trunk rotation	.97
Wrist adduction	.91	Hip flexion	.90
Forearm pronation	.95	Hip extension	.94
Forearm supination	.91	Hip abduction	.82
Elbow flexion	.95	Hip adduction	.89
Elbow extension	.94	Hip inward rotation	.95
Shoulder flexion	.94	Hip outward rotation	.95
Shoulder extension	.97	Knee flexion	.97
Shoulder horizontal flexion	.93	Knee extension	.94
Shoulder abduction	.94	Ankle dorsiflexion	.93
Shoulder adduction	.94	Ankle plantar flexion	.93
Shoulder inward rotation	.94	Ankle inversion	.86
Shoulder outward rotation	.93	Ankle eversion	.92

Coefficients of objectivity are those reported in Clarke HH: Cable Tension Strength Tests: A Manual. Stuart E. Murphy, Springfield, Massachusetts, 1959. They represent correlations for intertester reliability.

[a] Clarke,[15] in reporting these values, does not explain why he offers multiple coefficients for these motions.

"objectivity coefficients." The values ranged from .74 to .99. (For a complete list and the motions that were tested, see Table 3-1.[15])

Clarke states that coefficients of .90 or greater are "desirable," whereas coefficients as low as .80 indicate that the test "can be used for individual measurements."[15] He offers no rationale for setting these levels and does not explain what is meant by the phrase, "used for individual measurement." Assuming that the Pearson product moment was used for correlation, the coefficients may be squared to yield coefficients of variation.[18] Therefore, Clarke found it acceptable when 64 percent of the variability in the first measurement was accounted for by the variability in the second measurement. In other words, up to 36 percent of variation may occur, on the average, between first and second measurements for some tests. Cable tensiometer users should be aware of the potential variability (i.e., know the coefficients) associated with the tests they are conducting. However, Clarke's reliability levels can only be expected when his techniques are used. These procedures were developed as a result of considerable experimentation. For example, Clarke rejected some test positions and revised others on the basis of his studies.[19]

Alderman and Banfield, using far more elaborate experimental and statistical methods, tested the reliability of a cable tensiometer system for three sets of muscles.[13] They contended that the setup they used, which included a modified Hettinger chair, allowed for better limb stabilization than had been obtained previously. Knee extension, elbow flexion, and elbow extension were tested bilaterally in 32 male college freshmen. The reliability coefficients were determined from tests conducted 24 hours apart; however, it is not clear whether the same person conducted the tests on both occasions. Therefore, the study appears to involve intra-tester reliability and attempts to assess the variability between sessions solely as a function of changes on the part of the subject. Despite the differences between the methods of Alderman and Banfield and those of Clarke, the results are reasonably in agreement. This would indicate that the use of the chair for stabilization did not improve reliability.

Currier, in assessing the influence of joint position on elbow extensor performance, examined the reliability of the cable tensiometer with the elbow flexed 60°, 90°, and 120°.[12] His method of testing was quite different from that of Clarke. Currier's reliability coefficients were in the range of .723 to .775. Reliability did not depend on elbow position.

The literature on cable tensiometers contains protocols for reliability testing of normal subjects. However, it has yet to be determined whether the patients seen in physical therapy clinics can be reliably tested. Because the training of examiners was never described by Clarke, we may also ask whether the average physical therapist can obtain reliable results when using a cable tensiometer.

Clarke demonstrated that normal subjects can reasonably replicate their performance if they are tested twice during a single session. He did not consider whether performance changed if the inter-test interval was longer. This question has been discussed previously in this chapter and is of greater significance when we measure muscle performance in patients who may be influenced by a variety of nonmuscular factors that can alter muscular output (e.g., attitude or general health status).

Validity

As has been discussed earlier in this chapter and in Chapter 1, validity is a complex issue. In its simplest form, validity deals with whether a measurement reflects whatever element is supposed to be measured.[9] A more useful definition of validity relates the measurement to the inferences that can be made, in other words, how the measurement can be used to make judgments.[9]

The narrow definition of validity was dealt with by several investigators who compared cable tensiometer measurements to those obtained by other methods. Clarke compared the following instruments: a cable tensiometer, a Wakim-Porter strain gauge, a spring scale, and a Newman Myometer.[10] Comparisons were made on the basis of which instruments were the most reliable and whether the measurements obtained with the different devices were equivalent. Finger flexion, wrist dorsal flexion, shoulder "outward rotation," neck extension, knee extension, and ankle plantar flexion were examined. Clarke categorized these actions as being strong or weak, with knee extension and ankle plantar flexion constituting the strong category.

The cable tensiometer and the strain gauge were used for all tests, while the spring scale was used to examine only shoulder rotation and neck extension. The myometer was used only for the wrist and finger tests. The choice of what to test with each device was based on the limitations of force that could be recorded with each instrument. Under the conditions studied, no instrument appeared to be more reliable than the others, although the myometer tended to have poorer reliability than either the strain gauge or the tensiometer for the finger and wrist measurements.

Clarke correlated the values obtained with the strain gauge, the myometer, and the spring scale with those taken with the tensiometer. The weak motions correlated poorly between the tensiometer and the strain gauge (coefficients ranged from .14 to .43), while for the stronger motions of knee extension and plantar flexion the values were .89 and .90. The correlation of the tensiometer and spring-scale measurements was .58 for shoulder rotation and .80 for neck extension. The correlation of the tensiometer and myometer was .14 for finger flexion and .36 for wrist dorsiflexion. However, it was pointed out by Clarke that the myometer utilizes a "break test" (see Ch. 2), whereas the tensiometer tests isometric contractions.

Despite the minimal differences in reliability coefficients, Clarke argued that the strain gauge was less useful because it was too sensitive. He also argued that because the other two devices had limited applications and could not be used for many muscles, the tensiometer was the best overall instrument. This conclusion is clearly based on his subjective observations relative to the ease of application of the various instruments rather than on reported data.

Wakim et al., simultaneously measured elbow flexion forces with a strain gauge and a cable tensiometer.[16] The strain gauge and the tensiometer were the same types as those used by Clarke. Measurements on 24 normal subjects were made at various positions; as a result 200 simultaneous measurements were obtained. Because the average strain-gauge measurement was 61.1 pounds while the average tensiometer value was 57.0 pounds, Wakim and his colleagues concluded that the tensiometer readings were erroneously low because of "friction" within the tensiometer. No evidence or discussion was offered to support this conclusion. These authors apparently believed that the strain gauge was the standard by which all other instruments should be judged. As will be discussed later in this chapter, such a statement is not justified by the available data. Although strain gauges can be highly accurate and useful in measurement, their reliability is on a par with that of the tensiometer.

Kennedy, using a different type of strain gauge but the same type of cable tensiometer previously described, examined measurements of knee flexion and extension bilaterally.[17] The measurements were essentially interchangeable, leading Kennedy to conclude that the devices were equally good. He also stated that both the strain-gauge and cable tensiometer measurements were highly correlated with the maximum weight that a subject could lift. However, correlation coefficients were not reported.

The three studies described above attempted to compare cable tensiometer measurements with those taken by means of other devices. It is also reasonable to ask, "Can cable tensiometers meaningfully reflect the performance of a given muscle or a muscle group?" If stabilization has been achieved, the cable represents the only resistance to limb movement, and therefore the tensiometer should reflect the isometric performance of the muscles being tested.

Some of the previous discussion has dealt with whether cable tensiometers have a sound theoretical basis (a form of construct validity) to be used to "reflect" muscle tension. The studies discussed dealt with whether tensiometer measures correlate with other measurements. This can be considered a form of criterion-related validity, i.e., does one type of measurement have the ability to predict another? However, what does it mean to say that several devices similarly reflect muscle performance? What does that tell us about a subject's ability to perform and function? Obviously we might seem justified in using the cable tensiometer to measure focal weakness (i.e., is the muscle being tested able to generate a lot of tension?). Other inferences may not be legitimate. On what basis can we say that someone is weak? This question is not only applicable to cable tensiometers. Throughout this chapter and this volume, it has been noted that we lack standards that can be used to place measurements in a meaningful context. What measurements can we consider to be too low when using a cable tensiometer? No normal values have been published based on the use of cable tensiometers to measure clinically relevant populations.

Clarke cited the opinions of various medical experts in an effort to make a case for the validity of cable tensiometers.[15] Clinical use of tensiometers at three hospitals led Clarke to observe that tensiometer measurements were compatible with "physicians' impressions." He also noted that patients tolerated the procedure without ill effect. Clarke's terms (e.g., clinical impressions) remained undefined and data to support the conclusions were not offered. At best, Clarke has presented a case for the face validity of his device being used in medical settings.

Summary and Conclusions

Cable tensiometers have been used for muscle evaluation for nearly 40 years, yet they are a clinical rarity. There is impressive evidence for the reliability of the device when it is appropriately used on normal subjects. A comprehensive instruction manual is available and the tensiometer itself is not very expensive. Evidence that the device can be used on patients with various disabilities is clearly lacking. Because this deficit is not uncommon in devices that measure muscular performance, it is probably not the reason for the failure of tensiometers to win widespread clinical acceptance. Clinicians apparently have not accepted its value as a tool for the evaluation of patients. The following factors may have contributed:

1. Few clinicians are exposed to the device or are taught its use during their professional training;
2. Tensiometers are not readily available in most clinical settings;
3. Special equipment is required for accurate testing (e.g., permanent fixation, straps and harnesses, pulleys);

4. Testing is time-consuming because of the exacting positions required; often two testers are needed, and;

5. Cable tensiometers can only be used for testing and not for exercise.

Tensiometer-obtained measurements, although they may agree with those obtained with other devices, still may be perceived as less meaningful by some clinicians than "dynamic measurements" of muscle performance. In fact (as discussed below), neither dynamic testing nor tensiometer testing really reveals whether a muscle may be used during functional activities. Measurements obtained with a tensiometer would be far more useful if we knew that patients could be measured reliably and if there were published norms that could be used to determine whether specific patients are weaker than would be expected. These deficits are, as noted previously, not unique to tensiometer measurements. In view of the existing body of research on cable tensiometers, it appears that this instrument has some potential usefulness. It is clear that further research is needed to show how cable tensiometers can be used in clinical practice and to examine the clinical reliability and validity of this measurement tool.

STRAIN-GAUGE DEVICES

The Devices

Strain-gauge devices designed to measure muscular performance vary greatly in their methods of application, design, and electronics. However, all are based on common principles. Loads (i.e., tension, compression, or shear) applied to materials cause a change in the geometric configuration of the material.[20] Strain is the deformation in the material caused by a load. Strain can be measured.

Strain gauges are made of electroconductive material and are usually applied to the surfaces of finely machined metal rings or rods. When the load is applied to the ring or the bar, the metal deforms with an accompanying deformation of the strain gauge. Deformation of the gauge leads to a change in the electrical resistance of the gauge. Therefore, a voltage or a current passed through the gauge will vary (because of Ohm's Law) as a function of the applied load.[21] Changes in voltages or currents may be shown with a variety of devices (e.g., strip-chart recordings, digital displays, volt meters).

Strain-gauge devices have been most often used for muscle evaluation by having the metal ring attached to an object that a limb segment can either push or pull against (creating either compressive or tensile strain). If the device is appropriately calibrated, the voltage or current change can be converted into measurements of force.

The major difference between the various types of strain-gauge devices that have been used to measure muscle performance are:

1. The manner in which the voltage or current change is displayed;

2. The way in which the devices are applied to limb segments (e.g., whether the subjects push or pull); and

3. The types of interfaces used to connect limb segments (e.g., cuffs, pads, straps).

The variability in display characteristics may relate to whether clinicians find the devices easy to use. Other factors, including the method of application and the type of interface, can seriously affect the quality of measurements.

History

Strain gauges are widely used for materials testing and biomechanical studies. Physiologists have used them to define basic properties of muscles, such as the length–tension and force–velocity relationships. Ralston and Inman appear to have been the first to use strain gauges for the in vivo study of human muscle.[3] Their measurements of the muscle tension developed by patients who were cineplastic amputees are among the very few studies in which human muscle tension was directly measured (most often we measure rotary forces because the muscle acts through a lever system). Despite the use of strain gauges in research, it appears that these devices are rarely used in clinical settings.

Strain gauges have been added to existing clinical devices such as the Cybex II or specially designed test equipment so that each can be used to obtain measurements.[22,23] Although these strain-gauge devices may have been used for clinical measurements, there are at present no widely used commercial instruments that are based on strain-gauge technology. Despite this, clinicians still should be aware of strain gauges because they are potentially useful.

Reliability

Many strain-gauge devices have been described in the research literature, but few of the authors have addressed the issue of reliability. Most investigators seem to believe that because the instruments have a sound theoretical basis, consistency (i.e., reliability between sessions and examiners) can be assumed.[16] These assumptions ignore the need for population-specific and user-specific demonstrations of reliability. These issues are discussed by Rothstein in Chapter 1.

Only Asmussen and his colleagues attempted to demonstrate that force measurements obtained with a variety of strain-gauge devices were replicable.[24] They constructed five different strain-gauge dynamometers, each designed for a different part of the body, and assessed four of these for reliability. Six muscle groups in 50 normal young men were tested twice. In the words of the report, the six muscle groups were responsible for: forward trunk flexion, backward trunk flexion, "downward pull of the arm," handgrip, knee extension, and

Table 3-2. Reliability of Strain Gauge Measurements for Six Motions

	Motion					
	Trunk Movement		Pulling Downward of the Arm	Knee Movement		
	Forward Flexion	Backward Flexion		Extension	Flexion	Hand Grip
Differences between first and second tests	7.5%	5.0%	3.7%	9.8%	5.9%	5.3%
Reliability Coefficients	0.91	0.92	0.96	0.91	0.95	0.94

Data from Asmussen E, Heeball-Neilsen K, Molbech SV: Methods for evaluation of muscle strength. Comm Dan Natl Assoc Infant Paralysis 5, 1959

knee flexion. Reliability coefficients ranged from .91 to .96 (Table 3-2). The statistical methods used to generate these coefficients were not described.

Clarke compared the reliability of cable tensiometers and the Wakim-Porter strain gauge for the measurement of six muscle groups in 64 nondisabled male college students (Table 3-3).[10] For some of the muscles, tests were also performed with a spring scale and a myometer. Clarke reported that test–retest correlations (''objectivity coefficients'') ranged from .81 to .94 and were very similar to those he obtained with the cable tensiometer.

The two studies described above show that when experts test normal subjects under controlled conditions, strain-gauge devices can reliably measure forces generated by some muscles. Does this mean we can assume that there would be equal reliability in clinical settings? There are several reasons why the assumption could be unwarranted. The devices used are not necessarily the same clinicians would use. The subjects did not reflect patient populations. Strain gauges are known to be sensitive and require frequent calibration. In addition, they are sensitive to temperature variations.[10]

There are other potential sources of errors when strain gauges are used. *The limb must either push or pull against the device in the same way (in the same line) that the calibration weights were applied to the instrument, or the measurements will be inaccurate.* For reliability, the application during different tests must be identical (in the same line). Stabilization of the limbs must

Table 3-3. Comparisons of Objectivity Coefficients for the Wakim-Porter Strain Gauge and the Cable Tensiometer

Motion	Cable Tensiometer	Strain Gauge
Finger flexion	.90	.94
Wrist dorsal flexion	.92	.85
Shoulder outward rotation	.91	.91
Neck extension	.92	.87
Knee extension	.96	.81
Ankle plantar flexion	.94	.94

The coefficients are those reported in Clarke HH: Comparison of instruments for recording muscle strength. Res Quart 25:398, 1954 be maintained so that force measurements reflect only those muscles being tested (i.e., there is no substitution). Unless the interface (the place where the patient makes contact with the device) is comfortable, the patient is not likely to push or pull maximally. The interface must be designed so that forces are delivered to the strain gauge.

The lability of the patient, i.e., whether what is being measured is stable as a result of subject characteristics, is an issue for all types of muscle evaluations. The users of strain gauges, like the advocates of other electronic measurement devices (such as the Cybex II) frequently appear to ignore this issue because of their belief in the technology they are applying. However, the true meaning of reliability is thus ignored, making it possible that obtained measurements will be made less meaningful.

Validity

The comparison of strain gauges with cable tensiometers has been described under the section on tensiometers. Some investigators imply validity because strain-gauge instruments accurately reflect applied loads.[25] The comparisons with loads and tensiometers have been used to justify the use of strain-gauge devices to measure muscle performance. Another rationale offered is that the strain gauge can be applied in the manner of manual muscle testing (MMT) and can therefore "objectify" an otherwise "subjective" test.[16] Validating one test by comparing it with another test is legitimate. However, MMT has limited validity, especially in terms of predicting functional performance (see Ch. 2). The most justifiable inference from MMT is whether or not a muscle is innervated, and there is certainly no need for a strain gauge at the force levels examined to determine denervation.

Normative data obtained with strain gauges have not been published, and relationships between force levels and functional performance have not been demonstrated. Almost all of the conceptual problems that relate to muscle testing that have been discussed in this book are relevant to strain gauge devices.

Summary

Clinically useful instruments that employ strain gauges are, at best, a rarity. The technological problems associated with such a device do not appear insurmountable. Development of a small device that uses strain gauges is feasible, as is the possibility of clinically testing such an instrument.[26,27] Whether stabilization and interfacing difficulties can be overcome will need to be studied. If such devices are developed, reliability studies in clinical settings on relevant patient populations must be conducted. Like the cable tensiometer, the strain gauge is not in widespread clinical use, but there is potential applicability that should be explored.

ISOKINETIC DEVICES

The Devices

Until recently, only a limited number of devices have been available to provide isokinetic (constant velocity) loading (i.e., the Cybex, Orthotron, Kinetron, and Fitron).* Of these, only the Cybex II could be considered an instrument designed for measurement. Recently many other devices, most notably the Kincom,† have been introduced and promoted as measurement tools. However, reports describing the measurement capabilities of these machines have not yet appeared in scientific literature. This section will therefore focus on the use of the Cybex II for measurement. Most of the issues raised will be equally relevant for other devices. Isokinetic exercise will not be discussed here.

The Cybex II consists of a movable lever arm controlled by an electronic servomotor that can be set for angular velocities from 0° to 300° per second. The lever arm is attached to a subject's limb and the subject is then asked to move as fast as possible. When the subject attempts to accelerate beyond the pre-set machine speed, the machine resists the movement. The machine is designed to maintain limb movement at a constant angular velocity and provide accommodating resistance.[28] A hydraulic load cell within the machine measures the torque (the angular analog of force) needed to keep the limb from accelerating beyond the machine's pre-set speed. The torque is registered on a strip-chart recording. Many of the machines are equipped with a second recording channel that provides goniometric data. Recently, a Cybex computer has been introduced that provides a digital printout, modifies data, and permits measurement of other variables such as power and work. Because there are no publications describing the characteristics of the computer and the algorithms used for data handling have not been published, the computer will not be discussed here.

The strip-chart recorder provided with the Cybex II allows for various gain settings and for signal conditioning through the use of a damp (a filtering network). This latter mechanism, which can have a dramatic effect on torque measurements, will be considered later.[29,30] There are other unique characteristics of the Cybex II system that must be understood before the devices can be used.

Torque measurements are normally derived by multiplying a force by its perpendicular distance from the axis of rotation.[31] With the Cybex II, this computation is not necessary. When a limb is attached to the Cybex, the axis of rotation for that limb must be aligned with the mechanical axis of the Cybex. Thus, the lever arms for the limb and the machine are equal and the distance from the axis does not have to be measured and used in calculations. In other

---

* Cybex Division of Lumex, Inc, 2100 Smithtown Ave, Ronkonkoma, NY 11779.

† Chattex Corporation, 101 Memorial Dr, PO Box 4287, Chattanooga, Tenn, 37405.

words, *when the axes are aligned, the limb and the machine act upon each other with the same moment arm eliminating the need to consider this variable (i.e., measure the length of the lever arms).*

A second characteristic deals with the level of measurement in isokinetic testing (see Ch. 1 for a discussion of levels of measurement). Torque measurements are usually considered ratio-scaled because a zero normally indicates an absence of the quantity being measured. Therefore, it is not surprising that many clinicians assume that Cybex II torque readings are ratio-scaled. However, consider what happens when a subject moves a limb at a speed slower than the machine's set speed. No torque will be registered on the strip chart recording. *The Cybex II records only the resistive force needed to keep the limb from accelerating.* When the limb speed is below the machine speed, the muscles being measured are developing tension and are creating a moment (a torque) that causes the limb to move. That torque must be sufficient to accelerate the limb and the attached lever arm against the force of gravity.[32] The Cybex II does not start measuring torque of muscular origin until a certain critical value is exceeded; a value that will vary depending on the limb's weight and length and the machine's speed setting. Because the zero measurement does not reflect a true absence of the quantity being measured, Cybex II torque values are interval scaled. Interval-scaled data cannot legitimately be used to create ratios.[33,34] Downward motions are also not ratio scaled, because when a limb is moved in the direction of the gravitational force, the zero torque level on the machine can be exceeded without muscular effort (i.e., when the limb accelerates down as a result of gravity). Therefore, motions in the direction of gravity do not have a meaningful zero point for the measurement of torque of muscular origin.

The Cybex II has been commonly used for the measurement of knee flexor- and extensor-generated torques. Attachments for the machine that permit almost any movement to be tested are available. Data dealing with the measurement characteristics for all of these movements are not available.

Isokinetic devices were the first instruments commercially available for the measurement of dynamic muscular activity. This is probably the reason why the devices have generated so much excitement in the last two decades. The ability of these instruments to measure torques reciprocally and to be used for exercise as well as testing are features that have apparently contributed to their widespread clinical acceptance.

History

The concept of isokinetic exercise was introduced by Hislop and Perrine in 1967,[28] and later were elaborated on by others[32,35,36] Moffroid et al described the use of the Cybex I, which had a speed range of 0 to 25 RPM for measurement.[35] Moffroid and her colleagues examined whether recorded torque was in agreement with expected torque levels (i.e., they loaded the machine with weights). Although this study is commonly used as a reference for Cybex II reliability and validity, the machine tested was radically different from present-day models in terms of speed range, stabilization, and recording systems. This study will be discussed when reliability and validity are considered.

During the last decade, clinical interest in isokinetic testing has blossomed. There is little doubt that the Cybex II is now the most commonly used instrument for the clinical measurement of muscular performance. Cybex II torque measurements are also commonly used in research conducted by physical therapists and other members of the profession. However, despite the plethora of publications that describe the use of the Cybex II, there have been very few articles that critically examine the measurement characteristics of the system, especially in terms of clinical practice.

Reliability

Some users of the Cybex II have conducted reliability studies as a part of their research,[22,37,38] and some investigators have even modified the device for these studies.[22,38] Such results cannot be generalized. Because they do not directly address the issue of the reliability that can be expected in clinical practice, they will not be discussed here.

Moffroid et al examined the reliability of the Cybex I by attaching weights to the machine's lever arm. The arm was set so that it was parallel to the ground, and therefore the weights were at a right angle to the gravitational vector. With the speed set at 0° per second, various loads were applied (60, 57, 40, 30, 20, 10, and 5 lbs) on a two-foot-long lever arm.[35] According to the authors, ten test–retest sessions using these loads produced a coefficient of reliability of $r = .995$. Because the method did not appear to yield sets of paired scores (which are normally used for correlation), it is unclear how this statistic was calculated. Fundamental design limitations also limit the usefulness of this "reliability study." What is most obvious is that isokinetic movement was not tested. All testing was done statically; the procedure assessed the reliability of the device for the static measurement of weights.

The study described above has been cited as evidence for the reliability of the Cybex II, yet the Cybex I was tested and the study did not involve people, let alone patients. Reliability cannot be generalized from weights to people. The problems inherent with stabilization, motivation, subject comfort, and axis alignment cannot be addressed by studies with weights. The variability of patient performance in general and stability over time, specifically, was not considered. The original paper dealt with a machine that is no longer available, utilized the static testing of inanimate objects, and offered confusing statistical evidence. In view of these observations, it is hard to imagine why this article has become the standard reference for Cybex II reliability.

The inter-machine reliability of the Cybex II has never been documented. That is, are the measurements obtained with one machine the same as those that would be obtained with another? Rothstein et al (unpublished observations) has found that different machines will yield different torque measurements even when weights are measured. Each machine was observed to have a consistent error that could be corrected with a linear regression equation specific to that machine, however. Some of the devices consistently measured too high, whereas others measured too low. Some also measured too high or too low at one torque level (e.g., low levels), whereas the opposite error was found at the other end of the spectrum. The potential error caused by inter-machine variability can be minimized if the calibration procedures suggested by Olds and associates[43] are used (these are discussed in the section on validity, below).

Johnson and Siegel examined whether a Cybex II could reliably measure knee extensor peak torque in 40 presumably healthy women (ranging in age from 17 to 50 years).[39] Subjects were tested at 180° per second on six consecutive days. On each occasion, subjects were allowed three submaximal warmup contractions that were followed by six maximal contractions. There was a 20-second rest period between successive contractions. After a preliminary statistical analysis, Johnson and Siegel determined that reliability was best when the mean values from the last three contractions were used. Therfore, *the reliability reported is for a protocol that calls for use of a mean value of three contractions obtained after three submaximal and three maximal warmup contractions, with 20 seconds of rest between contractions.*

Using their protocol, Johnson and Siegel obtained high indices of reliability. An analysis of variance based intra-class correlation coefficient was used for statistical analysis. This statistic assesses how closely multiple scores agree with each other. These correlations ranged from .93 to .99. The authors concluded that if their protocol was followed on similar subjects, excellent reliability could be expected. This study documents method precisely and even reports how the lever arm was attached to the subject and where straps were placed for hip stabilization.

The Johnson and Siegel study represents the most carefully designed and fully documented investigation into the reliability of Cybex II measurements of knee extensor peak torque. However, the following factors should guide generalizations from this study:

1. Healthy subjects were tested;
2. One speed was examined;
3. Only knee extension was tested;
4. Movement was tested in one direction;
5. A precise protocol was followed; and
6. Mean data were used.

Special attention should be paid to the fact that these researchers achieved a very high level of reliability by testing motion in only one direction. Although the Cybex II allows for reciprocal movements, and although this may be useful in exercise training, *there is no published evidence that tests using reciprocal contractions are reliable.* Asking subjects to reverse their direction immediately after a maximal effort does not seem likely to increase the reproducibility of test results. Any use of the time interval between reciprocal contractions as a measure of neuromuscular performance must be similarly questioned. The reliability of measurements such as the time between contractions has not been discussed in the literature. As will be shown later, reciprocal measurements and time measurements are especially questionable if a damp is used on the recorder.

Reliability over time and the need for warmup contractions were other issues examined by Mawdsley and Knapik in a study of knee extensor peak torque at 30° per second.[40] Sixteen subjects (12 men and four women ranging in age from 20 to 50 years) were tested with the Cybex II on three occasions with a two-week interval between sessions. The protocol called for six maximal knee extensor contractions, with a one-minute rest between contractions. It is unfortunate that correlation coefficients or intra-class correlation coefficients were not reported. However, based on a trend analysis using analysis of variance methods, the authors concluded:

1. Measurements did not change significantly over the six-week period (although from the method it appeared subjects were only tested over a four-week period); and
2. Only one maximal warmup contraction is needed to ensure reliable measurements.

These findings appear to disagree with those of Johnson and Siegel, but differences in methodology and subjects (the earlier study was on young women) make comparisons inappropriate. Mawdsley and Knapik demonstrated stability of the measurements over a longer period of time. This adds to the usefulness of Cybex II measurements. Because stability over a period of six weeks was demonstrated, it can be assumed that when similar subjects are tested under similar conditions, changes in peak torque measurements represent meaningful variation in muscle performance.

Emphasis must be placed on the methods used by Mawdsley and Knapik to obtain reliability. Their population was different from that tested by Johnson and Siegel. Although this may explain why only one warmup was necessary, a more likely explanation lies in the fact that a slower speed was used for testing. Johnson and Siegel examined the reliability of peak torque for knee extensors at 180° per second, whereas Mawdsley and Knapik investigated reliability at 30° per second. Two different testing situations were under study and the requirements for reliability need not be identical for both. Movements at the slower speed may be more easily replicated by subjects without warmups than movements at higher speeds. Clinicians may want to take this observation into account when testing patients, and they should also remember that both studies were performed on healthy subjects. The two studies demonstrate that reliability for one group of subjects, or at one particular speed, does not assure reliability when different groups are tested or when other speeds are used.

Molnar et al used a Cybex II to examine the reliability of bilateral peak torque measurements in children for the following motions: shoulder flexion, extension and abduction, hip flexion, extension and abduction, knee flexion and extension, and elbow flexion and extension.[41] Between 40 and 100 school children (ranging in age from 7 to 15 years) were subjects in most parts of the study and 60 mentally retarded children of similar ages were also tested. The authors did not report the speeds tested or whether motions were tested reciprocally. Four physical therapists tested subjects. The authors stated that intra-test variability was examined by having subjects make three successive efforts, but there is no description of the time interval between contractions.

The authors concluded that intra-test variability was minimal (never exceeding more than 8%). No correlation was reported, although it was stated that no statistical difference existed between the three trials. Although this does indicate some stability in the measurements, the absence of statistical evidence of differences between groups after repeated measures is a crude assessment of reliability. There was no discussion of whether the measurements of any muscle group was more reliable than any other.

The examination of inter-test reliability was not clearly described in the paper. Forty school children and a similar number of mentally retarded children were retested after seven to ten days, apparently by the same examiner. Once again, the authors did not report correlation coefficients, but based on variations of between 3% and 12%, they concluded that there was excellent inter-test reliability. No mention is made of the ways in which the different movements were analyzed. The most confusing aspect of the analysis is the use of a Chi-square test by the authors to determine whether there was a significant difference between the results of the various sessions. Why the authors used a nonparametric statistic for parametric data and why they did not use the same statistics they used previously (an analysis of variance) was never explained.

Molnar et al also examined inter-tester reliability on 40 normal boys and girls and 40 mentally retarded boys and girls. Two different therapists tested the children with a seven- to 10-day interval between sessions. Once again, differences were reported as being minimal for both groups of children (they did not exceed 12%). Differences between the groups were found not to be significant (a *t* test was used in this analysis), but no correlation was reported.

The results of Molnar and her colleagues would seem to suggest that the Cybex II can yield reliable measurements for many motions in both normal and mentally retarded children. However, the methodology is poorly reported. Replication is therefore impossible. The statistical analysis was less than complete. A failure to: (1) report the torque levels generated, (2) state the speeds tested, and (3) describe the reliability for each muscle group further impairs the usefulness of the study. Torque levels are particularly important because of the lack of adequate statistical analysis; i.e., the main measure of reliability was percentage differences. Children generate very low levels of torque and the range of their measurements is therefore quite truncated. This would make large percentage differences between repeated measures unlikely unless the measurement instrument was very sensitive. Despite the incredible effort that must have gone into data collection for this study, the report does little to document the reliability of the Cybex II measurement system.

One article that is repeatedly cited as containing evidence for the reliability of Cybex II peak torque measurements is an investigation by Thorstensson et al.[42] Subjects were 25 healthy normal men ranging in age from 17 to 37 years of age. Measurements of knee extensor torque were made at 15°, 30°, 60°, 90°, and 180° per second. In addition, isometric torque was measured with the knee flexed 90°, 75°, 60°, 45°, 30°, and 15°. The Cybex II recorder was not used; data were recorded with a UV recorder.

An often-cited aspect of this study was the analysis of the movement characteristics of the Cybex II lever arm. An initial period of nonconstant velocity movement was found. This will be discussed when we consider validity. Another unique methodological feature of this study is often overlooked. In order to prevent what the authors termed "inhibitory reflexes" at the end of ROM, a rubber bumper was used. This prevented an abrupt end to the extension movement and presumably minimized anticipatory "braking" on the part of the subject at the end of knee motion. Whether or not this increased reliability cannot presently be determined.

Reliability was examined by Thorstensson and his colleagues by having three groups of subjects tested twice. One group performed all the contractions in a pre-set order (isometric contractions from large knee angles to small angles, and slow isokinetic speeds to fast). A second group was given a random presentation of the conditions, while the third group used the same order as the first, but testing was done on two separate days. Although correlations were not reported, based on 900 "duplicate determinations," the average difference between repeated measures was reported to be 10 percent. The group tested on two different days had an average 13.7 percent difference whereas the two groups tested twice on the same day showed a difference of approximately 8.5 percent.

Clinicians should note that even when healthy subjects are tested, a variation of as much as 13.7 percent can be expected simply because measurements are taken on different days, and a variation of as much as 8.5 percent can be expected when subjects are tested twice on the same day. However, since we have noted that isokinetic measurements are not ratio scaled, the use of percentages is inappropriate; and the "true" variability seen in this study cannot really be discerned. It is unfortunate that there was no discussion by Thorstensson and his colleagues about whether there was a different amount of variation for the various speeds and the isometric positions. Reporting average variability for 11 different types of contractions does not permit clinicians to know the variability (measurement error) associated with any one speed or contraction type. However, the observed variability in normal subjects (8.5 to 13.7 percent) raises the question of how much change is necessary in peak torque measures before clinicians can assume that a patient is "stronger" or "weaker." Because the Cybex II appears to represent advanced technology, users of the device seem to assume that it is reliable for clinical measurements. Evidence for reliability of this instrument for clinical measurement is lacking. To date, no studies have examined meaningful samples of any type of *patient population* for reliability.

In view of the many types of measurements that can be obtained with the Cybex II, clinicians must consider whether there is evidence demonstrating reliability for the measurement they are using. For example, there is the study of Johnson and Siegel dealing with knee extensor peak torque in normals, but can that be used to legitimize testing of other joints such as the hip? Can fatigue tests be considered reliable in the absence of studies dealing with this test's reliability? *Each measurement obtained with the Cybex II for each joint and each speed should be examined for reliability.* Only in this way can we know if Cybex II measurements really yield clinically meaningful data. Such studies must be performed on clinically relevant populations, i.e., the types of patients that clinicians test. In view of the widespread use and availability of the Cybex II instrumentation, such studies are feasible. The absence of reliability data does not mean that the Cybex II is not a reliable instrument for measuring muscle performance, but it does mean that caution must accompany interpretation of test results until reliability is known.

Validity

The term, "validity," was used repeatedly by Moffroid and her colleagues[35] to describe various studies designed to examine whether the Cybex I could "accurately" measure peak torque, angle-specific torque, and work at various velocities. The criteria used for accuracy was a comparison of obtained (and in the case of work, calculated) values and those values anticipated, because known loads (weights) were applied to the lever arm. Correlation coefficients for these three measurements were exceedingly high—.946 to .999—and there can be little doubt that at the speeds tested (4, 8, and 12 rpm), measured values reflected predicted values. It must be emphasized again that this study examined an earlier model of the Cybex and tested only up to 12 rpm.

As has been noted previously, the ability of a system to measure a quantity is only the narrowest interpretation of validity. Moffroid et al may have demonstrated the validity of the Cybex I for the measurement of weights, but did they demonstrate that the device could validly measure muscle performance?

The clinician must know what evidence there is that measurements can be used to make judgments (inferences) about muscle performance. Before this can be known, we will attempt to consider some general issues relevant to the interpretation of Cybex II measurements.

Olds and associates have essentially challenged the Cybex II manufacturer's suggested calibration protocol, which is based on the use of weights at a single speed.[43] After 2,880 trials with a variety of weights at nine different speeds, Olds and his colleagues concluded that, "It is necessary to calibrate the Cybex II isokinetic dynamometer every testing day and at every test speed." The loads applied to the Cybex II lever arm ranged from 6 to 75 Nm. The speeds tested were 0°, 15°, 30°, 45°, 60°, 75°, 90°, 105°, and 120° per second. Testing was performed in both directions (i.e., loads were applied in clockwise and counterclockwise directions), and the authors concluded that, "The only test mode that does not require a recalibration is a rotational direction change." Based on the observations of Sinacore et al that damp settings affect measured torque values, it seems logical that all calibrations should also be carried out with the damp set at the same level that will be used for subject testing.[30] Olds et al did not address this issue because they used an undamped signal.

Thorstensson et al used microswitches triggered by the Cybex II lever arm every 15° as it moved through its arc of motion to test the machine's speed.[42] An electronic timer revealed that, at lower angular velocities (which were not specified), the measured speed was the same as the set speed. However, at the highest velocity tested (180° per second), the lever arm moved faster than the set speed for the first 0.5 seconds of torque registration. This accounted for an arc of approximately 5° to 10°. During movement through this arc, the authors concluded, there was a period in which the lever arm accelerated. The authors suggested that termination of this acceleration phase resulting from the machine's resistance to further acceleration led to the formation of a ''bump'' on the torque curve. Subsequent authors have referred to this ''bump'' as ''torque overshoot.''[29] Although this study did not deal with speeds in excess of 180° per second, it is commonly believed that ''overshoot'' is speed dependent and becomes more evident at higher isokinetic speeds.

According to Sapega et al, overshoot results in an erroneously high torque recording because the machine is arresting the inertia developed by the moving limb. Therefore, overshoot creates more error in measurement when: (1) large limb segments are tested; (2) large amounts of torque are developed, or (3) small arc of movements are tested. For some tests, such as hip movements, all three of these factors may combine. Sapega and his colleagues based their observations on experiments that used weights and human subjects at various speeds. Cinemagraphic analysis of the lever arm's movement was used and recordings were compared to calculated values. The reader should consult this work for a complete understanding of the methods used. This study confirmed Thorstensson's observations that there was a period of acceleration during part of the lever arm's movement.

An alternative explanation of ''overshoot'' has been offered by Perrine and Edgerton[44] and by Gregor et al.[45] These authors believe that the bump described by Thorstensson[42] is caused by the ''inherent initial energy oscillations through the total (muscle instrument) system.'' This explanation implies that the ''bump'' represents a biological as well as a mechanical phenomenon. Sapega and his colleagues rejected this explanation because they found overshoot present when testing inanimate objects, i.e., weights.

Sapega's group made several suggestions regarding strategies for eliminating the measurement error caused by overshoot. One suggestion involves the use of an undamped signal, noting that ''artifact free data can be sampled in the portion of the range following the resolution of the torque oscillations.''[29] This technique had been used previously by Rothstein and his associates.[37,46] However, as Sapega's group has pointed out, this technique may not be useful at higher speeds (180° per second for example), at which the oscillations may continue late into the arc of movement and may actually obscure peak torque measurements.

For higher velocity testing, Sapega et al suggested that use of a damp may be unavoidable. Based on their observations, the authors suggest that a damp

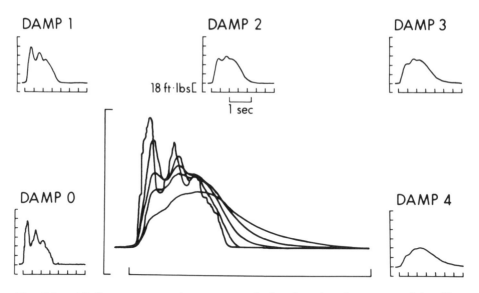

Fig. 3-2. All five torque tracings were made by dropping the same weight. Note changes in the torque curve as damp setting varies. The central figure is an overlay of all five tracings. Note how torque diminishes as damp increases and how the torque curve is shifted to right (i.e., later in time) (From Sinacore DR, Rothstein JM, Delitto A, et al: Effect of damp on isokinetic measurements. Phys Therap 63:1248, 1983.)

setting of 2 may be used, but they caution that even this affects the torque curve to some extent. In their opinion, however, routine clinical tests in the lower velocity range will not be excessively influenced by damp-induced artifact.

Although Sapega and his co-workers did not actually study the damping characteristics of the Cybex II system, they stated, "Increasing the damping beyond a setting of 2 in an attempt to suppress any remaining overshoot has not provided an acceptable solution because this suppresses grossly appreciable quantities of true muscular torque in addition to the overshoot and this simply substitutes one artifact for another."

The effect of damp on isokinetic measurements was studied by Sinacore et al, using weights dropped at various velocities (30°, 75°, and 180° per second) and recording with damp settings 0 through 4.[30] The results clearly demonstrate that measured torque decreases as the damp setting is increased (Fig. 3-2). The authors also observed that the damp caused a shift in the torque curve to the right, i.e., torque recordings appeared later in time. This second finding has great clinical and experimental significance. If a damped torque curve is accompanied by a goniometric tracing, the torque values will appear to occur later in the range of motion than it should. In other words, damp delays the registration of torque, making angle specific measurements questionable. The greater the damp, the greater the effect. Clinicians can observe this effect for themselves by testing patients with a highly damped signal (Fig. 3-2). For example, with reciprocal motions on the part of the patient, the torque from knee extension may be aligned over a goniometric measurement showing knee flexion. This phenomenon can also be seen if a weight is dropped so that it hits the floor. If the signal is heavily damped, torque registration will persist after the movement has stopped, i.e., after the weight is resting on the floor.

Sinacore and his colleagues suggested that because damp affects measurement, clinicians must report damp and consider its effect on obtained values. However, maintaining damp at one setting may only appear to eliminate errors produced. Because damp has the effect of delaying the torque signal for a period of time, even the use of a single damp setting will have a variable effect when different speeds are being used for testing. A similar delay, which probably occurs when a given damp is used, leads to a different amount of displacement in the torque recording relative to the goniometric recording at different speeds. The amount of ROM that occurs during a given time delay is a function of the speed. In other words, the higher the speed, the more the torque curve will be shifted as compared to the goniometric tracing, even when a single damp setting is used for all speeds.

Damp will distort any measurement that involves temporal elements or the need to relate the torque curve to the goniometric tracing. Angle-specific measurements may not be accurate if a damp is used because torque readings will not relate to the goniometric trace (e.g., they are displaced so that they appear later in ROM). The error will increase with the size of the damp and will always be greater at higher speeds. For example, when the damp is used and knee peak torque is measured at 45° of knee flexion at speeds of 30° and 180° per second, the torque readings *do not reflect measurements of the torque at the same angle.* The displacement of the torque curve is greater at 180° per second.

The effect of damp has been discussed primarily as it relates to peak torque and other torque measurements. When Cybex II torque curves are integrated (i.e., the area under the curve is measured), damp becomes an even greater potential source of error since the entire curve is distorted. Because measurement of work or power require integration of the curve, use of the damp can be expected to distort power and work measurements.*

Rothstein et al have attempted to avoid problems by using a "window" with undamped torque curves at speeds up to 120° per second.[37,46] This window

---

* Power and work may be calculated from isokinetic torque curves. First, the area under the torque curve must be calculated. This is usually measured with a planimeter or a digitizer. The area measurement is then used in one of the following formulae: Area × Torque per Unit of Vertical Displacement × Speed/(Time × Chart Speed) = Power. Because the Cybex II records in English units, the following formula is suggested because it will convert to metric units and power will be expressed in Nm × radians/s. Area (in inches^2) × (25.4 mm^2/in^2) × (ft × lb/mm) × (1.356 Nm/ft × lb) × (speed in radians/s)/((time in seconds) × (chart speed in seconds)) = Power. The factor (ft × lb/mm) of the above equation represents the calibration (i.e., how many foot × lbs per mm on the recording). The factor (1.356 Nm/ft × lb) is the conversion to Nm. Work is obtained from the above by multiplying the power figure by time.

excludes the torque artifact that invariably occurs within the first 10° of knee extension motion at these speeds.

Their window involves the measurement of only the central 70° in a 90° arc of knee extension. Elimination of the first 10° is designed to exclude the torque overshoot. Elimination of the last 10° is designed to exclude the part of the ROM in which subjects have been known to decelerate their limbs (i.e., make less than maximal efforts) in preparation for stopping movement. The observation of Rothstein and his colleagues was similar to that of Thorstensson, who also believed that subjects might not manifest maximal effort at the end of the motion.[42] Thorstensson believed the effect to be caused by reflex inhibition and used a rubber bumper to allow for comfortable deceleration at the end of motion. Because he was not measuring area under the curve, this was an acceptable solution for his investigations.

The method developed by Rothstein and his colleagues[37,46] represents an effort on the part of a group of researchers to eliminate the effect of overshoot without creating errors caused by the use of damp. Clinicians and other researchers must be aware of the effects of overshoot and damp. Strategies for eliminating these two sources of error will depend on what the Cybex II is being used to measure.

A previously unpublished observation by Rothstein and his colleagues may help those who wish to use an undamped signal. When attempting to measure patients even at slow speeds, they noticed that at times there could be multiple artifacts or overshoots, not just the single "bump" observed by Thorstensson. This made use of an undamped signal impossible. However, it was found that when the Cybex II was fully stabilized, and no movement of the whole device occurred as the subject attempted to move the lever arm, only a single overshoot was present. To achieve this level of stabilization, great care was taken to find a flat surface for the Cybex II. All fittings had to be perfectly aligned and tightened. On some occasions, the investigators had to stand on the device to ensure that it would not move when subjects attempted to extend their knees.

Rothstein and his colleagues believed that such stabilization was absolutely essential if a Cybex II measurement was to be meaningful; however, only when an undamped signal was used could the full effect of poor stabilization be readily observed. They hypothesized that when the machine moved in the same direction as a moving limb, the subject's movement actually lifted the dynamometer up. They believed that the following sequence of events was taking place: (1) the subject accelerated to the machine speed and an overshoot was recorded; (2) as the machine attempted to decelerate the limb, the subject's movement actually began to accelerate the machine (i.e., move it); and (3) the machine then needed to decelerate the subject again. With an unstable dynamometer, they felt that the process of acceleration and deceleration occurred more than once during a given arc, and each time an overshoot of lesser magnitude was created.

Methods of calibration, overshoot, and damp have all been proven to be potential sources of error and can threaten the validity of Cybex II measurements. Winter et al have described another major problem associated with isokinetic testing—the failure to account for gravitational factors.[32] Noting that Moffroid and her colleagues attempted to establish a form of validity without measuring subjects on the dynamometer[35] Winter's group questioned much of the published work concerning use of the Cybex II. The complexity of the mechanical analysis applied by Winter's group makes a complete description within this chapter impossible. Readers are advised to examine the original article to critically review the methods used and the basis from which conclusions were drawn.

In essence, their analysis demonstrates that the torque added to downward movements by the force of gravity is not trivial. Similarly, their work shows that when movement is against gravity, the torque not recorded is also significant. As has been noted previously, this added torque with downward movements and missing torque with upward movements means that Cybex II data is not ratio scaled.

Winter and his colleagues noted that peak moments (torques) may not only be distorted in amplitude because of gravitational factors, but may appear up to 15° out of their true positions. The following represents the summary of findings as quoted from the original article:

> In summary it can be said that uncorrected joint moments due to gravitational forces acting on the leg whilst using an isokinetic dynamometer can:
>
> 1. Introduce large errors into calculations of mechanical work. This problem is especially severe in flexion during low level contractions;
> 2. Substantially alter the value of the knee moment recorded during flexion or extension, especially near full extension. Again, this percentage error increases as the contraction becomes lighter; and
> 3. Alter inferences drawn about muscle function based on the fatigue index.
>
> To overcome these problems, a relatively simple solution is presented which compensates for the effect of gravity over a full range of motion.[32]

Note that Winter and his associates state that almost all of the errors in measurement are larger when torque values are low. When healthy athletes are tested, the large torque values may minimize the effect of some of these errors. But when patients are tested, even if they are athletes, the lower torque levels will certainly be affected by gravitational factors. Some testing protocols magnify the errors. For example, at low speeds, subjects will generate more torque than at high speeds. For a given patient, there will be more distortion in the high-speed torques than in the low-speed torques. Comparing torque values across speeds may therefore be questionable. Neither are comparisons of repeated contractions by a single subject justified. As a subject becomes fatigued, torque becomes lower and the error factor becomes larger. The new Cybex II computer is supposed to eliminate problems resulting from gravity, overshoot, and damp, but documentation or experimental evidence supporting this contention has not yet appeared in the literature.

Special attention should be paid to Winter's comments regarding the "fatigue index." This test, which was apparently developed by Thorstensson and Karlson,[47] has been widely used but, to date, reliability studies on meaningful clinical populations have not been described. The validity of the test in terms of functional inferences (other than muscle fiber predictions), has never been established. The criticism offered by Winter further calls into question the value of this test.

The Cybex II has been used to measure many different muscle groups. Reliability studies have been performed almost exclusively on knee motions. Inherent differences in the joints, weights of limb segments, and methods of stabilization must raise doubts about whether reliability can be assumed for other joints. In the absence of reliability, validity is not possible.[9] Even if the measurements were reliable, many joints seem unlikely to be good candidates for the isokinetic approach. As was noted previously, torque is the magnitude of a force multiplied by the perpendicular distance from the axis of rotation. With isokinetics, the distance is the same when the anatomical axis of the subject's joint is aligned with the axis of the machine. When the two are not aligned, one or the other has a mechanical advantage, and readings that are not corrected can be erroneously high or low. In the absence of research that examines this issue, clinicians should consider whether stabilization and adequate joint alignment can be attained when various joints are tested, e.g. the shoulder or ankle.

For some uses of isokinetic devices, such as for the measurement of low back muscle torque, it has been suggested that a single (L_5-S_2 articulation) axis can be used to represent multiple axes[48]; it remains for research or mathematical modeling to validate this concept. However, it is interesting that other groups who measure back muscles place the mechanical axis at the hip joint[49] or at the iliac crest.[50] It is obvious that the three different approaches will yield different measurements. Axis placement as well as problems with stabilization threaten the validity of isokinetic measurement of many different muscle groups.

Some of the major elements that threaten the validity of isokinetic measurements have been delineated. The effect of ignoring these issues and the potential for inappropriate clinical decisions may be illustrated by considering published studies.

Wyatt and Edwards measured the knee flexor and extensor peak torques of 50 men and 50 women between the ages of 25 and 34 years.[51] The purpose of this study was to describe various characteristics of this group because many similar subjects have knee injuries. The authors felt that by doing this they could generate criteria that could be used to decide when a patient could return to normal activity. Such data would certainly be useful and could serve as a guide in the rehabilitation process—if the data were meaningful.

Subjects were allowed to practice knee flexion and extension movements at 120° per second to become accustomed to the device. Five to ten practice contractions were then performed at each of the following speeds: 60°, 180°, and 300°, per second. After a two-minute rest period, subjects were tested during maximal reciprocal contractions. Half of the subjects were tested at the fast speeds first, while the other subjects were tested at the slow speeds first. Peak torque values were read from the strip-chart recording. The authors do not state how many contractions were made, but it appears that all data represent the values obtained from a single contraction.

Before considering the results and conclusions of Wyatt and Edwards, let us examine potential sources of error in this study. Calibration is never described, although Olds et al demonstrated that significant measurement errors can be caused by a failure to calibrate the device properly.[43] The use of a damp setting is not mentioned and, as a result, the distortion caused by either overshoot or damp may be present. Reciprocal high-speed contractions were tested even though there is no evidence that adults can be reliably measured using reciprocal contractions, and there are no reports examining reliability for the speeds used. Reliability was never discussed at all in the article.

Based on the results obtained, the authors state that the information provided by this study should be helpful to clinicians who are examining similar populations of non-athletes. For example, at higher speeds, the authors found that the hamstring-quadriceps ratio approached 1, and that at all speeds, the ratios were different. They postulated that since the ratio increased with speed, the possibility exists that at speeds above 300° per second the hamstrings might be "stronger" than the quadriceps.

None of the above observations can be considered valid in view of the evidence supplied by Winter et al demonstrating measurement errors caused by gravitational factors.[32] As has been pointed out, the use of ratios only compounds the errors resulting from gravity in torque measurements.

The problems described above are not unique to that study. Similar problems can be found in many reports. Because these authors failed to consider threats to reliability and validity, their conclusions are highly questionable. Clinicians may appreciate how similar failures on their part could lead to misinterpretation of data obtained during patient testing. Depending upon the clinical question, the erroneous conclusions could result in diminished quality of patient care or in the incorrect evaluation of patient disability.

Attempts have been made to use Cybex II torque tracings to make inferences about pathological processes in the knee. Such studies, although they may have admirable intent, could result in incorrect evaluations if threats to the quality of measurement are not considered. Hoke et al tried to demonstrate a relationship between patellofemoral compression testing (which was supposed to indicate changes in patellofemoral articular cartilage), and isokinetic measurements.[52] After patients were tested for pain on patellofemoral compression, isokinetic testing was performed at 30° per second. Reciprocal knee motions were examined. The authors stated that a torque curve was: "regular" or "irregular." Few or no visible deflections meant a regular curve, whereas multiple deflections of the curve were said to represent an irregularity.

Although data exist that describe procedures for ensuring the reliability of testing knee motions in a single direction, the authors chose to test reciprocally, thereby using a method of unproven reliability. The possible effect of the damp on the distortion of the curve was never discussed. A thorough, and therefore universally useful, operational definition of "curve irregularity" was not provided, and it is not clear whether examiners judging the torque curve to be irregular were aware of the results of the compression testing. Reliability for the assessment of the curve was not reported. We know of no studies that validate the use of isokinetic torque curves for diagnostic purposes.

The use of isokinetic measurements for various inferences is obviously desirable in that clinicians would be able to make greater use of such instruments for evaluation and treatment planning. However, unless evidence for such inferences is carefully obtained, clinical science is not served by such claims. For example, because it has been suggested that a 75% torque level can be used with other measurements to infer that patients who have had knee surgery are ready for normal activities, the clinician may feel that they now have a useful criterion to guide patient management.[53] However, because no documentation is offered for this inference and the type of testing suggested is of questionable validity and reliability, the clinician may actually be guided into incorrect judgments. This is not to suggest that the 75% criteria is wrong, but rather to state that suggestions such as these should be accompanied by evidence that demonstrates the validity for such inferences. (See Rothstein elsewhere in this volume for a further discussion of these criteria and related issues.)

Isokinetic measurements seem to have potential validity for many types of inferences. Previously, some researchers have used isokinetic measurements to infer something about the nature of the muscle fibers within a subject's limb.[37,54] It is beyond the scope of this chapter to consider whether these biological inferences were correct. However, these studies demonstrate the potential of the Cybex II as an instrument that can be used to examine basic biological properties of muscle.

The usefulness of isokinetic testing may be a function of the type of measurement that is obtained. Most of this section has focused on peak torque, angle-specific torque, and power measurements. Examples of inappropriate measurements were described, such as ratios and some versions of fatigue tests. Clinicians should realize that each measurement must be examined relative to its reliability and validity. For example, Rothstein et al have shown that in steroid-treated rheumatic disease patients, who presumably have type II muscle fiber atrophy, there is a deficit in power production.[37] These authors argued that measurements of power and power–velocity slopes can be used to infer something about type II muscle fiber atrophy. They demonstrated that peak torque values and peak torque–velocity slopes did not allow for such inferences. A full discussion of the biological significance of this finding is inappropriate here, but this study does illustrate how some isokinetic measurements may have more appropriate uses than others. All measurements derived from the use of the same instrument—even on the same patients—cannot therefore be assumed to have the same reliability or inferential capacity.

At times there may be reasons for substituting one isokinetic measurement for another. For example, peak torque is much easier to measure than is power or work. Can one variable be inferred or derived (i.e., mathematically predicted) from another? The initial part of this chapter dealt with definitions of terms; it must be emphasized, however, that in order for clinicians to infer one variable from another, there must be evidence to justify the substitution. The evidence must be based on research that uses appropriate definitions to describe the variables. Strength-testing literature sometimes contains a use of terms that is less than precise. Misuse of terms is particularly rampant in the isokinetic literature. Moffroid and Kusiak, for example, suggested that torque measures could be used to infer power measurements. They used definitions for some forms of power that are incompatible with physical laws.[55] Rothstein et al defined variables in accord with classical physical laws and generated population-specific equations that allowed for the prediction of power and work from peak torque measurements.[46]

The need for population-specific equations indicates that the relationship between peak torque and power is not the same for all types of subjects. Substitution of peak torque for power would not be valid unless the nature of the relationship were known for the patient being tested. Clinicians must, therfore, be wary when they attempt to derive one isokinetic measurement from another.

Similar problems with clinical judgments may arise because of the nomenclature used by various promoters of isokinetic testing. The term, "strength," as was noted earlier in this chapter, needs an operational definition, whereas the term "power" has a definition that originates in Newtonian physics. To state that one isokinetic speed tests something called "strength" while another tests something called "power" is to assume such inferences can be made. *There is no evidence to support the assumption that different speeds test different muscular characteristics and can, therefore, be used to make different inferences.* Examination of most torque–velocity curves actually demonstrates a linear relationship across speeds. Therefore, there is a strong relationship between performance at any one speed and performance at other speeds.[46] This suggests that measurements taken at any speed may reflect the same qualities measured at any other speed.

Several investigators have attempted to examine whether there is a relationship between isokinetic (dynamic) measurements and isometric (static) measurements.[38,56,57] These studies have led to disparate conclusions, with Osternig et al stating that a relationship is almost nonexistent, and Fugl-Meyer[58] describing strong relationships. A middle ground is taken by Knapik and Ramos,[56] who suggest that relationships are strongest with low-speed isokinetic contractions. These studies have decidedly different methodologies and deal with different musle groups. Although these factors alone may account for the differences in conclusions, all of the studies fail to establish reliability within the context of the investigations. All of them may also be questioned because of the issues that have been discussed in this chapter (e.g., effects of gravity, calibration, and damp). Expected relationships between isokinetic and isometric contractions are based on the understanding of muscle biology. To comprehend such relationships fully, clinicians should review the physiology of dynamic and static contractions and how both have been related to muscle fiber populations.[59–62]

Some sophisticated issues have been discussed relative to what limitations may be placed on judgments derived from isokinetic measurements. The most obvious inference a clinician may draw is that a muscle is not as "strong" as it should be. To make this inference, the clinician may want to compare isokinetic measurements between affected and unaffected limbs when it is possible. This issue applies to isokinetic tests as well as to any muscle force measurement, or for that matter, goniometry. Are such comparisons always appropriate? Miller has questioned the value of such comparisons in regard to goniometric measurments (see Ch. 4). Those questions are equally relevant here. Should we expect measurements to be equal bilaterally? Can unilateral disease alter patterns of muscular use in the so-called nonaffected limb, leading muscles in that limb either to increase or to decrease in force-generating capacity? What range is acceptable before limbs are considered to be essentially equal?

Some of the problems associated with interlimb comparisons could be eliminated if isokinetic measurements were compared to accepted norms. Such norms, as has been discussed elsewhere in this volume, must meet logical requirements relative to being derived from samples that reflect meaningful populations (i.e., samples that reflect patient types). Several reports have attempted to describe various isokinetic measurement characteristics in aged subjects, multiple sclerosis patients, children, elite female athletes, high school football players, and elite amateur ice hockey players.[38,41,63–65] Norms for these groups would be useful. However, all of these studies failed to evaluate adequately the reliability of the measurements for the populations tested. In addition, methods were in some cases poorly described, and in almost all cases, consideration was not paid to the validity issues that would render questionable the values obtained. Sample sizes tended to be so small in most of these studies that "true norms" could not possibly have been generated.

Probably the most important inference that can be made from any evaluation of muscular performance concerns whether measurements can be used to predict function. Patient care would be greatly improved if we knew the critical levels of torque or power that was required by patients before they were capable of using their limbs for functional activities.

Critical levels of power or torque have not been determined for any activity, and in fact one might wonder whether muscularly generated forces can ever be used as predictors of functional performance. (See Ch. 6 for a discussion of this in regards to gait). Research to date has suggested that isokinetic torque measures do not predict athletic performance.[66] In terms of patient performance, muscles that are incapable of generating any tension will obviously lead to the patient losing function, but what levels of force are necessary to perform specific functional tasks? Until this question is answered, isokinetic measurements cannot be considered valid indicators for predicting patient performance in complex tasks or for functional recovery.

Because isokinetic devices test dynamic rather than static movements, clinicians may have assumed that these devices provide more meaningful (i.e., more functional) measurements than do strain gauge or cable tensiometers. The evidence in the athletic literature suggests that this is not the case. Relative to rehabilitation, there is no evidence to support the argument that dynamic testing is a better predictor of functional capacity than static testing (see Ch. 5 for a consideration of the needs for functional testing).

Future research may demonstrate some predictive use of isokinetic measurements, but at present, any suggestion that functional performance may be determined from isokinetic testing is conjecture.

Summary and Conclusions

Isokinetic testing, although first described in 1969,[35] has only recently become widespread in clinical practice. However, many questions remain about the reliability and validity of isokinetic testing. These have been discussed relative to the Cybex II, but are equally valid with regard to any of the isokinetic devices recently introduced.

The use of isokinetic devices for testing must be considered independently of the use of isokinetic exercise. Dynamic testing appears to be a concept strongly endorsed by the clinicians. The Cybex II has thus become the preferred instrument for testing patients. In view of the information presented in this section, clinicians are urged to review the manner in which they use isokinetic measurements.

Therapists must deal with isokinetic measurements, either in their practice or when reading the literature. Research is urgently needed that will guide therapists and others in the proper use and interpretation of isokinetic data. Such research must be more carefully carried out than has been the case in the past. As can be seen from the literature reviewed here, much of the work examining isokinetic measurements has promoted the use of isokinetics without regard to fundamental questions regarding the quality of these measurements.

HAND-HELD DYNAMOMETERS

The Devices

Hand-held instruments to measure muscle function vary in their methods of translating force into units, but the modes of application are similar. Therapists interpose the device between their hand and the limb to be tested and then perform a "break test." Most often the force of the patient pushing against the device is translated linearly by an oil-filled chamber to a pressure gauge.[67,68] Strain gauges are sometimes used.[26] Calibration is performed by loading the devices with known weights.

History

In 1949, Newman described a hand-held device called a "myometer," which consisted of a 3 ¼ inch long and 2 inch diameter cylinder, and which had a pressure-transmitting button at one end and a gauge at the other.[67] Encased within the housing was a hydraulic system. In order to measure different muscles, the device was designed to measure forces in three ranges, from 0 to 5 lbs, from 0 to 15 lbs, and from 0 to 60 lbs. Newman believed that if a muscle could exert more than 60 lbs of force, there was no need to measure the force with an instrument. A pressure-equalizing disc 2 ¼ inches in diameter was interposed between the pressure button and the subject's skin in order to distribute forces over large areas when limbs pushed on the device.

Newman used the myometer to test upper extremity muscles in standard manual muscle test positions. He noted the importance of applying the force at right angles to the limb being tested. He emphasized that the myometer always had to be applied to limbs in precisely the same way (keeping the line and point of application constant) if measurements were to be replicable. However, he did not describe any reliability tests.

Although Clarke compared the myometer's reliability with that of the cable tensiometer,[10] the two devices are different in their mode of application and in the type of muscle performance that they measure. The cable tensiometer measures isometric force as the subject attempts to move against the fixed resistance of the cable. The myometer measures force by having the subject push against the pressure button (through the disc), while the examiner pushes back. The reading is taken when the subject "breaks," i.e., when the subject is unable to resist the examiner's force and is moved in the direction away from the contracting muscle. As has been noted by Lamb (see Ch. 2), the "break test" may be a measure of isometric or eccentric muscle action. We do not yet know which measure it represents.

Reliability

Most articles that discuss the merits of hand-held devices focus on the utility and portability of the devices rather than on the reliability of the instruments. Without evidence for reliability, the devices cannot be used to make statements (i.e., inferences) about patient progress and disease status. Can we assume reliability based on what we know about other devices? The following are especially difficult to achieve with hand-held devices: (1) stabilization of the limb and the device, (2) control of the speed of contraction, and (3) the force needed by the examiner to break the contraction of the subjects.

Of the four devices he examined, Clarke found the myometer to be the least reliable. The "objectivity coefficients" for intra-tester reliability of .82 for finger flexion and .79 for wrist dorsiflexion were considerably lower than those for the cable tensiometer and the strain gauge. Clarke's results indicate that hand-held devices may be less reliable than other instruments, but to generalize from tests of two actions appears to be inappropriate at present.

Edwards and McDonnell have described the use of a myometer similar to the Newman device.[68] Force ranges between 0 and 12 kg can be measured. The authors argue that an examiner would not be strong enough to measure forces of greater magnitude. Hosking et al investigated the reliability of this instrument by testing the following muscles (and groups) in 19 children (ranging in age from 4 to 13 years): neck flexors, shoulder abductors, wrist extensors, hip flexors, knee extensors, and ankle dorsiflexors.[69] Calibration was performed with a load cell. The same examiner tested 18 of the subjects twice, with a one-month inter-test interval. Although correlation coefficients were not reported, the investigators said that variability between the sessions never exceeded 15 percent. The investigators reported difficulty in measuring quadriceps and hip flexor forces because they frequently exceeded the upper limit of the device. They concluded that measurement of large muscles was not possible with hand-held devices. We must emphasize that this was based on their measurement of children. The limitation will be even more widespread when hand-held devices are used with adults.

Stephen tested a hand-held device developed by Hack that used a strain gauge.[27] The device consisted of a cuff placed against a limb segment. The cuff in turn was attached to a strain gauge. After the subject pushed against the device, the force level was displayed digitally in relative units. The device could be calibrated with weights to obtain standard units. Details on the device's reliability were not reported. However, it was stated that the device was "accurate" when used by a single examiner to test the triceps brachii and hip abductors of ten normal college students over a one-week interval. The positions used for testing—whether a break test was used, how the device was applied, and results—were not described.

Validity

The proponents of hand-held dynamometers appear to imply that the devices will be valid since they can be used in the MMT positions to "objectify" an otherwise "subjective" test. As has been noted, MMT has limited validity and therefore cannot be used to justify most inferences derived from measurements obtained with a hand-held device. There are no normative data that can indicate the forces that would be normal in any of the MMT positions. The only study that attempted to compare hand-held devices with other instruments was that of Clarke, and he reported that they had the lowest reliability of all the devices that he tested.[10] Validity would also be limited for hand-held devices in view of the observation by Hosking and colleagues that they could only be used to measure low force levels. Measurements of powerful muscles would be limited not only by the construction of the device, but also by the requirement that the examiner exert a "breaking force."

Summary and Conclusions

Several hand-held devices have been described in the literature, and still others are commercially available. They all seem to be easy to use and adaptable for a variety of measurements, and to provide immediate force readings.

However, the reliability of these devices is questionable and has only been examined for a limited number of muscle groups and only on normal subjects.[10]

The argument has been made that the devices can be used in MMT positions, but perhaps they can be more effectively used in other positions, especially positions that include stabilization techniques. The technical limitations of the devices, (e.g., the low upper limit for measurement) should be surmountable with strain gauges and digital displays, but these improvements cannot change the test and overcome the inherent limitations in break tests.

Hand-held devices, like strain gauges and cable tensiometers, appear to have potential clinical usefulness. However, hand-held devices probably are less applicable. They can probably be applied only to patients who have very limited force-generating capabilities.

HAND DYNAMOMETERS

The Devices

Many instruments have been developed to measure the forces created during "gripping" and "pinching." Some authors have suggested that these instruments measure overall hand function[70] while others have used them to examine the progress of diseases[71–73] and the effects of maturation on muscle performance.[74] However, hand dynamometers are most commonly used to measure isometric grip. Many devices are available, though spring-scale and strain-gauge systems are the most common. Measurements are usually made with the hand and forearm in a standard position that involves some type of stabilization. The subject is asked to "squeeze and hold." The strain-gauge devices are usually attached to a strip-chart recorder or a digital readout. The spring scales have a needle that indicates force, and a pointer that remains at the highest value until it is reset.

History

Some investigators believe that the most important part of hand assessment is the measurement of forces exerted in functional positions.[70,75] Therefore, a variety of methods have been developed to measure forces created by muscles during "gripping" and "pinching." Other devices have been designed to measure isolated muscle performance. The discussion in this section will be limited to those devices that have been examined for reliability and validity.

Mundale developed a strain-gauge dynamometer that maintained the forearm in the neutral and stabilized position while finger flexion was measured in a position that he had determined would yield optimum force production.[75] This instrument is of special importance because investigators have used it to make inferences about the clinical course of dermatomyositis.[71,72]

Jones used an elliptical spring-scale instrument to measure the changes in grip forces in children over a six-year period.[74] Duvall et al examined the reliability of the spring scale using data supplied by Fischer.[76] Fowler and Gardner used a similar device to examine the grip forces of healthy subjects and patients with various forms of muscular dystrophy.[73] As has been noted previously, Clarke used a cable tensiometer to measure forces created by finger flexors and extensors as well as thumb abductors and adductors.[15]

Reliability

The reliability of measurements of grip forces and isolated finger actions has been assessed by several investigator. However, there are no reports on the reliability of pinch measurements.

"Objectivity coefficients" for the cable tensiometer were reported by Clarke for the following: finger flexion = .90; finger extension = .93; thumb abduction = .84; and thumb adduction = .91. He compared these to the coefficient of .82 obtained with the Newman myometer for measurement of finger flexion. Clarke believed that his results indicated that the cable tensiometer could reliably measure finger forces.

Fischer tested 13 healthy adults (11 women and two men) with a spring dynamometer.[76] Subjects were tested twice on the same day and again up to eight months later. Subjects were told to grip the device maximally; there was no attempt to control position. The report does not describe the positions the subjects used; thus, it is impossible to know exactly how the testing was carried out and replication of the technique is not possible. However, Duvall et al analyzed the data of Fischer and reported test–retest correlation coefficients of .97 when the "best" (greatest) values obtained from three trials in each session was compared. Because they demonstrated that use of the "best" value of ten trials yielded an *r* value of .99, they concluded that reliability was essentially the same for both conditions. They suggested that the best of three trials be used for clinical measurements. Although the reliability coefficients reported by Duvall et al and Clarke are not radically different, only Clarke's methods can be replicated.

Jones used an elliptically shaped spring dynamometer that fit into various frames to measure different muscle groups.[74] He examined the reliability of grip force measurements in children 11 to 17 years of age. Subjects were tested three times on each of two successive days and the highest values for each day were correlated. The correlation for the right hand was .915 and .934 for the left. This reliability study was a precursor of an investigation into the grip force changes that accompanied maturation in children. He described his testing procedure, subject selection criteria, and discussed the motivational problems that were encountered during testing.

Reliability for the device developed by Mundale has not been established, but the instrument is still of interest because of the way in which it has been used by researchers. Pilot studies led Mundale to design a strain-gauge device that maintained the metacarpophalangeal (MCP) joints in 150° of flexion and the proximal interphalangeal (PIP) joints in 110° of flexion. The forearm was stabilized by the instrument. When Mundale conducted 254 fatigue tests on ten normal subjects, he followed a standardized protocol which he described.

Validity

Several of the hand dynamometers are based on strain-gauge designs; therefore, all of the issues raised in that section also apply here. However, there is an additional concern when the strain gauges or any other devices are purported to measure "hand function." It is clear that an operational definition of "function" is needed before one can say that a hand is functional based solely on grip force measurements. Tables of normal values, which might indicate minimal acceptable force levels, would help the inferential process, but to date none have been published for the devices described above.

Two groups of investigators used Mundale's dynamometer to measure grip forces in order to infer something about the progress of dermatomyositis. Dinsdale et al examined the course of the disease in a 19-year-old athlete.[71] They demonstrated an inverse relationship between force measurements and serum levels of serum glutamic-oxaloacetic transaminase (SGOT), an enzyme that appears in increased quantities in the blood when muscle is damaged or destroyed. They also reported relationships between biopsy analysis of the patient's muscle and the force levels. These variables (force, tissue, and serum SGOT) were measured over a 15-month period. Dinsdale et al concluded that grip strength was a sensitive measure for assessing the progress of dermatomyositis.

A similar conclusion was drawn by Resnick et al, who studied six children with dermatomyositis for two to six years.[72] Serum levels of SGOT, creatine phosphokinase (CPK) and lactate dehydrogenase (LDH) were correlated with grip force measurements. Enzyme levels increased as the force measurements decreased. The authors concluded that the serum analysis was less useful in guiding therapeutic decisions than was the grip force data. They also noted that this demonstrated the inadequacy of MMT for such patients, because MMT had previously led investigators to believe that dermatomyositis was a disease of the proximal musculature. This last observation is of considerable importance and has broad implications for physical therapy. Resnick and his colleagues noted that they and Dinsdale were able to document disease-associated weakness only when they used instruments to measure muscle performance. We must ask whether other conditions may have been inappropriately described (i.e., in terms of the pattern and severity of weakness) because of the failure to use the proper measurement instruments.

Further evidence that diseases may be poorly understood because of improper measurement is provided by Fowler and Gardner. They used hand dynamometers to test patients with different forms of muscular dystrophy.[73] They observed distal weakness in these patients. Previously, proximal weakness had been the recognized clinical finding in such patients.

The studies of dermatomyositis and muscular dystrophy patients demonstrate the diversity of inferences that can be made from measurements of muscular performance. However, because the reliability of the device used in the dermatomyositis studies was not established, results must be cautiously interpreted, Replication of these studies is desirable. Probably more important is the need to consider how many other inferences can be made from force measurements *if* the proper instrumentation is used.

Summary

Despite the widespread use of hand dynamometers and the fact that they are readily available from many suppliers, there is little documentation about how they can be used, whether they are reliable, and what inferences can be made from obtained measurements. Of all the devices available to measure hand performance, only the spring scale used by Jones and the cable tensiometer used by Clarke have been shown to be reliable, and these studies have been limited to healthy subjects.

USE OF WEIGHTS TO MEASURE MUSCULAR PERFORMANCE

History

In 1945, DeLorme described measurement of muscle performance as part of a method called "heavy resistance exercise."[77] The exercise protocol called for the determination of the maximal weight that a subject could lift ten times in one session. To measure the quadriceps, for example, subjects would wear an iron boot that had a metal bar through its center (combined weight 5 lbs) where weights could be added. If subjects could lift the load, additional weights were added until the subject reached the maximum load that could be lifted ten times. In 1948, DeLorme renamed his technique "progressive resistive exercise." The method of determing the maximal load remained the same.[78]

Reliability and Validity

Studies on the use of weights to measure muscle performance have often failed to address the issues of reliability and validity. However, there have been some reports that can contribute to our knowledge in these areas, and they will be considered together here.

DeLateur has questioned whether the determination of the maximum for ten repetitions could be made reliably when weights are added one after another during a single session (i.e., without rest intervals).[79] Although this observation seems reasonable, data demonstrating that the problem really exists have not been presented.

Kennedy, as noted earlier, used a modified Elgin chair and compared measurements obtained with the use of weights, strain gauges, and cable tensiometers.[17] This procedure has been described previously. Kennedy stated that the testing with weights was reliable but offered no evidence. However, once again the possibility exists that with serial testing (i.e., one load after another), subsequent tests may not be valid. Kennedy also stated that there was a high correlation between the measurements made with cable tensiometers and strain gauges and the maximum weight a subject could lift. Data were not presented.

Summary and Conclusions

We have briefly described the way in which weights have been used to measure muscle performance. Although clinicians may not use the same type of formal protocols described above, most therapists informally or even subconsciously assess patients with weights. We frequently give patients weights and ask them to lift them. From this, we make judgments. Because we can keep notes on the limb's position, the type of contraction (e.g., isometric, isotonic), and the weight held, this method may be reliable and valid. In view of the ease with which such tests can be carried out, documentation of reliability and validity would be very useful. We need to know if stabilization, positioning, speed of contractions, and other variables can be held constant so that weights can measure muscle performance reliably.

SUMMARY AND CONCLUSIONS

In this chapter, we have reviewed the literature that describes the instruments that can be used clinically to measure muscle performance. We have put forth the argument that measurement of muscle performance must be made in a meaningful context. Measurement for the sake of obtaining numbers really does not permit therapists to say much about their patients or their treatments. There must be an understanding of why measurements are taken, why specific instruments are chosen, and why specific test modes are used. The therapist must consider the purpose of testing and the nature of the inferences they need to make. Reliability must also be considered by the therapist. As we have noted in this chapter, many of the procedures now being used to assess patients have questionable reliability.

In view of the paucity of research describing clinical measurement of muscle performance any review of the topic, such as the one presented here, might appear excessively negative. This reflects the state of the art, rather than any desire on our part. Throughout this chapter, we have pointed out areas in which further research is needed.

Examples of research needs are described throughout this chapter; however, we think one type of inquiry is particularly vital. We must consider whether we can legitimately use muscle performance tests to: (1) infer a patient's functional status, (2) describe diseases and disabilities, and (3) assess the effects of our treatments. Because these are validity questions, reliability is a prerequisite for any inquiry.

With better instruments and with reliable and valid protocols, it is possible that we will discover previously unappreciated phenomena that may change the way in which physical therapy is practiced. Consider how Resnick et al described distal weakness in a disease previously thought to manifest only proximal weakness[72] and that Fowler and Gardner had similar findings.[73] We are suggesting that our understanding of various diseases, syndromes, and disabilities may have been limited in the past because insensitive instruments, such as MMT, or unreliable or invalid measurements, such as isokinetic ratios, were used.

We have described the many weaknesses in our measurement systems, and we must conclude that there are presently no generally reliable or valid instruments available for the measurement of muscle performance in the clinic. Some of the existing instruments may yet be shown to be reliable or valid— but that will take considerable research. The most promising aspect of such a research effort will be the potential impact on patient care. We may not know enough about our patients and our treatments today because we have not had the proper measurement tools. When we have the proper tools, a new and more effective era of scientific physical therapy may begin. That observation leads us to believe that this chapter is neither negative nor pessimistic, but rather one that offers great hope for our profession.

REFERENCES

1. Webster's 3rd New International Dictionary, Unabridged, G. & C. Merriam, Springfield, Massachusetts, 1969
2. Kroemer KHE: Human strength: terminology, measurements and interpretation of data. Hum Factors 12(3):297, 1970
3. Ralston HJ, Inman VT, Strait LA, Shaffrath MD: Mechanics of human isolated voluntary muscle. Am J Physiol 151:612, 1947
4. Williams M, Lissner HR: Biomechanics of Human Movement. Saunders, Philadelphia, 1966
5. Watkins MP, Harris BA, Kozlowski BA: Isokinetic testing in patients with hemiparesis. Phys Ther 64:184, 1984
6. Singh M, Karpovich PV: Isotonic and isometric forces of forearm flexors and extensors. J Appl Physiol 21:1435, 1966
7. Fenn WO, Marsh VS: Muscular forces at different speeds of shortening. J Physiol (Lond) 85:277, 1935
8. Partridge LD: Muscle properties: a problem for the motor controller physiologist, p. 189. In Talbot RE, Humphrey DR (eds): Posture and Movement. Raven, New York, 1979
9. Kerlinger FN: Foundations of Behavioral Research, 2nd Ed. Holt Rinehart and Winston, New York, 1964
10. Clarke HH: Comparison of instruments for recording muscle strength. Res Q 25:398, 1954
11. Clarke HH, Bailey TL, Shay CT: New objective strength tests of muscle groups by cable-tension methods. Res Q 23:136, 1952

12. Currier DP: Maximal isometric tension of the elbow extensors at varied positions. Phys Ther 52:1043, 1972

13. Alderman RB, Banfield TJ: Reliability estimation in the measurement of strength. Res Q 40:448, 1969

14. Clarke HH: Objective strength tests of affected muscle groups involved in orthopedic disabilities. Res Q 19:118, 1948

15. Clarke HH: Cable Tension Strength Tests: A Manual. Stuart E. Murphy, Springfield, Massachusetts, 1953

16. Wakim KG, Gersten JW, Elkins EC: Objective recording of muscle strength. Arch Phys Med Rehabil 31:90, 1950

17. Kennedy WR: Development and comparison of electrical strain-gauge dynamometer and cable tensiometer for objective muscle testing. Arch Phys Med Rehabil 46:793, 1965

18. Linton M, Gallo PS: The Practical Statistician: Simplified Handbook of Statistics. Brooks/Cole, Monterey, California, 1975

19. Clarke HH: Improvement of objective strength tests of muscle groups by cable-tension methods. Res Q 21:399, 1950

20. Frankel VH, Burstein AH: Orthopaedic Biomechanics. Lea and Febiger, Philadelphia, 1970

21. Frost HM: Orthopaedic Biomechanics: Orthopaedic Lectures, Vol. V. Charles C Thomas, Springfield, Illinois, 1973

22. Murray MP, Baldwin JM, Gardner SM, Sepic SB, Downs WJ: Maximum isometric knee flexor and extensor muscle contractions. Phys Ther 57:637, 1977

23. Jensen RH, Smidt GL, Johnston RC: A technique for obtaining measurements of force generated by hip muscles. Arch Phys Med Rehabil 52:207, 1971

24. Asmussen E, Heeboll-Neilsen K, Molbech SV: Methods for evaluation of muscle strength. Comm Dan Natl Assoc Infant Paralysis 5, 1959

25. Darcus HD: A strain gauge dynamometer for measuring the strength of muscle contraction and for re-educating muscles. Ann Phys Med 1:163, 1953

26. Hack SN, Norton BJ, Zahalok GI: A quantitative muscle tester for clinical use (abstr). Phys Ther 61:673, 1981

27. Stephen GA, Norton BJ, Hack SN: Clinical reliability of a quantitative muscle tester (abstr). Phys Ther 61:673, 1981

28. Hislop HJ, Perrine JJ: The isokinetic concept of exercise. Phys Ther 47:114, 1967

29. Sapega AA, Nicholas JA, Sokolow D, Saraniti A: The nature of torque "overshoot" in Cybex isokinetic dynamomentry. Med Sci Sports Exerc 14:368, 1982

30. Sinacore DR, Rothstein JM, Delitto A, Rose SJ: Effect of damp on isokinetic measurements. Phys Ther 63:1248, 1983

31. Gowiztke BA, Milner M: Understanding the Scientific Basis of Human Movement, 2nd Ed. Williams and Wilkins, Baltimore, 1980

32. Winter DA, Wells RP, Orr GW: Errors in the use of isokinetic dynamometers. Eur J Appl Physiol 46:397, 1981

33. Stevens SS: Measurement, psychophysics and utility. In Churchman CW, Ratoosh P (eds): Measurments: Definitions and Themes. Wiley, New York, 1959

34. Campbell NR: An Account of the Principles of Measurement in Calculations. Longmans and Green, London, 1928

35. Moffroid M, Whipple R, Hofkosh J, et al: A study of isokinetic exercise. Phys Ther 49:735, 1969

36. Thistle HG, Hislop HJ, Moffroid M, Lowman EW: Isokinetic contraction: a new concept of resistive exercise. Arch Phys Med Rehabil 48:279, 1967

37. Rothstein JM, Delitto A, Sinacore DR, Rose SJ: Muscle function in rheumatic disease patients treated with corticosteroids. Muscle Nerve 6:128, 1983
38. Murray MP, Gardner GM, Mollinger LA, Sepic SB: Strength of isometric and isokinetic contractions. Phys Ther 60:412, 1980
39. Johnson J, Siegel D: Reliability of an isokinetic movement of the knee extensors. Res Q 49:88, 1978
40. Mawdsley RH, Knapik JJ: Comparison of isokinetic measurements with test repetitions. Phys Ther 62:169, 1982
41. Molnar GE, Alexander J, Gutfeld N: Reliability of quantitative strength measurements in children. Arch Phys Med Rehabil 60:218, 1979
42. Thorstensson A, Grimby G, Karlsson J: Force-velocity relations and fiber composition in human knee extensor muscles. J Appl Physiol 40:12, 1976
43. Olds K, Godfrey CM, Rosenrot P: Computer assisted isokinetic dynamometry. A Calibration Study, p. 247. Fourth Annual Conference on Rehabilitation Engineering, Washington, D.C., 1981
44. Perrine JJ, Edgerton VR: Muscle force-velocity and power-velocity relationships under isokinetic loading. Med Sci Sports 10:159, 1978
45. Gregor RJ, Edgerton VR, Perrine JJ, Campion DS, DeBus C: Torque-velocity relationships and muscle fiber composition in elite female athletes. J Appl Physiol 47:388, 1979
46. Rothstein JM, Delitto A, Sinacore DR, Rose SJ: Electromyographic, peak torque and power relationships during isokinetic movements. Phys Ther 63:926, 1983
47. Thorstensson A, Karlsson J: Fatiguability and fiber composition of human skeletal muscle. Acta Physiol Scand 98:318, 1976b
48. Davies GL, Gould JA: Trunk testing using a prototype Cybex II isokinetic dynamometer stabilization system. J Orth Sports Phys Ther 3:164, 1982
49. Hasue M, Fujiwara M, Kikuchi S: A new method of quantitative measurement of abdominal and back muscle strength. Spine 5:143, 1980
50. Suzuki N, Endo S: A quantitative study of trunk muscle strength and fatiguability in the low back pain syndrome. Spine 8:69, 1983
51. Wyatt MP, Edwards AM: Comparison of quadriceps and hamstring torque values during isokinetic exercise. J Orth Sports Phys Ther 3:48, 1981
52. Hoke B, Howell D, Stack M: The relationship between isokinetic testing and dynamic patellofemoral compression. J Orth Sports Phys Ther 4:150, 1983
53. Malone T, Blackburn TA, Wallace LA: Knee rehabilitation. Phys Ther 60:1602, 1980
54. Thorstensson A: Muscle strength, fiber types and enzyme activities in man. Acta Physiol Scand 443: suppl. 1, 1976
55. Moffroid MT, Kusiak ET: The power struggle: definition and evaluation of power of muscular performance. Phys Ther 55:1098, 1975
56. Knapik JJ, Ramos MU: Isokinetic and isometric torque relationships in the human body. Arch Phys Med Rehabil 61:64, 1980
57. Osternig LR, Bates BT, James SL: Isokinetic and isometric torque force relationships. Arch Phys Med Rehabil 58:254, 1977
58. Fugl-Meyer R, Sjostrom M, Wahlby L: Human plantar flexion strength and structure. Acta Physiol Scand 107:47, 1979
59. Burke RE: A comment on the existence of motor unit "types," p. 611. In Tower DB (ed): The Nervous System, Vol. 1, The Basic Neurosciences. Raven, New York, 1975
60. Edgerton VR: Mammalian muscle fiber types and their adaptability. Am Zoo 18:113, 1978

61. Rose SJ, Brooke MH: Muscle biology. Phys Ther (Special Issue) 62:1743, 1982
62. Salmons S, Henriksson J: The adaptive response of skeletal muscle to increased use. Muscle Nerve 4:94, 1981
63. Armstrong LE, Winant DM, Swasey PR, Seidle ME, Carter AL, Gehlsen G: Using isokinetic dynamometry to test ambulatory patients with multiple sclerosis. Phys Ther 63:1274, 1983
64. Gilliam TB, Sady SP, Freedson PS, Villanacci J: Isokinetic torque levels for high school football players. Arch Phys Med Rehabil 60:110, 1979
65. Smith DJ, Quinney HA, Wenger HA, Steadward RD, Sexsmith JR: Isokinetic torque outputs of professional and elite amateur ice hockey players. J Orth Sports Phys Ther 3:42, 1981
66. Genuario SE, Dolgener FA: The relationship of isokinetic torque at two speeds to vertical jump. Res Q 51:593, 1980
67. Newman LB: A new device for measuring muscle strength. Arch Phys Med Rehabil 30:234, 1949
68. Edwards RHT. McDonnel M: Hand-held dynamometer for evaluating voluntary muscle function. Lancet 1:757, 1974
69. Hosking GP, Bhat US, Dubowitz V, Edwards RHT: Measurements of muscle strength and performance in children with normal and diseased muscle. Arc Dis Child 51:957, 1976
70. An K, Chao E, Askew LJ: Hand strength measurements. Arch Phys Med Rehabil 61:366, 1980
71. Dinsdale SM, Cole TM, Zaki FG, Awad EA: Measurements of disease activity in dermatomyositis. Arch Phys Med Rehabil 52:201, 1971
72. Resnick JS, Mammel M, Mundale MO, Kottke FJ: Muscular strength as an index of response to therapy in childhood dermatomyositis. Arch Phys Med Rehabil 62:12, 1981
73. Fowler WM, Gardner GW: Quantitative strength measurements in muscular dystrophy. Arch Phys Med Rehabil 48:629, 1967
74. Jones HE: Motor performance and growth: developmental study of static dynamometric strength, University of California Press, Berkeley, 1949
75. Mundale MO: Relationships of intermittent isometric exercise to fatigue of handgrip. Arch Phys Med Rehabil 51:532, 1970
76. Duvall EN, Houtz SJ, Hellebrandt FA: Reliability of a single effort muscle test. Arch Phys Med Rehabil 28:213, 1947
77. DeLorme TL: Restoration of muscle power by heavy resistance exercises. J Bone Joint Surg 27:645, 1945
78. DeLorme TL, Watkins AL: Technics of progressive resistance exercise. Arch Phys Med Rehabil 29:263, 1948
79. DeLateur BJ, Lehmann JF, Fordyce WE: A test of the DeLorme axiom. Arch Phys Med Rehabil 49:245, 1968

4 | Assessment of Joint Motion

Peter J. Miller

The measurement of joint motion is an integral part of the physical therapy evaluation. Our profession and the modern approaches to joint assessment both have their origins in the World War I era. Today, assessment of range of motion (ROM) is probably the most commonly used evaluative technique of the physical therapist. As a result, it appears that the quality of the measurement is often taken for granted.

For a measurement to have value, it must be reliable and valid (see Ch. 1).[1] Reliability deals with the consistency of a measurement—whether we can expect the same measurements when they are taken at different times or by different people.[2] Validity deals with whether a measurement really tells us something.[2] These two essential qualities for a measurement, reliability and validity, should concern all clinicians who measure joint motion.

Many decisions regarding patient status, treatment, and prognosis are based wholly or in part on measurements of joint motion. For example, intervention may be chosen based on joint measurements. Judgments of vocational potential and disability status may also depend on goniometric measurements. Can such judgments be correct if goniometric measurements do not provide meaningful (i.e., reliable and valid) information? Perhaps because of the widespread use of goniometric measurements therapists have assumed that they are meaningful. However, we must ask whether we should place so much faith in goniometric measurements and whether we can improve the quality of these measurements.

The purpose of this chapter is to provide an overview of joint motion measurement methods, including discussions of normal values, techniques, devices, notation systems, recording methods, and reliability and validity studies. In addition, a protocol will be presented that can be used to examine goniometric reliability in clinical settings. This chapter attempts to provide clinicians with insights into both the applications and limitations of joint motion measurements so that clinical decisions can be made on a more scientific basis.

NORMAL VALUES AND JOINT MOTION STANDARDS

After a measurement is obtained, there is a need to judge it, to compare it with something in order to determine what the obtained value means. There are several standards that clinicians use to judge joint measurements. These standards are often used to assess the success of therapeutic interventions and are also used to determine what forms of treatment, if any, patients will undergo. These standards also help us determine what may be causing functional deficits and, in addition, the standards are used in medical-legal proceedings.[3,4] "Normal" ROM values have been reported by many authors.[3-19] These so-called normal values often serve as the standard when therapists determine whether patients have limitations in motion.

Early Studies

Normal ROM values were first reported in 1920 by Clark.[5] Reports by Cobe[6] and Hewitt[7] followed. These authors determined normal values for college students and also studied diurnal fluctuations in normal ROM. Hewitt reported on the wrist motion of women. She found that the activities in which the subjects engaged (e.g., pianists and athletes) influenced wrist ROM.

Symmetry of Range of Motion Values: Left *vs* Right

Leighton[10] found that there was essentially no difference for corresponding motions of the arms, legs, and trunk between the right and left side. Boone and Azen[16] and Roaas and Andersson,[19] in more extensive studies, also found that joint motions were essentially equal bilaterally in normal male subjects. Allender et al found a slight reduction in motion on the dominant side in normal subjects.[20] However, most authors have concluded that with unilateral involvement, the motion of the contralateral (noninvolved) joint can be used to judge the adequacy of movement for the affected limb. This view has been strongly supported by the American Academy of Orthopaedic Surgeons (AAOS) in their widely used handbook on joint motion[12] as well as by Salter,[21] Boone and Azen,[16] and Roaas and Andersson.[19] Although this approach seems logical, we question whether it is always appropriate.

After unilateral injury (or a disease affecting only one side), patients may alter the way in which they use their bodies. This may be done in an attempt to continue to perform functional activities. For example, a person with a unilateral above-the-knee amputation will have to use the remaining lower extremity in a way that differs from that used before amputation to ambulate and perform activities of daily living. The "noninvolved" limb may have been used for a swing-through gait for a period of time before the patient was examined by the therapist. If the therapist compares the amount of hip extension for the amputated limb with that of the other limb, the comparison may not be appropriate. The noninvolved limb has been subjected to an altered pattern of use. The gait may have altered the amount of limb extension.

There has been no documentation of whether altered patterns of use significantly change ROM in non-involved limbs. Until research addresses the issue, the concept may be questioned. However, the use of the contralateral extremity as a criterion is especially questionable in the presence of diseases that affect both sides of the body, or when preexisting conditions are factors (i.e., there was previously a problem with the non-involved limb).

Use of the contralateral limb as a standard for comparison may be appropriate in acute situations, when the patient has not had the opportunity to alter the pattern of use of the "uninvolved" extremity. This problem of comparing the involved extremity to the uninvolved extremity does not apply only to joint measurements; it is relevant to other situations in which comparative measurements are used, (e.g., strength testing).

Age and Sex Differences

Several studies have demonstrated that age and sex influence ROM. Bell and Hoshizaki[17] found that in the 17 movements of the upper and lower extremities, there was a gradual decline in joint motion as age increased. For most of the motions examined (in 190 subjects ranging in age from 18 to 88 years), there was a decline in motion from the ages of 20 to 30 years, then a plateau from 31 to 60 years, followed by a decline in those over 60 years. Several motions actually increased after the age of 55, such as shoulder rotation in men and women, shoulder flexion and extension in women, and knee flexion and extension in men. The authors also found that upper extremity joints retained more of their motion than did lower extremity joints as age increased. The authors hypothesized that this could be caused by the higher levels of activity involving the upper extremities that are maintained by elderly people in later life, and that this may delay physiological changes that lead to decreased joint motion. Boone and Azen[16] reported that normal male subjects (18 months to 54 years of age) showed decreased motion in upper and lower extremities as age increased.

Values for "normal" joint ROM are also dependent upon gender. Cobe[6] reported that women always had more motion for all wrist movements than men; however, Cobe examined only 100 men and 15 women. Clarke[22] found that, on the average, males had 92 percent of the motion that females had in gleno-humeral movements (120 subjects with ages from 20 to 80 years). Bell and Hoshizaki[17] found that women tended to have greater ROM in the upper and lower extremities than did men and that this was true throughout life.

"Normal Values" and Alternatives

Various authors have attempted to present tables that state what the normal ROM should be for various joints (Table 4-1). From an analysis of the data in Table 4-1, it is apparent that there are considerable discrepancies between suggested "normal values." There are many reasons for this variation.

Only one of the sources cited in Table 4-1 (Boone and Azen) described how and from what kinds of subjects (age, sex) their values were obtained. As has been noted previously, age and sex can influence ROM values. Therefore, it is unlikely that a single set of values can describe what is normal for both sexes throughout an entire lifetime. Because activity, especially vocation, can also influence ROM, it would also be useful to know whether the "normal values" were obtained from samples representing a diversity of backgrounds, or from a homogeneous sample. In Chapter 1 of this volume, there is a more detailed discussion of the logical requirements for normative data; however, it should be noted here that none of the sources cited in Table 4-1 meets all the requirements. This defect is most notable when the ubiquitous *American Academy of Orthopaedic Surgeons Handbook* is considered. Several authors have noted this deficiency in this widely cited handbook.[16,19,22] In summary, it is not possible to state with certainty whether any of the so-called normal values are applicable to a given patient because: (1) methods of measurements are not stated (except by Boone and Azen); (2) we do not know whether these values are for passive or active motions or in what positions they were taken; and (3) the relevant populations are unknown (what were the sex, age, and activity profiles for those measured?).

The values presented in Table 4-1 have been published and repeatedly cited despite their serious limitations. Although these "normal" values have been derived from scientific investigations that are less than thorough, they remain in use because they have become widely accepted (and are therefore traditional) and because no real, alternative values exist. The establishment of population- and method-specific normal values for joint motion should be a focus for future research. Although the work of Boone and Azen[16] and Hoshizaki[17] is promising, much must be done before we possess meaningful norms that can be used for clinical decision making.

The clinician who needs to know how much joint motion is acceptable for a patient is still faced with the problem of what to use as a standard for comparison. Should published normal values be used? Should the contralateral extremity be measured and that value used? Perhaps, in view of the previous discussion, neither of these methods is appropriate. An alternate method involves the use of functional criteria. For example, consider a 70-year-old man with a three-month history of adhesive capsulitis who has 90° of shoulder flexion. The clinician must ask how much shoulder flexion *this* patient needs. The therapist might consult tables of normal values (e.g., Gerhard and Russe) and decide that the patient needs 170° in order to be "normal" again. But once again, we must ask whether 170° of flexion is normal for a 70-year-old man since we do not know from whom Gerhard and Russe obtained their values.

Table 4-1. Published Normal Range of Motion Values, in Degrees

	Wiechec and Krusen[3]	Dorinson and Wagner[8]	JAMA[11]	Daniels and Worthingham[13]	Esch and Lepley[23]	Gerhardt and Russe[15]	Boone and Azen[16c]	AAOS[12]	CMA[24]	Clarke[5]
Shoulder										
Flexion	180	180	150	90[a]	170	170	167	180	170	130
Extension	45	45	40	50	60	50	62	60	30	80
Abduction	180	180	150	90[a]	170	170	184	180	170	180
Internal rotation	90	90	40[b]	90	80	80	69	70	60[b]	90[b]
External rotation	90	90	90[b]	90	90	90	104	90	80[b]	40[b]
Horizontal abduction	—	—	—	—	—	30	45	—	—	—
Horizontal adduction	—	—	—	—	—	135	140	135	—	—
Elbow										
Flexion	135	145	150	160	150	150	143	150	135	150
Pronation	90	80	80	90	90	80	76	.80	.75	.50
Supination	90	70	80	90	90	90	82	80	85	90
Wrist										
Flexion	60	80	70	90	90	60	76	80	70	80
Extension	55	55	60	90	70	50	75	70	65	70
Radial deviation	35	20	20	25	20	20	22	20	20	15
Ulnar deviation	75	40	30	65	30	30	36	30	40	30
Hip										
Flexion	120	125	100	125	130	125	122	120	110	120
Extension	45	50	30	15	45	15	10	30	30	20
Abduction	45	45	40	45	45	45	46	45	50	55
Adduction	—	20	20	0	15	15	27	30	30	45
Internal rotation	—	30	40	45	33	45	47	45	35	20
External rotation	—	50	50	45	36	45	47	45	50	45
Knee										
Flexion	135	140	120	130	135	130	143	135	135	145
Ankle										
Plantarflexion	55	45	40	45	65	45	56	50	50	50
Dorsiflexion	30	20	20	—	10	20	13	20	15	15
Inversion	—	50	30	—	30	40	37	35	35	—
Eversion	—	20	—	—	15	20	26	15	20	—

[a] These "normal" values are associated with manual muscle testing (MMT), and the authors list only the part of the movement attributable to the deltoid muscle.

[b] Tested with the shoulder in 0° of abduction.

[c] This is the only article in which the methodology for obtaining normal values was reported. The values presented represent the means of measurements taken on 109 men ranging in age from 18 months to 54 years.

The 170° of flexion may be normal for a 20-year-old or 40-year-old man. However, is it reasonable to expect a 70-year-old man to possess the motion of the younger man? In this case, and in many others, existing "normal" values may not be very useful. They may even lead to unrealistic expectations and inappropriate treatments. The therapist could, in this case, measure the contralateral shoulder. However, even if the clinician found it to have 170° of flexion, the possibility would still exist that the 3-month history of adhesive capsulitis caused the patient to use the "uninvolved extremity" more than he normally would have. In some cases, an "uninvolved extremity" might even lose ROM during a period of excessive use, possibly because the increased use exacerbated arthritic or inflammatory conditions (e.g., tendonitis or bursitis). Altered patterns of use, compensatory to supposed unilateral involvement might, therefore, lead to increases or decreases in ROM, causing use of measurements of this contralateral extremity for a standard to be of questionable value.

Because there are problems with the use of supposed normal values and use of the contralateral extremity, there must be a reconsideration of the way in which clinicians set standards for their patients. How much flexion does this patient really need in order to carry out functional activities? The clinician can attempt to determine what activities the patient has not been able to perform because of shoulder limitations. The clinician can then decide how much motion the patient needs to regain function. For example, if the patient cannot reach into a cupboard and grasp a plate with the involved extremity, the therapist can estimate how much flexion would be necessary for the patient to be capable of performing the task. This estimate would be the standard. If the clinician compiles a list of functional activities that a *given patient* cannot perform the therapist can determine how much ROM *that patient* really needs. In this way, goals are appropriate and meaningful for each patient. If, in the above example, the patient needs 140° of flexion to reach into the cupboard and no other functional activity requires more than that, 140° of motion is the value that the therapist attempts to obtain with the patient.

The use of functional activities to derive goals for joint motion offers two major advantages over other methods. First, it allows the goal of treatment to be based on the individual patient's age, sex, and activity level (the patient's individual needs). In this way, it insures that goals are not set too high or too low, which is always possible when using the "normal" value tables or when using the contralateral limb measurements. The second advantage is that use of functional standards permits more meaningful use of goniometric measurements in other areas of evaluation and treatment. In the above example, it was determined that 140° of shoulder flexion was required for the patient to remove a plate from an overhead cupboard. But, to perform this act normally, the patient must *also* have adequate muscle power and the ability to maintain proper posture (i.e., he must avoid the compensatory trunk movements that can become habitual in patients with shoulder joint restrictions). By focusing on function—and considering a functional goal—all three elements (motion, power, and posture) can be better considered by the therapist. The functional approach helps clinicians understand the existing problem and aids in the development of treatment strategies. Functional goals help the therapist focus on relieving a problem, rather than on the achievement of an arbitrary amount of movement.

The use of functional ROM values for goals would be enhanced if we knew how much motion was required for functional activities. Perhaps future studies will document how much motion is needed for various functional activities, much in the way that research has demonstrated the amount of lower extremity ROM necessary for normal gait. Increased reliance on functional standards rather than on the use of questionable "normal values" (which may not reflect a patient's needs) would allow clinicians to derive appropriate goals for patient treatment and would provide patients with a realistic view of their functional status and prognosis.

METHODS OF GONIOMETRIC MEASUREMENT

Moore stated that there had to be "one best way" to measure joint motion.[13] Despite this assertion, many methods appear to have been used.[4,8–12,15,23–28] These vary considerably, with some applicable to many joints[4,8,10–12,15,23,25,28] and others designed to measure only one joint.[26–28] Some of these methods have been painstakingly described in terms of technique, whereas others have been explained diagrammatically.[12,15] Instructions differ as to how the goniometer should be placed and even as to whether a goniometer should be used. Some of the methods require special devices[10,26,27] and are therefore not generally applicable for clinical use.

The AAOS (1963 and 1965 editions)[12] handbook states that when the bony landmarks of an extremity are obvious, a goniometer can be used accurately. When the landmarks are not easily noticeable, the manual states that the "experienced surgeon" can visually estimate ROM accurately. However, this statement is not substantiated in the handbook. The AAOS manual does not even mention how to use bony landmarks for goniometric measurements. Therefore, it is difficult to determine when the manual is suggesting that visual estimation, (or "eyeballing," as it is often called) is the preferred technique. The question of whether visual estimation of joint motion is better than goniometric measurement has been studied by others and will be discussed later.

Axis of Rotation

Accurate placement of the goniometer's axis of rotation has been thought to be essential for accurate measurement. Several authors provide precise instructions for the location of the axis for each joint to be measured.[8,23,26,27] It is apparent that the strategy is to make the goniometer an external representation of the limb being evaluated. The axis, therefore, is supposed to represent the center of rotation of the joint, and the arms of goniometer represent the proximal and distal bony structures. Several authors argue that axis placement, i.e., congruency with the joint axis, is absolutely essential for accurate measurement.[3,29] However, this assumption may be incorrect since most joints have no single identifiable axis. The universal goniometer has a simple hinge joint, whereas not even the knee or elbow has a simple hinge joint. There is probably no joint in the body with a simple hinge joint.

The axis of rotation for joints is known to change as a limb segment moves through its ROM.[30–34] Therefore, a goniometer cannot be placed in a given position in an attempt to align its axis with the joint axis. In addition, there are problems associated with finding the axis (i.e., in terms of anatomical landmarks). Placement of the axis in line with the joint axis therefore is difficult to achieve in clinical practice.[4,28,35] When therapists attempt to place the goniometric axis congruent with the perceived joint axis, they may actually be increasing the amount of error in the measurement.

What may seem like precise alignment of the goniometric axis may not (and often does not) coincide with the proper alignment of the goniometer's arms (relative to the suggested bony landmarks). After aligning the arms of the goniometer, a therapist may find the joint's axis of rotation lying above or below the location of the goniometer's axis. The therapist is then faced with the task of deciding which anatomical landmarks (the two for the arms or the one for the axis) to follow most closely. A compromise must be made. Because this involves a judgment on the part of the individual therapist, the process has introduced a subjective element into the measurement process. Therefore, the chance of clinicians obtaining similar measurements (inter-rater reliability) when measuring the same joint is lessened.

Robson[35] and Defibaugh[28] have described how ROM measurements can be affected by even slight variations in axis placement (Fig. 4-1). The issue is especially relevant for joints such as the hip or shoulder, in which it is often difficult to locate precisely the anatomical axis of rotation. To use Robson's example, if hip flexion is measured with a standard 10-in goniometer and the recorded motion is 80°, a 1-in variation in axis placement (in either direction) could result in readings from 73° to 89°. This 16° range represents a substantial error.

Although it is commonly emphasized that the axis of the goniometer must be congruent with the joint axis, it seems that this does not add to the accuracy of measurement, but rather may introduce a substantial source of error. Even if one consistent set of anatomical landmarks were to be used for placement of the axis, the problems identified by Robson might still exist. Robson felt that the problem was so severe that he advocated use of the pendulum goniometer, a non-axis basis device that will be discussed later.

The axis problem can be handled in a rather simple manner. Therapists can ignore the placement of the goniometer's axis after they have carefully aligned the movement arms. This approach has been implicitly suggested by several authors since their techniques either ignore the issue of axis placement or minimize its importance.[4,12,15] These authors contend that whether or not the arms intersect at the joint axis is irrelevant, since axis placement is always secondary to the placement of the goniometer's arms. Consistent placement would be achieved by emphasizing placement of the arms according to ana-

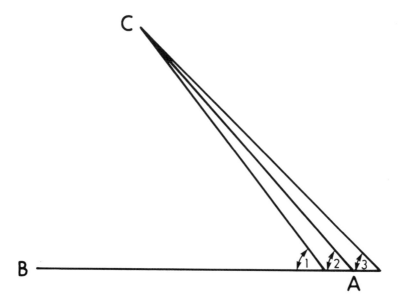

Fig. 4-1. Errors associated with malaligned goniometric axes are shown. Point A represents the initial placement of goniometer's axis in an attempt to make it overlie the joint axis. Points B and C are the anatomical landmarks used for placement of the goniometer's arms. When the original axis placement is at point A, angle 2 is obtained. If the axis is moved toward B, angle 1 is obtained, whereas angle 3 is obtained with movement in the opposite direction. Note that angle 1 > angle 2 > angle 3.

tomical landmarks. When the arms determine axis placement, as has been suggested above, it is unlikely that the goniometer's axis will be aligned with the joint's axis. Therefore, potentially, some accuracy may be sacrificed. However, when measurement is dependent on arm placement alone, and not on arm and axis placement, clinicians have a simpler and, theoretically, more reproducible technique. In a sense, some "potential" validity may be sacrificed to improve reliability. But, it is generally believed that reliability is a prerequisite to validity.[36,37]

GONIOMETRIC INSTRUMENTS

Through the years, many devices have been designed and used to measure joint motion. The best-known device is the goniometer (once known as an arthrometer or fleximeter[8,19]), which consists of a protractor with two arms attached to it (one stationary relative to the protractor and one mobile). Moore called this instrument the universal goniometer because it could be used to measure any joint.[26] Joint-specific goniometers have been designed for many different joints in the body.[38] There are also pendulum goniometers, fluid goniometers and, recently, electric goniometers that can be used to measure most joints. The simplest of all these devices, the universal goniometer, remains the instrument most commonly used clinically.

The Universal Goniometer

Although it is not known where the idea for the universal goniometer originated, designs and modifications were described between 1910 and 1930.[39] Many of the designs originated in France, where goniometers were used to evaluate World War I injuries. Contributions to the design of the goniometer were made by Silver,[40] who constructed a base and made both arms movable, and by Wiechec and Krusen,[3] who made the base adjustable. In 1949, Moore[9] argued that a universal goniometer with a stationary arm that extended in both directions from the axis was the best device for clinical use. She stated that the arms of the instrument should be from 12 to 16 inches in length to facilitate accurate alignment when the device was applied to joints with long limb segments.

Until the 1950s, most universal goniometers were made of wood or metal. Some had half-circle protractor scales whereas others had full-circle scales. There does not seem to be any significant advantage for either type of scale except that the half-circle scale goniometer can be applied more easily to joints when a patient is in a supine or prone position.

In 1952, Wainerdi[41] introduced a universal goniometer that was transparent and had sliding arms, much like a slide rule. He stated that opaque goniometers did not allow accurate alignment of the goniometer axis with the axis of the joint, and thus a transparent device should, theoretically, be more accurate. The sliding arms made the device easy to use on both large and small limb segments. The two parts of Wainerdi's goniometer were riveted. Most metal goniometers had locking nuts and threaded holes which often became worn with use, thus allowing excessive motion between the two arms. Wainerdi suggested that goniometeric scales be in 10° increments to make reading the scale easier. He stated that since there was an inherent error in goniometric measurements, changes of only a few degrees could not be significant. However, no data to support his hypothesis were presented.

Goniometric design has not changed much over the past 30 years, although universal goniometers vary considerably in fabrication and size. Plastic goniometers are widely used, probably because of their availability, portability, and low cost. Small goniometers (with arms as small as 6 in) are popular probably because of their convenience, despite Moore's assertions that the larger goniometers are more accurate. The relative merits of different types of universal goniometers have been investigated and will be discussed later.

Joint-Specific Goniometers

Because some joints (e.g., the metacarpal–phalangeal and interphalangeal joints) are difficult to measure with a universal goniometer, instruments designed to measure these joints have been developed. For example, the finger goniometer is placed over the dorsal aspect of the joint being measured, and readings are taken from a 180° scale. Although devices have been designed to measure almost every joint, few are used clinically today, in part because of the versatility of the universal goniometer. However, some devices such as the finger goniometer survive because of their practicality.

Joint-specific devices were first described in the 1920s and 1930s, soon after universal goniometers were described.[39] Cobe[6] used a flat table with protractors attached to measure wrist ROM in normal young adults. Hewitt[7] later used the same device to obtain normal values for wrist motion in college-age adults. However, since these values were obtained with a special device that is not in common use, it is likely that they cannot be used by clinicians who are using universal goniometers.

Wiechec and Krusen[3] reviewed the literature on joint measurement in 1939 and reported that many joint-specific devices were being used. Many of these were attached to the limb segments with straps. As a result, there were problems with alignment. Measurement error could also have been produced by variations in the amount of soft tissue in the person being measured. Pollock and Brooks[42] in 1942 described the design of an apparatus that simultaneously measured muscle strength and wrist ROM. In essence, the instrument was a spring-balance dynamometer activated by hand pressure on a hinged plate, to which was attached a protractor. According to the authors, the instrument could register muscle "strength" in grams while it also measured ROM. However, when a patient was found to have limited motion, it would have been difficult or impossible to discern with this instrument whether the limitation was caused by joint limitation or weakness.

The popularity of joint-specific devices declined in the 1950s, probably as a result of the classic work of Hellebrandt and her colleagues.[43] They reported that the universal goniometer yielded more reliable measurements than did any of the joint-specific devices. Following the publication of this finding, reports describing joint-specific devices declined. However, the use of some joint-specific devices persist. Bansil et al[44] reported in 1975 that adding a wheel with degree markings to a conventional shoulder wheel would allow measurements of glenohumeral joint motion. They argued that this type of device would eliminate trunk compensation, but they never explained how this modified shoulder wheel would do so. Ellis et al[45] modified a conventional, large, plastic goniometer by adding Velcro straps to each arm and by adding metal pointers to the scale. The device was then used to measure hip flexion and extension statically and dynamically (e.g., when the person walked). Hassellkus et al[46] described a two-axis goniometer that could be used to measure metacarpal–phalangeal joint flexion, extension, and radioulnar deviation.

Special Devices for Joint Measurement

The pendulum goniometer was introduced in the 1930s and was promoted by Leighton,[10] who in 1955 described the "Leighton fleximeter." The device consisted of a weighted pointer attached to a weighted 360° scale. The scale and the pointer were both influenced by gravity but operated independently. The dial was locked at the extreme of motion (e.g., full extension), and the arc of movement was registered under the pointer. The device was strapped onto the limb segment. The pendulum goniometer was also promoted by Robson,[35] who argued that it was more accurate than the universal goniometer. He argued that because the pendulum goniometer measured the angle that the limb segment makes with the horizontal plane, and that because this angle is the same at the joint and at the instrument, the device is accurate. However, this is true *only* if the person being tested is upright or if the scale is properly adjusted when the person is not upright. Defibaugh[28] used a pendulum goniometer attached to a mouthpiece to measure head motion, and recently Ekstrand et al[47] used a modified Leighton fleximeter for the measurement of lower extremity ROM.

The fluid goniometer (also known as the bubble goniometer or hydrogoniometer) introduced by Schenker[48] in 1956 incorporates a 360° scale in a flat, fluid-filled circular tube that contains a small air bubble. The device is strapped on the limb and as the segment is moved, the scale can be rotated while the bubble remains stationary. At the point at which the scale is stopped, ROM is read. The fluid goniometer has been tested and used by several authors.[14,22,49-52]

Though pendulum and fluid goniometers have an advantage over universal goniometers in that they are not subject to errors in estimating anatomical landmarks, they have disadvantages. These instruments have the same problems that joint-specific devices have. When the device must be strapped on, it is subject to variations in placement caused by soft tissue variability, and it is also prone to slip during movement. For example, the device is likely to be positioned differently on an endomorphic person than on an ectomorphic person. The problem of reliable positioning is not only present between different types of people, but may also be present within the same person. When the circumference of a limb under the strap changes (such as occurs during a muscle contraction), this change can affect the readings obtained. The presence of edema can also alter soft tissue architecture and affect the measurement. A second disadvantage is that for the readings to be accurate, the proximal segment of the joint being tested must lie exactly in the horizontal or vertical planes, depending on the technique. This problem can be overcome somewhat by adjustable scales, but precise adjustments must then be made if the measurement is to be meaningful.

Electric Goniometers

The electrogoniometer was introduced by Karpovich and Karpovich in 1959.[53] Although there have been many designs for electrogoniometers, almost all are based on the same principle. A potentiometer is attached to two arms, which are strapped to the proximal and distal limb segments. Movement of the arms causes the resistance in the potentiometer to vary. After the device has been calibrated, variations in voltage (or less often, current) may be used to represent joint excursions. The potentiometer must normally be aligned so that limb movements move the arms and therefore alter the resistance in the potentiometer. Some electrogoniometers have three potentiometers so that they can measure motion in all three cardinal planes.[55] Alignment, however, is still difficult to achieve. Electrogoniometers appear to be especially useful for the measurement of dynamic ROM, e.g., kinematic variables during gait. The electrogoniometer is being used in biomechanical and physical therapy research.[54–56]

The cost of electrogoniometers and the equipment needed to use them (e.g., strip-chart recorders, digital displays) has mitigated against their use in the clinic. The time needed to attach the goniometer and align it, and the need to have the patient attached to a recording device, have also limited the clinical usefulness of electrogoniometers. The devices also appear to be more accurate for the measurement of joint excursions (i.e., the total arc of movement) than they are for the measurement of absolute limb position. However, advances in technology such as miniaturization and telemetry may make electrogoniometers clinically useful for the assessment of both static and dynamic joint function.

NONGONIOMETRIC METHODS OF JOINT MEASUREMENT

From the 1920s through the 1950s, a large number of alternative methods of joint measurement were reported. As previously discussed, there were goniometers adapted to specific joints.[39] In addition, there were (and still are) many ways to measure joint motion without the use of a goniometer. Few of these techniques are being used today; most of them were impractical, inaccurate, and unreliable.

Visual Estimation

Visual estimation is a common form of nongoniometric measurement. Probably every clinician "eyeballs" joint motion, if not actually to record a number, then at least to quickly gauge the effects of treatment. There is no record to show how or when this became a common practice. "Eyeballing" is obviously the easiest technique to use, since no equipment is needed, and it is practical when no goniometer is handy.

The practice of visual estimation has been described by several authors,[12,21,25] and has been promoted by the AAOS, whose handbook has probably contributed more than anything else to the widespread acceptance of visual estimation. The merits of this technique will be considered in the section on reliability.

Radiography and Photography

Radiography is the most accurate means of assessing joint motion. On a radiograph, bony structures are visible and ROM can be accurately measured.[57] However, radiography is clearly impractical clinically because of the radiation exposure, the expense, and the time required.

Double-exposure photography of joints (taking pictures of a joint at each extreme of motion on one negative) was suggested by Wilson and Stasch.[58] The technique eliminates the need to place the goniometer accurately, yet angles must still be measured from lines drawn on the photograph. Placement of lines can probably be no more reliable than measurements dependent on goniometric arm placements. Photography, although more practical than radiography, is not widely used clinically. This is probably because the method is time-consuming and expensive. In some clinics, copy machines have been used to "photograph" joint movement, although the method has not been described in the literature. Copy machines can be used to measure finger and wrist motions. The joint to be tested is positioned so that the proximal and distal segments are parallel to the glass screen after full ROM has been achieved. However, as with photographic methods, lines must be drawn on the copy before an angle can be measured.

Linear Measurements

Recording motion in terms of linear measurements (i.e., distances) rather than angular measurements (i.e., degrees) is widely used when motion involving several joints is measured.[12,15] Measuring the fingertip to palm distance for gross finger flexion or the fingertip to floor distance for forward or lateral flexion of the spine are common example of such recordings. When using this technique, differences are noted by changes in linear measures (e.g., centimeters or inches).[15]

Optical Methods

Wilmer and Elkins[59] designed an optical goniometer that was essentially a circular scale imposed on a concave reducing lens. The tester looked through the device (which was aligned perpendicular to the plane of motion) at the joint being examined. Alignment and movement of the limb could be measured by using landmarks indicated on the skin. The optical device was shown to be inaccurate for joints such as the subtalar joint, where small arcs of motion occurred. Zankel[60] projected a circular scale from a photographic slide onto the joint being measured, and the limb segment served as the "indicator" of the degrees of motion on the scale. The main problem with this method was that the slide projector had to be precisely aligned in all three planes in order to measure the motion accurately. The constant need for adjustment made this technique impractical and potentially inaccurate.

Schematography, which was described by Wiechec and Krusen,[3] also used optics to measure joint motion. In this technique, lights and mirrors were used

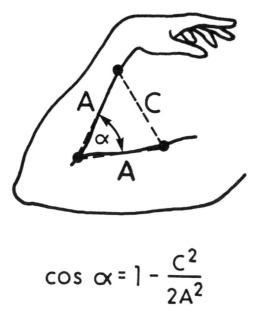

$$\cos \alpha = 1 - \frac{C^2}{2A^2}$$

Fig. 4-2. Angle of elbow flexion may be calculated trigonometrically. For elbow measurements, it has been suggested that points 20 cm from the ventral crease should be marked. The distance from the crease to these points is A. The distance between the two points C is then measured, and the angle is calculated from the equation.

to reflect an image of a segment onto a piece of paper, where it was traced on successive occasions to record joint motion. As in the previous method, the necessity for very precise adjustment of the equipment made this method impractical.

Trigonometry

Williams[61] suggested using trigonometric calculations for determining joint position. In this method, the triangle formed by the proximal and distal segments moving about an axis (Fig. 4-2) is measured. The angle is then calculated.

The angle can also be obtained by using a graph on which the angle has been plotted against linear measures. Although this concept is interesting, there are some potential sources of error. A point must be located and three distances (proximal A, distal A, and C) must be measured. Williams did not discuss whether body type (e.g., obesity, hypertrophy, edema) could affect accuracy. There are no reports describing the accuracy or reliability of this method. With trigonometric methods, there are four potential sources of error (location of the origin at the joint, measurement of the proximal and distal segments and in calculation) whereas use of the universal goniometer would appear to have only two sources of error (placement of the two goniometric arms). The trigonometric technique cannot be used for movements such as rotation (e.g.

external rotation of the hip) or pronation–supination. Measurements made with trigonometric techniques require calculations or the use of references tables or the drawing of graphs for each position measured. Therefore, this method would take considerably more time than conventional methods.

NOTATION AND RECORDING

In the 1940s and 1950s, there were not only many devices for measuring joint motion, but there were also many methods of documenting ROM. Two topics will be discussed in this section: *notation*, which is how motion is described in terms of degrees, and *recording*, which refers to the forms, tables, or graphs used for charting. Today, many clinicians use one system of notation, although numerous methods are in use. Methods of notation and recording should be a concern for the clinician because they guide the ways in which physical therapists present the results of an evaluation to other disciplines. If the notation and recording methods used are not logical and concise, those who are unfamiliar with joint motion evaluation are likely to have difficulty in relating to the evaluations. Therefore, it is imperative that clinics have standardized systems for the notation and recording of joint motion.

Notation

0-180 System. One of the most widely used systems of notation was first described by Silver[40] in 1923 and later by Cave and Roberts,[62] and has been endorsed by others.[15,23] The widespread acceptance of the 0-180 method results largely from the recommendation of the two most widely consulted sources in the field, Moore[9] and the AAOS.[12] In the 0-180 system, the starting position for all movements is considered to be 0°, and movements proceed toward 180° (Table 4-2).

180-0 System. The 180-0 System was described by Clark[5] in 1920 and later by Wiechec and Krusen.[3] In this system, movements toward flexion approaches 180°, and extension approaches 0°. Various rules are used for the

Table 4-2. Hip ROM Represented by Three Different Notation Systems

	0–180	180–0	360
Flexion	125	55	55
Extension	15	165	195
Abduction	45	45	135
Adduction	45	15	195
Internal rotation	45	135	45
External rotation	45	135	45

Using "normal" values taken from Gerhardt JJ, Russe, OA: International SFTR Method of Measuring and Recording Joint Motion. Huber, Bern, 1975.

other planes of movement. Movements past the neutral position toward extension (e.g., shoulder "hyperextension") approach 0° (Table 4.2). This system is rarely used today.

360 System. The 360 system was introduced by West[29] in 1945 and was later used by Wilmer and Elkins,[59] Dorinson and Wagner,[8] and Esch and Lepley.[23] Although it is similar to the 180-0 system, in the 360 system movements of extension or adduction past the neutral position approach 360° (Table 4-2). Different rules are used for the other planes of motion. This system is also not widely used today, partly because, like the 180-0 system, the notations are more difficult to interpret than those of the 0-180 system.

Recording Methods

Joint motion has been recorded in the form of tables or charts,[3,7,12,15] sketches,[4,9] and graphs.[9] All of these methods can be useful, but tables and charts are probably the easiest to use and interpret. The major disadvantage of tables and charts is their length. Using the 0-180 notation system, each movement must be listed separately, as shown in Table 4-3.

Gerhardt and Russe[15,63] have proposed a different method of recording joint motion within the 0-180 system of notation; it is called the SFTR (for sagittal–frontal–transverse–rotational) recording method. This method records all motion in a given plane together, which shortens the length of the record. Three numbers are used for each plane of motion. Two numbers represent the extremes of motion, and the other numbers (listed in the middle) represent the starting position (0° for normal motion). Extension, movements away from the body, and lateral flexion and rotation to the left are recorded first; the reciprocal movement is listed last. For example, in SFTR, shoulder motion is recorded:

Shoulder ROM (in degrees)

S	45–0–180
F	180–0–0
T	45–0–135
R (F90)	90–0–90

Shoulder flexion–extension is in the sagittal plane (S), abduction is in the frontal plane (F), and horizontal abduction–adduction is in the transverse plane (T).

Table 4-3. Joint Motion Using the 0-180 Notation System

Right Shoulder	ROM (in degrees)
Flexion	180
Extension	45
Abduction	180
Internal rotation (abduction at 90°)	90
External rotation (abduction at 90°)	90
Horizontal abduction	45
Horizontal adduction	135

Rotation (R) is recorded separately, and the "F90" indicates that rotation is being measured with the arm in 90° of abduction (in the frontal plane). This system provides a means for recording the motion of all extremity joints, spinal motion, and also positional deformities such as genu valgus or genu recurvatum.

The SFTR system has several advantages. First, when using this recording method, it is easy to describe the proximal limb position, as seen in the above example. Limb position is important since the position of one joint can influence the ROM for the adjacent joint, either proximally or distally. For example, the position of the hip can influence knee ROM because of the effect of the two-joint muscles spanning the hip and knee. A second advantage of the SFTR system is that positional deformities can be easily described. For example, a fixed genu valgus of 20° is recorded as F20-0, because valgus occurs in the frontal plane. Genu recurvatum of 10° is recorded as S10-0-130. Note that in the example of the valgus recording only two digits were used. Two digits, in the SFTR system, indicates a fixed deformity (i.e., a nonmovable positional deformity). A three-digit recording, as in the recurvatum example, indicates a nonfixed deformity. In the example given, this means that the knee can be flexed to 130° but that extension can continue past the neutral (zero) position to 10° of recurvatum. If there was a valgus laxity and the knee could be moved from 20° degrees of valgus to neutral, this would be recorded as F20-0-0. The third advantage of the SFTR system is that the starting position is clearly noted without the use of negative numbers. This makes descriptions of contractures very clear. If a patient lacked 30° of knee extension (i.e., had a 30° knee flexion contracture) but could flex to 120°, this would be written as S0-30-120. The middle number, when it is not zero, indicates that the starting position was not neutral; i.e., there is a contracture.

SFTR recording facilitates standardized recording and permits the use of abbreviations without the loss of clarity. The SFTR system is not familiar to most clinicians and has not been taught in most schools. Although the system is used in Europe, where it was developed, it is rarely used in the United States. However, the system is easy to learn and is clearly the most concise and logical recording method.

VALIDITY AND RELIABILITY

A measurement cannot yield meaningful information unless it is reliable and valid. A measurement must also be practical and easily obtained, if it is to be clinically useful. There can be little argument that goniometry, when compared to other methods, is the most practical means of measuring joint motion. This sections examines the reliability and validity of the methods used to measure joint ROM.

Reliability

In clinical settings, patients may be evaluated several times and sometimes even by different therapists. Therefore, the consistency of this measurement becomes a critical concern. Research on goniometric reliability has been directed into two main areas: inter-tester and intra-tester reliability and device reliability. Each will be discussed here.

Tester reliability refers to the consistency of the measurement as it is affected by the person taking the measurement. Two categories may be identified, intra-tester and inter-tester. Intra-tester reliability deals with how well a person can reproduce his or her own measurements when they are taken at a different time (this is sometimes referred to as test–retest reliability or stability over time). Inter-tester reliability deals with how well a person can reproduce another person's measurements. For a complete discussion of these terms and associated concepts, see Chapter 1 in this volume. Theoretically, intra-tester reliability should be better than inter-tester reliability because errors resulting from individual differences in those taking the measurements are not present. Intra-tester reliability can be expected to be greater than inter-tester reliability because a person is more likely to reproduce his or her own method rather than that of someone else.

The first studies to deal with the reliability of goniometric measurement were reported in 1928 by Cobe[6] and Hewitt,[7] who examined normal wrist motion in hundreds of adults, most young. Both found that goniometric measurements of normal wrists varied considerably within the same subjects. These authors recommended taking several measurements and recording the average value. Hellebrandt et al[43] described the first major study of goniometric reliability in 1949. They found that individual testers could reproduce their own measurements on patients and that a "highly skilled" tester (in terms of experience and training) was even more reliable than the average tester. They recommended that a single therapist take all the measurements on a particular joint unless inter-tester reliability in that setting was determined.

Defibaugh[28] examined the intra-tester and inter-tester reliability of measuring head motion of 30 normal subjects by eight testers and found moderate to high reliability ($r = .660$ to $.939$). An unexpected finding in this study was that inter-tester reliability was better than intra-tester reliability. This result may partially be explained by the fact that the interval between intra-tester measurements was between one and seven days whereas the intertester interval was less than two hours. Any comparison between the two types of reliability is therefore difficult to make. Another drawback of this study lay in the method of data reduction. Three measurements were taken for each head position, and the two or three that varied 5° or less from each other were averaged to obtain a single value. Disregarding measurements that varied too much from the others probably led to better reliability than one can actually expect clinically.

Ahlback and Lindahl[57] compared different methods of measuring flexion and extension of normal and osteoarthritic hips and found good inter-tester reliability for two testers (a difference of 5° or less in 74% of the measurements). Hamilton and Lachenbruch[64] studied finger joint motion (metacarpal–phalangeal [MCP], proximal interphalangeal [PIP], distal interphalangeal [DIP]) on normal hands and found that intratester reliability was better than intertester reliability. Mitchell et al[65] examined reliability of knee measurements for both patients and normals with two testers and found intra-tester and inter-tester reliability both to be high. It should be noted, however, that the testers used a standardized method and not the individual techniques they would normally use in the clinic. Mitchell's group also discovered that a diurnal variation in the amplitude of knee motion did not exist in groups of normal subjects or in rheumatoid arthritis patients.

Low[66] examined reliability using 50 testers to measure one normal subject's wrist and elbow joints; he found that intra-tester reliability was better than inter-tester reliability. In this study, the testers used their own goniometric techniques and not a standardized method. Based on these results, Low recommended that one person take all the measurements for a particular joint. In addition, Low examined the effect of using the average of several measurements. The use of the mean of several measurements had been previously recommended for increasing reliability in clinical practice.[67] Low found that use of the average measurement improved goniometric reliability.

Boone et al[68] also found that intra-tester reliability was better than inter-tester reliability for four testers examining normal upper and lower extremity motions under standardized conditions ($n = 12$). The standard deviation for inter-tester measurements of the knee joint was 5.2°, and they postulated that when measurements are taken by different testers they would have to differ by more than 5.2° if an actual change in knee motion was to be demonstrated. However, their data were obtained from normal subjects. It is questionable whether this finding can be extrapolated to patient testing. The 5.2° SD reported by Boone et al could represent error in measurement, but it could also reflect the normal variability that is expected when different subjects are measured. Therefore, the statement that variation must exceed 5.2° to be meaningful is really debatable.

Boone and her colleagues also examined the effect of averaging several measurements and showed that use of one measurement led to reliability that was as good as that obtained by taking the average of several measurements. This disagrees with Low's findings. Boone and her colleagues also reported that lower extremity movements were more difficult to measure reliably than were upper extremity movements.

Rothstein et al[69] studied reliability on 24 patients using unstandardized methods (allowing the 12 therapists involved to use their own clinical measurement methods) and found reliability high for both intra-tester and inter-tester measurements of knee and elbow movements with the exception of inter-tester reliability of knee extension. A post-hoc analysis of their data showed that when therapists used different test positions, the inter-tester reliability for knee extension measurements was much lower than when the therapists used the same test positions. This indicates that test position can be a major factor leading to variation in ROM measurements. In measuring knee extension, the influence of two-joint muscles (i.e., the hamstrings) could alter the amount of knee extension available because of the hip position. For this reason, it is recommended that the patient's position should be routinely described as part of the goniometric record. Rothstein et al also showed that averaging measurements did not improve reliability, confirming the findings of Boone et al.

When goniometric reliability studies are reviewed, use of a standardized method in the testing must be noted. It is important because it can be argued that individual variation in method (e.g., positioning, placement of the goniometer), could account for a large part of the variability in measurement, especially when inter-tester reliability is being examined. Ashton et al[70] found that giving specific, standardized instructions to the testers did not improve the inter-tester reliability of hip measurements on spastic cerebral palsy children, while Ekstrand et al[47] found that intra-tester reliability in normal hip motion testing was improved by the use of standardized techniques. Grohmann[71] compared two methods of goniometric measurement (lateral and over-the-joint) on a normal elbow, using 40 physical therapy students as testers, and found that there were no significant differences in the readings obtained with the two methods for the elbow.

Clinicians who are concerned with the quality of their clinic's goniometric measurements should pay particular attention to the issue of whether studies used standardized methods. The reliability estimates (in terms of percentage of agreement or correlation coefficients) obtained with the use of standardized (prescribed) techniques can only be expected clinically when all therapists follow the same standardized techniques described in the literature being cited. Studies that permit therapists to use whatever technique they choose have more global application, in that the reliability estimates are not dependent on the use of a single agreed-upon technique. Clinical applicability of findings from the various studies will therefore depend on whether all therapists in a clinic use exactly the same methods (and whether those were the ones used in a given study) or whether therapists tend to use their own techniques.

Device Reliability.   Some studies have examined whether different devices used in goniometry lead to the same results. This form of reliability is analogous to the "equivalence of forms" reliability that has been discussed by Rothstein in Chapter 1. The issue is whether different goniometers can be used and the results being the same?

The first study dealing with "inter-device" reliability was that of Hellebrandt et al.[43] These investigators found that in the hands of a "highly skilled tester", the universal goniometer was more reliable than joint-specific devices.

Leighton[10] found that a pendulum goniometer (previously described) was reliable for measuring the upper extremity, lower extremity and spinal motion in 120 normal young subjects, (r = .913 to .996). Defibaugh[28] also used a pendulum goniometer in his reliability study on head motion, and these two studies supported the use of the pendulum goniometer as an alternative to the universal device. However, the device must be strapped to the body segment, which makes it liable to move with changes in soft tissue architecture during movement. Pendulum devices are still in use today.[47]

Hamilton and Lachenbruch[64] found three devices used to measure finger motion (a dorsal finger goniometer, a small universal goniometer, and a pendulum finger goniometer) to be equally reliable for measuring finger joint (MCP, PIP, DIP) motion on normal hands. In 51 subjects with rheumatoid arthritis, Hasselkus et al[46] found that a two-axis goniometer (described previously) for the metacarpophalangeal joints was reliable for both intra-tester and inter-tester measurements when two testers were involved.

Rothstein et al[69] showed that three commonly used goniometers (large metal, large transparent plastic, and small transparent plastic) were all equally reliable in measuring knee and elbow motion in 24 patients.

Visual estimation of joint motion (i.e., "eyeballing") has also been investigated for reliability. Low[66] compared goniometric measurement to visual estimation for 50 testers (their level of experience was not described) and found that using the goniometer was more reliable (for normal joints). Marks et al,[72] in studying knee extension and flexion in rheumatoid arthritis patients, showed that visual estimation was a reliable method for both intra-tester (all r values > .91) and inter-tester testing (all r values > .90).

The effect of the size of the goniometric scale increments on reliability has been examined. Wainerdi[41] asserted that because of an inherent error in measurement, scales should have graduations of 10° to allow for better reliability. His argument seems logical. With fewer numbers on the scale to read from, a clinician stands a better chance of taking reliable measurements (e.g., readings are more likely to agree). This is because there are fewer values to choose, and small variations in the alignment of a device would probably not affect the reading. Many goniometers in clinical use have scales in increments of 2° or 5°, and measurements are frequently rounded off to the nearest 5°.[19,57] However, Rothstein, Miller, and Roettger (unpublished data) found that rounding off readings from a large metal goniometer (2° incremented scale) and a large plastic goniometer (1° incremented scale) to the nearest 5° did not result in better reliability than not rounding off the readings. Using a goniometer with 5° increments does not improve reliability. Thus, it is suggested that using a goniometer with a finely incremented scale does not sacrifice reliability; in fact, it gives better resolution in measurement (more detail).

Overview of Reliability.   Goniometric research has been as diverse as the methods used for the measurement itself. The most important goniometric study was clearly that of Hellebrandt et al.[43] This study, along with Moore's previous works,[9,38] proved to be highly influential in the clinical use of goniometric measurements. Suggestions from these studies formed the basis for a "conventional wisdom" that could be followed uniformly by the clinical community. Until then, there was very little standardization in goniometry. There were differences in the methods of measurement, variation in the normal values used, and in notation systems and devices used clinically. The wide diversity of methods and recording made it difficult to prove the value of goniometry as a measurement tool. After the studies of Moore and her colleagues, there was a decrease in the number of reports dealing with joint-specific devices, and the use of the 180-0 or 360 notation systems declined. There appeared also to be a decrease in the use of nongoniometric systems of joint motion measurement. The focus of many studies that followed those of Moore and her associates was on reliability. Therefore, it is important to review what Moore and her associates observed and suggested:

1. A standard method of measurement was recommended for use in the clinic.

2. Normal values were presented (taken from Daniels, Williams, and Worthingham[13]).

3. The 0-180 notation system was deemed to be the most logical and convenient.

4. The universal goniometer was proven to be the most reliable and practical clinical device.

5. Therapists were shown to be reliable in taking goniometric measurements.

This review of goniometric reliability demonstrates that although trends are apparent, there are still some questions about the clinical reliability of goniometry. Clinicians committed to investigating the quality of their measurements might be interested in determining their own reliability in their clinical setting (this will be discussed later in this chapter). Performing goniometric reliability studies has been shown to be feasible in the clinic and can provide valuable information.[69] Studies can also point out areas of deficiencies in goniometric evaluations and provide the basis for remediation. The necessity for the provision and documentation of quality assurance is growing in health care, and reliability studies are an excellent source of providing quality assurance for a basic evaluative tool. Last, better knowledge of the value of the measurement allows the clinician to use it in clinical decision making with more accuracy and confidence, which ultimately benefits the patient.

Validity

When a limb segment moves through an arc of motion, it forms an angle with the limb segment with which it articulates. The goniometer appears to describe joint motion. The question relative to goniometry is whether the goniometer can adequately measure the angle formed by the limb segments and therefore accurately measure joint motion?

There is no mention of the subject of validity in most of the early goniometric studies.[6,7,40] Authors apparently assumed that goniometry was valid and did not test this. In 1949, Moore[43] stated that goniometry was only "a grossly quantitative technic," though she argued that the use of a goniometer was better than visual estimation of joint motion, and she strongly urged that therapists use goniometers. Robson[35] showed, through the use of trigonometry, that the error of measurement caused by misplacement of the goniometric axis could be reduced by using goniometers with long arms instead of short ones. Ahlback and Lindahl[57] devised a method of measuring hip flexion and extension and found that measurements taken with a hip-joint-specific goniometer agreed closely with radiographic measurements. Baldwin and Cunningham[73] conducted a validity study on the measurement of elbow and radioulnar motions (flexion, extension, pronation, and supination) in normal children and children with rheumatoid arthritis, using 62 testers with experience varying from six months to 25 years. Baldwin and Cunningham found that visual estimation of elbow motion was more accurate than goniometric measurement of normal children, but that goniometry was more accurate for measurement of children with rheumatoid arthritis. A limitation of this study is that accuracy (validity) was tested by comparing the therapist's measurements with those taken by one experienced therapist. Comparisons with radiographs were not made. The accuracy of the experienced therapist's measurements was assumed, but never tested.

Ellis et al[45] found that a special hip goniometer (described previously) produced readings that were within 4 percent of measurements taken from high-speed motion picture films (the subject's skin was marked in order to measure joint motion from the film). This is surprisingly accurate considering that the goniometer took dynamic measurements, i.e., during gait. Chao and Hoffman,[54] and Chao,[55] in studies using a triaxial electro-goniometer, found it to be highly accurate in measuring angular motion when attached to a joint motion simulator.

The Issue in Validity Studies

Determining the validity of goniometric measurement is of major importance because if the measurement is to be useful, it must be possible to infer something from it. In other words, how valid is the information gained from goniometric measurements? If the goniometer does not accurately reflect joint motion, it serves no purpose.

There are limited inferences that can be made from goniometric measurements alone. Goniometry does reveal whether or not there is a limitation in the arc of motion for a joint, but does not indicate the cause of dysfunction—this must be discerned by other tests (e.g., radiography, MMT).

Certain inferences can be made about joint motion by comparing results from active and passive ROM tests. Active range of motion (AROM) can reveal information concerning the capability of the neuromuscular complex to produce movement around a joint. Functional deficits in the neuromuscular complex can include weakness (resulting from neuropathic or myopathic changes) in the prime movers and synergists, or inappropriate activity in the antagonists or synergists (e.g., spasticity). AROM measurements then serve as the first step in determining the cause of dysfunction for a physical impairment (loss of motion).

Passive ROM (PROM) testing can yield information concerning the joint structures (bone, soft tissue) and their ability to allow motion. Testing for "end feel" can also help determine what kind of structures might be implicated in restricted motion. However, neuromuscular deficits such as spasticity can also affect PROM, and thus the two types of tests (PROM and AROM) can yield inconclusive information. But PROM serves as a further or second step in determining the cause of an impairment. For example, if active range of shoulder flexion is 90° and passive motion is 180°, it can be inferred that the cause of the dysfunction is probably not caused by a loss of elasticity in the soft tissue structures in the shoulder but rather is caused by a dysfunction in the neuro-muscular complex. Further evaluation (e.g., MMT, reflex testing) is then nec-essary to reveal the exact nature of the problem. If active and passive flexion of the shoulder are both limited, there could be a neuromuscular dysfunction such as "spasticity" limiting the motion, but there could be elastic factors (soft tissue tightness) also limiting motion. In this case, further testing becomes an absolute necessity. Differences between active and passive motion can be used to help create hypotheses as to why a joint has limited motion, but this must be confirmed through the use of other tests.

ESTABLISHING GONIOMETRIC RELIABILITY IN A CLINICAL SETTING

Despite all of the studies dealing with goniometric reliability, questions remain as to the quality of this ubiquitous physical therapy measurement tech-nique. Clinicians can conduct studies in the setting in which they work and demonstrate the reliability of the measurement as it is used in their clinic. Establishing reliability is akin to the process laboratories use to develop stan-dards (and values) for their own procedures so that measurement error can be accounted for when test results are interpreted.

Clinicians, who are interested in examining goniometric reliability can deal with the following clinically relevant questions:

1. Can therapists reproduce their own measurements (intra-rater relia-bility)?
2. Can therapists reproduce the measurements obtained by a colleague (inter-rater reliability)?
3. Can various goniometers (large, small, metal, plastic, pendulums, etc.) be used interchangeably?
4. Is reliability improved by using the means of multiple measurements?
5. Must clinicians all use a standard protocol to obtain reliable (inter-changeable) measurements or may they use whatever techniques they prefer?
6. Can inexperienced therapists take measurements as reliably as expe-rienced therapists?
7. Can visual estimations of joint excursions be as reliable as measure-ments taken with a goniometer?
8. Can some joints be more reliably measured than others?
9. Can various patient types be measured with equal reliability (e.g., are measurements taken on spastic patients as reliable as those taken on flaccid patients or normal patients)?

The following section presents a method for performing a clinical goniom-etric reliability study that can be modified to examine any of the above ques-tions.

Design

A clinical reliability study should deal with the questions pertinent to the clinic where the study is conducted. For example, in a large department with several therapists, inter-tester reliability should be a concern if different therapists are likely to measure the same patient. In a similar way, if many different goniometers are used in a clinic, inter-device reliability would be important. A meaningful, clinically relevant protocol can only be devised when these clinic-specific issues are identified.

Although many published reliability studies have dealt with normal subjects, a clinical study should be performed on patients. Although studying normal individuals yields some information, it must be asked whether the results of such studies can be extrapolated to a patient population. Boone et al[68] examined goniometric reliability on healthy individuals, but their results cannot necessarily be used to make inferences about goniometric reliability for patients, because of the differences in physical function between healthy and patient populations. A patient may have a complicating condition such as spasticity or may be incapable of being positioned correctly. Such factors can make goniometric reliability more difficult to achieve in patients. The patients selected for participation in the study should represent a true cross-section of the types of patients seen in that clinic (a representative sample). If the study is to examine overall reliability, enough patients must be included so that all of the diagnostic classifications seen in the clinic are included. For example, the testing population should not be made up of patients with orthopedic problems if the patient population seen in the clinic consists equally of patients with orthopedic, general medical, and neurological problems. In addition, the therapists selected for the study (in theory, all therapists involved in patient treatment should be included, but this is not always feasible) should represent all levels of experience and expertise within the clinic. One cannot make judgments about the goniometric reliability of the whole clinic if all of the therapists do not participate. If all therapists cannot participate, those who do should be representative (i.e., be a good sample) of all the therapists in the clinic.

If it is decided that the reliability of various goniometers is to be investigated, the devices that are chosen should all be in common use if their reliability is to be compared with each other. If a new device is to be investigated, the therapists should be given a chance to become accustomed to the device before the study, to insure that the results of the investigation are not influenced by the therapist's lack of familiarity with the device.

If the purpose of conducting an investigation is to test true clinical goniometric reliability, therapists must use their own technique when taking readings in order for the testing to replicate actual clinical conditions. If it is to be determined if unstandardized methods are as reliable as standardized methods, the segment of the investigation in which the therapists use standard methods should be conducted last, unless the clinic's protocol calls for use of a standard technique (and therapists actually do this).

Implementation

A protocol must be devised and rigidly adhered to if the study is to yield meaningful results. The protocol should give precise directions for the following:

1. Patient selection: Patients selected for the study should be persons for whom goniometric measurement of the joints to be tested is appropriate. Joints that are selected must also be appropriate for the diagnostic categories chosen.

2. Therapist selection: It is preferable that therapists should be selected randomly. If intra-tester reliability is to be determined, one therapist should be selected to measure a patient. If inter-tester reliability is investigated, two or more therapists must be selected and randomly paired.

3. Supervision: The test should be monitored by one person. If other persons are also used to supervise tests, it must be insured that they administer the test in the same way.

4. Testing sequence: If repeated measurements are taken on a joint, it is conceivable that the motion could change after repeated movements. Therefore, it is necessary that measurements be carried out by each therapist in the same sequence each time.

5. Blinding the goniometer: Devices to be used should have their scales covered so that the testing therapist cannot read the scale; it is possible that this could influence subsequent readings. Readings should be taken by whoever is monitoring (or supervising) the testing. If a device is to be used for repeated measurements, it should not be used twice consecutively if there are other devices also being used.

6. Recording: A data sheet should be used by the monitor to record all information, including the patient's name (or number), date, diagnosis, extremity tested, the tester or testers involved, and the monitor for the test. The makeup of the rest of the data sheet depends on the issues being investigated. Spaces must be included for the tester's number, each device, and the number of measurements. Whether or not the joint motion is carried out in the cardinal plane, and what the patient's position was during testing should also be recorded. Patient positioning, especially with regard to the joints adjacent to the one being tested, can influence the readings. However, no attempt should be made to standardize positioning unless this is an intended part of the study.

An example of a goniometric data sheet is shown in Figure 4-3. In this example, reliability of measurements of the shoulder joint are being tested. This sheet allows for the recording of measurements for one patient, examined in two testing sessions. There is room for the measurements of two therapists on the sheet. The first therapist's data is on the left, and the other therapist's data is on the right. This allows recording of data to examine intra-tester and inter-tester reliability. The form allows two goniometers to be used (large and small) for inter-device reliability, with each therapist using each goniometer twice, so that the effect of taking multiple measurements on reliability can be examined. Space is provided so that the monitor can note whether or not the

Patient _____ Hospital number _____ Date _____

Diagnosis _____ Extremity tested   Right   Left   Supervisor_____

First therapist number _____ Second therapist number_____

Session I

goniometer	1	2	c.p.	elbow pos.	pt. pos.	1	2	c.p.	elbow pos.	pt. pos.
					Flexion					
large			Y N		S P Sit			Y N		S P Sit
small			Y N		S P Sit			Y N		S P Sit
					Extention					
large			Y N		S P Sit			Y N		S P Sit
small			Y N		S P Sit			Y N		S P Sit
					Abduction					
large			Y N		S P Sit			Y N		S P Sit
small			Y N		S P Sit			Y N		S P Sit

Session II
Horizontal Abduction

large			Y N		S P Sit			Y N		S P Sit
small			Y N		S P Sit			Y N		S P Sit

Horizontal Adduction

large			Y N		S P Sit			Y N		S P Sit
small			Y N		S P Sit			Y N		S P Sit

External Rotation

large			Y N		S P Sit			Y N		S P Sit
small			Y N		S P Sit			Y N		S P Sit
	measured in		degrees abduction			measured in		degrees abduction		

Internal Rotation

large			Y N		S P Sit			Y N		S P Sit
small			Y N		S P Sit			Y N		S P Sit
	measured in____degrees abduction					measured in____ degrees abduction				

Fig. 4-3. A data sheet for goniometric reliability for all shoulder movements is shown. The sheet has space for two measurements to be recorded by two different therapists. In addition, space is provided for measurements made by two different types of goniometers (i.e., small and large). The first therapist uses the spaces on the left. The columns to the right of the space for the ROM data permits the therapist to check off whether motion was in a cardinal plane (c.p.). The following columns permit notation of the patient's elbow position and whether the patient is standing (S), prone (P), or sitting (Sit). For measurement of rotation, space is provided to indicate how much the shoulder was abducted.

movement is being carried out in the cardinal plane (CP), and the patient's position is recorded (supine [S], prone [P] or sitting [SIT]). Elbow position is noted because there are two-joint muscles (biceps brachii, triceps brachii) that span both the elbow and shoulder joints; these muscles can affect shoulder motion depending on their overall length. Modifications of this form can be used to record data for almost any type of clinical reliability study.

Data Analysis

Reliability is frequently analyzed by means of the Pearson Product Moment (*r*) which is an assessment of covariance.[74,75] Correlation examines the degree of association between two sets of paired measures. Another statistic that can be used is the intra-class correlation coefficient (ICC).[76,77] The ICC examines the degree of agreement between two or more sets of measures. The ICC is probably more appropriate for determining goniometric reliability because it is possible to have high product-moment correlations (approaching 1) even with large discrepancies between two sets of paired measurements. For example, if every measurement in one set (by one therapist) were 10° higher than the value of the corresponding measurement in another set (taken by a second therapist), the degree of association (covariance) would be perfect (and the correlation would be 1), but the degree of agreement (as measured by the ICC) would be lower. Because the purpose of reliability in clinical goniometry is to permit measurements to be used interchangeably, the ICC statistic is probably more meaningful (see Chapter 1 for a discussion of statistics used in reliability studies).

Data from goniometric measurements in a clinical reliability study can be analyzed in many ways depending on the issues in question:

1. Intra-tester reliability: One therapist's first measurement of a joint is compared with that therapist's second measurement.

2. Inter-tester reliability: One therapist's measurement is compared with another therapist's same measurement. (Note: in these correlations, it is very important to make sure the same phenomena are being compared—e.g., one therapist's first measurement cannot necesssarily be compared with another therapist's second measurement, even if they are measuring the same joint with the same device).

3. Device reliability: Correlations for devices within themselves (requiring two or more measurements) can be made or correlations between devices can also be done. Comparison of the correlations achieved with each device can also be made.

4. Average of measurements: The mean of several measurements can be correlated with only the first measurement. This can be done only when examining inter-tester reliability, because when testing intra-tester reliability, there is nothing with which to correlate the average of several measurements.

From these basic analyses, other issues, depending on the research design, can be examined; for example, visual estimation can be compared with goniometric measurements, or a comparison can be made of experienced therapists and inexperienced therapists. The possibilities are limitless, but for the study to be clinically relevant, the design should relate to the issues that are important in the clinic in which the study is being conducted.

SUMMARY AND CONCLUSIONS

Conclusions about "one best way" (to use Moore's phrase) to assess ROM are difficult to make. The existing literature does not lend itself to simple statements. However, the present body of research permits some general observations to be made.

The *universal goniometer* has been compared to other devices and it is clearly the most reliable, versatile, and clinically feasible instrument for assessing joint motion. Devices such as the pendulum and bubble goniometers appear to have some value, but they are not as easy to use as the universal goniometer. Electrogoniometers appear to have great potential, but at the present time they are not practical for routine clinical applications.

Visual estimation (or "eyeballing") is widely used clinically, but it is not clear whether this technique is as reliable as goniometric methods. In view of the widespread clinical use of visual estimations, there is an obvious need for research that will determine whether this technique is reliable.

Although several *notation systems* exist, the 0-180 method is most widely used because its inherent logic facilitates ease of interpretation and really eliminates any need to use the 180-0 or 360 degree systems of notation.

Different *recording systems* abound; each has merits, but none appears more reasonable than the SFTR system. Only this method provides for a succinct and complete method of recording, because it provides a system of abbreviations and a standardized recording format. Because the system requires only a few minutes to learn, it has the further advantage of providing a potentially universal system for recordings that can save time in the clinic and minimize confusion.

Despite the wide variation in methods, *reliability* studies have shown that goniometry is basically reliable, certainly for some joints and especially for intra-tester reliability. Inter-tester reliability is less clear. Because joint motion can be measured with so many different devices and by different methods, it is really up to clinicians to determine the reliability of the measurement as obtained in their settings. A method for doing this has been presented. The investment of time and effort in reliability studies will yield valuable scientific knowledge, provide a means of documenting a measurement for quality assurance and, most important, will give clinicians an indication of the strengths and weaknesses of an important clinical measurement.

Although the *inferences* that can be made from measuring joint motion are limited (i.e., *validity*), the measurement itself is invaluable as a basic indicator of patient status. If we, as a profession, commit ourselves to learning more about the measurement of joint motion, even if it is at the level of small clinical studies, we will increase the value of that measurement for our profession, and we will have advanced our profession.

REFERENCES

1. Michels E: Evaluation and research in physical therapy. Phys Ther 62:828, 1982
2. Ghiselli EE, Campbell JP, Zedeck S: Measurement Theory for the Behavioral Sciences. Freeman, San Francisco, 1981
3. Wiechec FJ, Krusen FH: A new method of joint measurement and a review of the literature. Am J Surg 43:659, 1939
4. Moore ML: Clinical assessment of joint motion. In Basmajian JV (ed) Therapeutic Exercise. 3rd Ed. Williams and Wilkins, Baltimore, 1978
5. Clark WA: A system of joint measurement. J Orthop Surg 2:687, 1920
6. Cobe HM: The range of active motion at the wrist of white adults. J Bone Joint Surg 26:763, 1928
7. Hewitt D: The range of active motion at the wrist of women. J Bone Joint Surg 26:775, 1928
8. Dorinson SM, Wagner ML: An exact technic for clinically measuring and recording joint motion. Arch Phys Med 29:468, 1948
9. Moore ML: The measurement of joint motion. Part II. The technic of goniometry. Phys Ther Rev 29:256, 1949
10. Leighton JR: An instrument and technic for the measurement of range of joint motion. Arch Phys Med Rehabil 36:571, 1955
11. A guide to the evaluation of permanent impairment of the extremities and back. JAMA (Special Ed.) 1, 1958
12. Joint Motion. Method of Measuring and Recording. American Academy of Orthopaedic Surgeons, Chicago, 1965
13. Daniels L, Worthingham C: Muscle Testing. Techniques of Manual Examination, 3rd Ed. Saunders, Philadelphia, 1972
14. Clarke OR, Willis LA, Fish WW, Nichols PR: Preliminary studies in measuring range of motion in normal and painful stiff shoulders. Rheumatol Rehabil 14:39, 1975
15. Gerhardt JJ, Russe OA: International SFTR Method of Measuring and Recording Joint Motion. Huber, Bern, 1975
16. Boone DC, Azen SP: Normal range of motion of joints in male subjects. J Bone Joint Surg 61-A:756–759, 1979
17. Bell BD, Hoshizaki TB: Relationships of age and sex with range of motion of seventeen joint actions in humans. Can J Appl Sports Sci 6:202, 1981
18. American Rheumatism Association: Dictionary of the Rheumatic Diseases. Vol. I: Signs and Symptoms. Contact Associates, New York, 1982
19. Roaas A, Anderson GJ: Normal range of motion of the hip, knee, and ankle joints in male subjects, 30–40 years of age. Acta Orthop Scand 53:205, 1982
20. Allender E, Bjornsson OJ, Olafesson O, et al: Normal range of joint movements in the shoulder, hip, wrist and thumb with special reference to side: a comparison between two populations. Int J Epidemiol 3:253, 1974
21. Salter N: Methods of measurement of muscle and joint function. J Bone Joint Surg 37-B:474, 1955
22. Clarke GR: Measurement in shoulder problems. Rheumatol Rehabil 15:191, 1975

23. Esch D, Lepley M: Evaluation of Joint Motion: Methods of Measurement and Recording. University of Minnesota Press, Minneapolis, 1974
24. Evaluation of Industrial Disability (Commission of California Medical Association and The Industrial Accident Commission of the State of California). Oxford University Press, New York, 1960
25. Rowe CR: Joint measurement in disability evaluation. Clin Orthop 32:43, 1964
26. Hurt SP: Joint measurement. Am J Occup Ther 1:209, 1947
27. Hurt SP: Joint measurement—part II. Am J Occup Ther 1:281, 1947
28. Defibaugh JJ: Measurement of head motion. J Am Phys Ther Assoc 44:157, 1964
29. West CC: Measurement of joint motion. Arch Phys Med 26:414, 1945
30. Panjabi MM, Goel VK, Walter SD, Schick S: Errors in the center and angle of rotation of a joint: an experimental study. J Biomech Eng 104:232, 1982
31. Poppen NK, Walker PS: Normal and abnormal motion of the shoulder. J Bone Joint Surg 58-A:195, 1976
32. Frankel VH, Burstein AH: Orthopaedic Biomechanics. Lea and Febiger, Philadelphia, 1970
33. Morrey BF, Chao EY: Passive motion of the elbow joint. J Bone Joint Surg 58-A:501, 1976
34. Frankel VH, Nordin M: Basic Biomechanics of the Skeletal System. Lea and Febiger, Philadelphia, 1980
35. Robson P: A method to reduce the variable error in joint range measurement. Ann Phys Med 8:262, 1966
36. Payton OD: Research: the Validation of Clinical Practice. Davis, Philadelphia, 1979
37. Michels E: Measurement in physical therapy: on the rules for assigning numerals to observations. Phys Ther 63:209, 1983
38. Moore ML: The measurement of joint motion. Part I—introductory review of the literature. Phys Ther Rev 29:195, 1949
39. Rosen NG: A simplified method of measuring amplitude of motion in joints. J Bone Joint Surg 20:570, 1922
40. Silver D: Measurement of the range of motion in joints. J Bone Joint Surg 21:569, 1923
41. Wainerdi HR: An improved goniometer for arthrometry. JAMA 149:661, 1952
42. Pollock GA, Brooks G: An apparatus to measure muscle recovery and range of joint movement. Br Med J 2:220, 1942
43. Hellebrandt FA, Duvall EN, Moore ML: The measurement of joint motion. Part III—reliability of goniometry. Phys Ther Rev 29:302, 1949
44. Bansil CK, Joshi JB, Singh S: Modification to the conventional wheel for measuring the range of movements of the shoulder joint. Med J Zambia 9:111, 1975
45. Ellis MI, Burton KE, Wright V: A simple goniometer for measuring hip function. Rheumatol Rehabil 18:85, 1981
46. Hasselkus BR, Kshepakaran KK, Houge JC, Plautz KA: Rheumatoid arthritis: a two-axis goniometer to measure metacarpophalangeal laxity. Arch Phys Med Rehabil 62:137, 1981
47. Ekstrand J, Wiktorsson M, Oberg B, Gillquist J: Lower extremity goniometric measurements: a study to determine their reliability. Arch Phys Med Rehabil 63:171, 1982
48. Schenker WW: Improved method of joint motion measurement. NY J Med 56:539, 1956

49. Buck CA, Dameron FB, Dow MJ, Skowlund HV: Study of normal range of motion in the neck utilizing a bubble goniometer. Arch Phys Med Rehabil 40:390, 1959

50. Bennett JG, Bergmanis LE, Carpenter JK, Skowlund HV: Range of motion of the neck. J Am Phys Ther Assoc 43:45, 1969

51. Inman VT: The Joints of the Ankle. Williams and Wilkins, Baltimore, 1976

52. Bower KD: The hydrogoniometer and assessment of glenohumeral joint motion. Aust J Physiother 28:12, 1982

53. Karpovich PV, Karpovich GP: Electrogoniometer. A new device for study of joints in action. Fed Proc 18:79, 1959

54. Chao EY, Hoffman RR: Instrumented measurement of human joint motion. ISA Trans 17:13, 1978

55. Chao EY: Justification of triaxial goniometer for the measurement of joint rotation. J Biomech 13:989, 1980

56. Knutzen KM, Bates BT, Hamill J: ELectrogoniometry of post-surgical knee bracing in running. Am J Phys Med 62:172, 1983

57. Ahlback SO, Lindahl O: Sagittal mobility of the hip joint. Acta Orthop Scand 34:310, 1964

58. Wilson GD, Stasch WH: Photographic record of joint motion. Arch Phys Med 26:361, 1964

59. Wilmer HA, Elkins EC: An optical goniometer for observing range of motion of joints: a preliminary report of a new instrument. Arch Phys Med 28:695, 1947

60. Zankel HT: Photogoniometry: a new method of measurement of range of motion of joints. Arch Phys Med 32:227, 1951

61. Williams PO: The assessment of mobility in joints. Lancet 263:169, 1952

62. Cave EF, Roberts SM: A method for measuring and recording joint function. J Bone Joint Surg 18:455, 1936

63. Gerhardt JJ, Russe OA (eds): Instructions in Application of the AFTR Pocket Goniometer in Measuring Joint Motion with the Neutral-Zero Method and SFTR Recording. Orthopedic Equipment Company, Bourbon, Indiana, 1978

64. Hamilton GF, Lachenbruch PA: Reliability of goniometers in assessing finger joint angle. Phys Ther 49:465, 1969

65. Mitchell WS, Millar J, Sturrock RD: An evaluation of goniometry as an objective parameter for measuring joint motion. Scot Med J 20:57, 1975

66. Low JL: The reliability of joint measurement. Physiotherapy 62:227, 1976

67. Myers H: Range of motion and flexibility. Phys Ther Rev 41:177, 1961

68. Boone DC, Azen SP, lin CM, et al: Reliability of goniometric measurements. Phys Ther 58:1355, 1978

69. Rothstein JM, Miller PJ, Roettger RF: Goniometric reliability in a clinical setting: elbow and knee measurements. Phys Ther 63:1611, 1983

70. Ashton BB, Pickles B, Roll JW: Reliability of goniometric measurements of hip motion in spastic cerebral palsy. Dev Med Child Neurol 20:87, 1978

71. Grohmann JL: Comparison of two methods of goniometry. Phys Ther 63:922, 1983

72. Marks JS, Palmer MK, Burke MJ, Smith P: Observer variation in the examination of knee joints. Ann Rheum Dis 37:376, 1978

73. Baldwin J, Cunningham K: Goniometry under attack: a clinical study involving physiotherapists. Physiother Can 26:74, 1974

74. Winer BJ: Statistical Principles in Experimental Design, p. 285. 2nd Ed. McGraw-Hill, New York, 1971

75. Kerlinger FN: Foundations of Behavioral Research, 2nd Ed. Holt Rinehardt and Winston, New York, 1973
76. Bartko JJ, Carpenter WT: On the methods and theory of reliability. J Nerv Ment Dis 163:307, 1976
77. Lahey MA, Downey RG, Saal FE: Intraclass correlation: there's more there than meets the eye. Psychol Bull 93:586, 1983

5 | State of the Art in Functional Status Assessment

Alan M. Jette

The scientific study of any health phenomenon must start with the careful examination of the nature of the phenomenon itself. It is only after a clear conceptual foundation has been laid that one can proceed to measure and interpret meaningfully information on the frequency, distribution, and change in the phenomenon under study.

The restoration of the disabled to their highest level of physical, vocational, and social function is an important treatment objective for the physical therapist. Yet physical therapists have traditionally focused on observable physical signs such as range of motion (ROM) and muscle strength and subjective symptoms such as pain relief in evaluating the extent to which interventions are effective. Focusing on physical signs and symptoms to evaluate interventions that purport to have an impact on functional status is narrow and much too limiting. It runs the risk of diminishing the importance of this investigative process. If we are sincere in our desire to evaluate critically the broad goals of physical therapy, we must focus more attention on examining the extent to which our efforts actually influence a patient's functional status. There remain, however, some important conceptual barriers in our path.

There is no clear consensus on what is meant by the terms "function" or "functional status" either within physical therapy or in related health fields. The term "function" has assumed numerous and diverse meanings in the health literature.[1-6] Function has been used to describe the characteristic action of body parts, e.g., the function of the shoulder; the performance of organs, e.g., kidney function; as well as the performance of the individual, e.g., as functioning in activities of daily living. The ambiguous use of this ubiquitous health term has led to considerable conceptual and semantic confusion. This in turn has hindered both the scientific study of functional status as well as the practice of physical therapy.

Conceptual clarification is a necessary first step on the path toward establishing the extent to which physical therapy interventions actually achieve their purported objectives. These efforts will contribute to the profession's scientific foundation, thereby enhancing the ability of physical therapy to grow and mature. In its absence, physical therapists run the risk of being denied full professional status and of being relegated to the role of technician.

A DEFINITION OF FUNCTION

To understand the concept of "functional status," we must begin with a discussion of the broader concept of health. The World Health Organization (WHO) defines health as a state of complete physical, mental, and social well-being, not merely the absence of disease and infirmity.[7] Such a global definition, although sufficient for communicating an ideal to the public, has been severely criticized as being overly simplistic, abstract, and difficult to measure.[8] The WHO definition of health has limited utility for researchers or clinicians who are seeking ways to study this concept scientifically.

Investigators who have attempted to define health in measurable terms have focused traditionally on one or more of three concepts: (1) physical manifestations, (2) symptoms or feeling states, and (3) functional status.

Physical Manifestations

Physical manifestations are directly observable events or characteristics of a host that can be observed or assessed by another individual, frequently a health professional. Laboratory blood analyses, body temperature, and blood pressure are all examples of observable, measurable characteristics of the host. Health professionals traditionally assume the responsibility of selecting the appropriate physical manifestations to assess under certain circumstances. A physical therapist, for example, decides if and when to assess muscle strength, joint ROM, or other physical manifestations during the course of a patient's initial evaluation and/or treatment. This selection is dictated by the accepted norms of professional practice and by past experience and professional judgment. Any deviation is interpreted as objective evidence of abnormality or ill health. Evaluation is made by comparing the patient's scores on each measure to a set of norms that presumably reflect ideal scores on those indicators. Treatment usually involves efforts to restore the individual to the normal range of score values.

Impairment

Most physical manifestations of concern to physical therapists fall into the category of impairment. Impairment refers to an anatomical or physiological abnormality or loss in an organ or system of the body.[2,9] The musculosketetal, neurological, pulmonary, and cardiovascular systems, for instance, are of great interest to physical therapists, primarily because impairments in these systems have a profound impact on functional status. In each body system, certain physical manifestations assume a predominant role as health indicators of patients undergoing therapy. In the musculoskeletal system for example, joint ROM and muscle strength are key treatment planning and evaluation parameters assessed by physical therapists.

Symptoms

Symptoms differ from physical manifestations in that they are relatively subjective phenomena experienced by an individual and are usually not observable by another person. Symptoms frequently arise from or accompany a disease or illness and are used as evidence of it. Pain, dizziness, and nausea are examples of symptoms. Symptoms are viewed as "softer" indicators of health status because they are "subjective" as compared with observable physical manifestations; they become known through the report of the individual who is being assessed. Symptoms involve the interpretation, feeling, and personal judgment of the patient. Symptoms are essential health parameters to physical therapists. The reduction of pain, for instance, is one of the most important treatment goals for many patients with chronic disorders.

The exclusive emphasis on physical manifestations and/or symptoms as indicators of health reveals an underlying assumption that health represents the absence or eradication of illness. Under such a definition, the student with spina bifida or an active school teacher with rheumatoid arthritis could never "qualify" as healthy. Until recently, signs and symptoms have been the primary health indicators of what is frequently called the "medical model" approach to defining health.

There is growing dissatisfaction with such a narrow definition (as revealed by WHO's definition). Some have gone so far as to define health exclusively in sociological terms. Parsons, for example, defines health as a state of optimum capacity of an individual for the effective performance of roles and tasks for which he or she has been socialized.[10] For Parsons, the concept of health is defined with reference to the individual's participation in the social system, not from the perspective of the state of the organism. From this perspective, then, illness is characterized by some generalized disturbance of the capacity of the individual for role-performance that is normally expected.

Functional Status

In physical therapy, in which the emphasis frequently is on helping people with relatively stable residual impairments such as nonprogressive paralysis, amputation, or aphasia, a definition of health based exclusively on observable physical manifestations and subjective symptoms is narrow and much too limiting. The broad goals of rehabilitation demand that attention be paid to defining health with respect to an individual's function. In helping the amputee, for instance, the therapist must know more than the nature of the impairment; he or she must know how the impairment affects the amputee's function. Measures of *function* or *functional status*, used in this context, reflect a more sociologic interpretation of health. An individual's functional status reflects his reaction to a biological condition; it represents the interaction of the individual with his or her environment. In assessing function, attention is paid to the individual, not to the "pathological" state of the organism.

In this chapter, the term "functional status" refers to the normal or characteristic performance of the *individual*. The individual is the unit of analysis in functional assessment, rather than body parts or organ systems. Thus defined, the functional status of the individual represents one aspect or dimension of health. Physical manifestations and symptoms, are related but distinct dimensions. An indicator of overall health would demand an assessment of all three dimensions: physical manifestations, symptoms, and functional status.

To define an individual's functional status for clinical or research purposes adequately, an individual's function is subdivided into four conceptually distinct categories. In keeping with previous conceptual work, I use the term *physical function* to represent the category of sensory-motor performance of the individual.[2,5,6] Physical function is the dimension of functional status that has received most attention from physical therapists. Walking, climbing stairs, the ability to perform housework, to shop, and to prepare meals are all examples of physical performance. Tasks concerned with fundamental daily activities, such as self-care or basic mobility, are usually defined as "basic" activities of daily living (ADL). More complex tasks are called "instrumental" ADL.[11,12] *Mental function*, the second functional category, represents the intellectual, cognitive or reasoning capabilities of the individual. Memory is one example of mental function. A person's affect and effectiveness in coping psychologically with life's stresses represent the *emotional function* dimension. Level of anxiety, life satisfaction, and happiness, are all indicators of emotional function. *Social function*, the final dimension, encompasses an individual's social interactions and performance of social roles or obligations. Parenting or being employed outside of the home are two of the many examples of an individual's function in social roles. The term "handicap" is frequently used when referring to disruption in an individual's ability to perform accepted social roles.[13,14]

In this chapter, the terms "disability" and "dysfunction" are used synonymously to refer to *any* deviation from the normal or characteristic function of an individual within any of the four categories just discussed. A disability or dysfunction may be *physical* (e.g., difficulty with or inability to walk), *mental* (e.g., difficulty with or unable to recall time or place), *emotional* (e.g., thinking sad thoughts), or *social* (e.g., not performing one's occupation). Disability refers to a *diminished capability* of the individual in function or performance. As such, disabilities (which refer to dysfunction at the level of the person) can be clearly differentiated from impairments (aberrations in organs or bodily systems).

MEASUREMENT OF PHYSICAL FUNCTION

An individual's functional status is a complex and multifaceted concept. A thorough review of existing approaches to measuring all four functional categories (i.e., physical, social, mental, and emotional) is beyond the scope of this chapter. I focus instead on the measurement of physical function, the sensory-motor performance of the individual, the functional category of greatest interest to physical therapists. I have restricted my review to instruments that have undergone some degree of formal development and that have been designed for use in clinical settings, to provide the physical therapist with an overview of what measurement tools are available to assess physical function, and the relative strengths and weaknesses of each.

This review focuses on each instrument's purpose, conceptual focus, measurement dimension, reliability, validity, and mode of administration.

1. *Purpose*: There are three common purposes for which functional status instruments have been developed.

   A. Description. Description involves the collection of information or data to establish a body of information about the concept under investigation. A description of physical function is usually performed to establish normative standards that can be used to determine community needs, to set goals for patient treatment or goals against which to test hypotheses about the effectiveness of specific health interventions.

   B. Screening and Assessment. Screening and assessment refers to a detailed review of physical function leading to conclusions about the nature of the problem and specific treatment plans. A measure designed for screening and assessment must be more detailed than one designed to describe the phenomenon. Assessment instruments, therefore, are frequently multidimensional and are time-consuming to administer.

   C. Monitoring. Monitoring involves repeated measurement to detect change in the phenomena over time. Monitoring physical function seldom requires the same level of detail as assessment, provided that the parameters expected to change can be identified. Monitoring instruments must be sufficiently precise, however, to detect the level or degree of change anticipated. Monitoring instruments are frequently used to test hypotheses about specific treatment effects on function.

2. *Conceptual Focus:* Does the instrument focus solely on physical function or does it include an assessment of other dimensions or concepts? What area (or areas) of physical function is (are) addressed? Does the measure address areas of basic ADL (e.g., walking, dressing), instrumental ADL (e.g., cooking, meal preparation, grocery shopping), or both?

3. *Measurement Dimension:* What aspect or characteristic of the concept is measured? The most common characteristic is degree of assistance or help used in performing a certain activity. Other characteristics, however, have been

addressed. They include, among others, time taken to perform the activity and degree of difficulty or pain perceived in performing the activity.

4. *Reliability:* Some degree of error is inevitable in virtually all forms of measurement. A measure of systolic blood pressure, for example, can differ markedly because of anxiety level, time of day in which the measure is taken, and body position, among other factors. Reliability is the extent to which score variability reflects "true differences" rather than random error. Reliability is determined by assessing the extent to which scores derived from measures are stable or reproducible or the degree to which items within a scale are inter-related (see Chapter 1).

5. *Validity:* A measure that produces stable, reproducible scores is not necessarily valid. From one perspective, validity refers to the degree to which an instrument actually measures what it purports to measure. For instance, scores from a particular measure of functional status, may be reliable and still not actually measure the concept of function (see Chapter 1 for a complete discussion of validity).

When we speak of a measure's validity, we are asking about the appropriateness of inferences drawn from the test results. A measure that is valid for one purpose may not be for another. Grip strength, for instance, has substantial face validity as a measure of hand function; however, it has questionable validity as a measure of global health status. All too frequently when evaluating clinical physical therapy outcomes, we assess what is easily measured (e.g., reliable) instead of attempting to assess what is most meaningful or valid. In rheumatology, for instance, few intervention studies attempt to assess complex functional activities related to social roles. Occupational status, parenting, and sexual function, which are of critical importance to many persons with arthritis are infrequently assessed when evaluating the impact of health interventions. Instead, more easily measured but potentially less valid indicators are used, such as morning stiffness or walking time.

6. *Mode of Administration:* Most functional status instruments rely on one or more of the following methods for collecting information: direct observation, structured interviews, self-administered questionnaires, clinical judgment, or timed performance. No one technique is inherently better than the other; each has its advantages and disadvantages. Directly observing an individual's function under standardized circumstances can produce reliable scores and can have substantial validity depending on how well the test is constructed and administered. Direct observation, however, is time-consuming and very costly. Direct observation is limited, moreover, to assessing basic ADL. It is rarely used to assess more complex instrumental ADL. Clinical judgment and a patient's self-report derived from questionnaires or structured interviews are less direct measurement approaches than observation; they involve more subjectivity. Each of these approaches has a greater chance of introducing error into the measurement process as compared with direct observation. The chief advantages lie in their cost and ability to assess more complex dimensions of function. All three approaches must be admin-

istered under highly standardized circumstances to derive reliable and valid scores.

STATE OF THE ART IN ASSESSING PHYSICAL FUNCTION

Katz ADL Index

The Katz ADL Index first attempted standardized assessment of physical function.[15,16] The original Katz Index includes a dichotomous rating of six basic ADL: bathing, dressing, going to the toilet, transfers, continence, and feeding. A score of 1 is given for each activity that is performed without human help; a score of 0 is given if the activity is performed with human assistance or is not performed. Used in this manner, the items are combined to form a cumulative, or Guttman Scale, in order of decreasing dependency.

Guttman scaling is a method of determining whether a set of items, here the six basic ADL, form a unidimensional, ordinal score. If they do, knowing an individual's score indicates the exact pattern of responses across all items. A score of B in the Katz Index, for instance, means that the individual is independent in performing all but one the six basic ADL. Table 5-1 displays the content of the original Katz ADL Index.

The original Katz scale has been adapted for scoring as a Likert-type scale.[17] Likert-type scaling is an approach to forming summated scales. As such, individuals respond to each item in terms of several graded choices. In Likert-type scaling of the Katz Index, for example, each ADL activity is given a score which ranges from 0 to 3, where 0 equals complete independence, 1 equals use of a device, 2 equals use of human assistance, and 3 equals complete dependence in the performance of the activity. Used in this manner, scores are summed to develop an overall score for the performance of basic ADL.

The Katz ADL Index has been used to standardize professional judgment, patient self-report, and data abstracted from chart reviews. The Katz ADL Index, originally developed for use with hospitalized patients, has been adapted for use in community and long-term care, institutionalized populations.[18,19] The community-based version of the Katz Index includes an assessment of walking and grooming. Continence is not assessed, although it is assessed in the original version.

The Guttman Scale version of the Katz ADL Index has demonstrated coefficients of reproducibility of .948 for elders in a home-care study and .976 for those in a sheltered housing study.[20] Reliability coefficients for the Likert-type version of the Katz Index are not available. The Likert-type version of the Katz Index does not have exhaustive categories and this may reduce the reliability of the instrument. There is no category for patients who use both a device and human assistance. The Katz Index has been used extensively over the past 20 years with institutionalized populations to assess clinically significant changes in function over time.[19–22]

Table 5-1. Katz ADL Index

The Index of Independence in Activities of Daily Living is based on an evaluation of the functional independence or dependence of patients in bathing, dressing, going to the toilet, transferring, continence, and feeding. Specific definitions of functional independence and dependence appear below the index.

A	Independent in feeding, continence, transferring, going to toilet, dressing, and bathing.
B	Independent in all but one of these functions.
C	Independent in all but bathing and one additional function.
D	Independent in all but bathing, dressing, and one additional function.
E	Independent in all but bathing, dressing, going to toilet, and one additional function.
F	Independent in all but bathing, dressing, going to toilet, transferring, and one additional function.
G	Dependent in all six functions.
Other	Dependent in at least two functions, but not classifiable as C, D, E, or F.

Independence means without supervision, direction, or active personal assistance, except as specifically noted below. This is based on actual status and not on ability. A patient who refuses to perform a function is considered as not performing the function, even though he is deemed able.

Bathing (sponge, shower, or tub)
  Independent: assistance only in bathing a single part (as back or disabled extremity) or bathes self completely.
  Dependent: assistance in bathing more than one part of body; assistance in getting in or out of tub or does not bathe self.
Dressing
  Independent: gets clothes from closets and drawers, puts on clothes, outer garments, braces, manages fasteners, act of tying shoes is excluded.
  Dependent: does not dress self or remains partly undressed.
Going to toilet
  Independent: gets to toilet, gets on and off toilet, arranges clothes, cleans organs of excretion (may manage own bedpan used at night only and may or may not be using mechanical supports).
  Dependent: uses bedpan or commode or receives assistance getting to and using toilet.

Transfer
  Independent: moves in and out of bed independently and moves in and out of chair independently (may or may not be using mechanical supports).
  Dependent: assistance in moving in or out of bed and/or chair, does not perform one or more transfers.
Continence
  Independent: urination and defecation entirely self-controlled.
  Dependent: partial or total incontinence in urination or defecation, partial or total control by enemas, catheters, or regulated use of urinals and/or bedpans.
Feeding
  Independent: gets food from plate or its equivalent into mouth (precutting of meat and preparation of food, as buttering bread, are excluded from evaluation).
  Dependent: assistance in act of feeding (see above), does not eat at all or parenteral feeding.

Katz S, et al: Studies of illness in the aged. The Index of ADL: a standardized measure of biological and psychosocial function, JAMA 185:94, 1963. Copyright 1963, American Medical Association.

PULSES Profile

Moskowitz and McCann are the original architects of the PULSES instrument, a multidimensional assessment tool that includes a section on physical function.[23] The original instrument, adapted and used extensively by Granger and Greer, examines six different conceptual dimensions: P, physical condition or basic health/illness status; U, upper limb functions; L, lower limb functions; S, sensory components (i.e., sight and communication); E, excretory function (i.e., control of bowel and bladder); and S, support factors (i.e., psychological, emotional, family, social, or financial support).[24] Each dimension is assessed along a four-point ordinal scale, which ranges from no abnormality to severe abnormality. Table 5-2 describes the components of the PULSES instrument.

The PULSES tool has been used to record professional judgment also with data abstracted from medical records. An examination of each dimension of PULSES reveals that a number of different concepts are contained in each item. For example, the upper limb function dimension includes an assessment of both level of independence in upper extremity self care and an assessment of impairment of the upper limbs. This mixing of dimensions within the same assessment item may affect reliability adversely. No scientific evidence of the reliability of the PULSES instrument could be found. A number of articles, however, have demonstrated a high correlation between PULSES scores and other measures of functional status, evidence of construct validity. The PULSES instrument has been shown to be more useful in detecting changes in hospitalized patients.[25] It has been used in a variety of patient groups, including stroke patients, spinal cord injury patients, patients with amputations, and the neurologically impaired.[23-25] Clarifying the conceptual content would improve the PULSES meaningfulness and utility. It appears to be more useful in situations in which a substantial degree of change in function is anticipated.

Barthel Index

Mahoney and Barthel developed a weighted index for assessing dependence in basic ADL for use with chronically disabled patients.[26] Health professionals award points to patients according to the amount of help needed to perform a particular activity. This assessment is based on professional knowledge of the patient supplemented by information from the medical record. Help is defined as use of personal assistance to perform an activity; use of adaptive equipment is not considered to be use of personal assistance. A person who used human help in eating, for example, would receive 5 points; independence in eating would receive a score of 10 points. Scores for 12 different activities are summed together to form an overall index that ranges from 0 to 100, where 0 equals completely dependent in all 12 activities and 100 equals completely independent in the performance of all 12 activities. The Barthel Index examines independence in feeding, transferring from wheelchair to bed, personal toilet, getting on and off the toilet, bathing self, walking on level surface, ascending and descending stairs, dressing, controlling bowels, and controlling bladder. Table 5-3 displays the Barthel Index along with the item weights.

Granger and Greer demonstrated a high correlation between the Barthel Index scores and the discharge status of persons treated in an acute-stroke care unit.[24] Wylie, in his work with stroke patients, also demonstrated substantial concordance between the Barthel Index and clinical judgment, length of stay, age, and place of discharge.[27] Although the reliability of the Barthel Index has not been reported, it includes extensive instructions that should facilitate standardized assessment. These instructions, however, do include an

Table 5-2. Modified PULSES Profile

P—*Physical condition:* includes diseases of the viscera (cardiovascular, gastrointestinal, urologic, and endocrine) and neurologic disorders:
1. Medical problems sufficiently stable that medical or nursing monitoring is not required more often than 3-month intervals.
2. Medical or nurse monitoring is needed more often than 3-month intervals but not each week.
3. Medical problems are sufficiently unstable as to require regular medical and/or nursing attention at least weekly.
4. Medical problems require intensive medical and/or nursing attention at least daily (excluding personal care assistance only).

U—*Upper limb functions:* Self-care activities (drink/feed, dress upper/lower, brace/prothesis, groom, wash, perineal care) dependent mainly upon upper limb function:
1. Independent in self-care without impairment of upper limbs.
2. Independent in self-care with some impairment of upper limbs.
3. Dependent upon assistance or supervision in self-care with or without impairment of upper limbs.
4. Dependent totally in self-care with marked impairment of upper limbs.

L—*Lower limb functions:* Mobility (transfer chair/toilet/tub or shower, walk, stairs, wheelchair) dependent mainly upon lower limb function:
1. Independent in mobility without impairment of lower limbs.
2. Independent in mobility with some impairment in lower limbs; such as needing ambulatory aids, a brace or prosthesis, or else fully independent in a wheelchair without significant architectural or environmental barriers.
3. Dependent upon assistance or supervision in mobility with or without impairment of lower limbs, or partly independent in a wheelchair, or there are significant architectural or environmental barriers.
4. Dependent totally in mobility with marked impairment of lower limbs.

S—*Sensory components:* Relating to communication (speech and hearing) and vision:
1. Independent in communication and vision without impairment.
2. Independent in communication and vision with some impairment such as mild dysarthria, mild aphasia, or need for eyeglasses or hearing aid, or needing regular eye medication.
3. Dependent upon assistance, an interpreter, or supervision in communication or vision.
4. Dependent totally in communication or vision.

E—*Excretory functions* (bladder and bowel):
1. Complete voluntary control of bladder and bowel sphincters.
2. Control of sphincters allows normal social activities despite urgency or need for catheter, appliance, suppositories, etc. Able to care for needs without assistance.
3. Dependent upon assistance in sphincter management or else has accidents occasionally.
4. Frequent wetting or soiling from incontinence of bladder or bowel sphincters.

S—*Support factors:* Consider intellectual and emotional adaptability, support from family unit, and financial ability:
1. Able to fulfill usual roles and perform customary tasks.
2. Must make some modification in usual roles and performance of customary tasks.
3. Dependent upon assistance, supervision, encouragement or assistance from a public or private agency due to any of the above considerations.
4. Dependent upon long-term institutional care (chronic hospitalization, nursing home, etc.) excluding time-limited hospital for specific evaluation, treatment, or active rehabilitation.

Granger C, Albrecht G, Hamilton B: Outcome of comprehensive medical rehabilitation: measurement by PULSES Profile and the Barthel Index. Arch Phys Med Rehabil 60:145, 1979.

Table 5-3. Barthel Index

	With Help	Independent
1. Feeding (if food needs to be cut up, help)	5	10
2. Moving from wheelchair to bed and return (includes sitting up in bed)	5–10	15
3. Personal toilet (wash face, comb hair, shave, clean teeth)	0	5
4. Getting on and off toilet (handling clothes, wipe, flush)	5	10
5. Bathing self	0	5
6. Walking on level surface (or if unable to walk, propel wheelchair)	10 0[a]	15 5[a]
7. Ascend and descend stairs	5	10
8. Dressing (includes tying shoes, fastening fasteners)	5	10
9. Controlling bowels	5	10
10. Controlling bladder	5	10

Mahoney F, Barthel D: Functional evaluation: The Barthel Index. Maryland State Med J 14:61, 1965.

[a] Score only if unable to walk

assessment of the time it takes for a subject to perform a particular task as a dimension of independence, thus exposing the assessment to considerable interpretation that might reduce its reliability. The Barthel Index has repeatedly achieved high correlations with other measures of functional status.[25]

The Barthel Index is a quick, standardized approach to assessment of basic physical function. It is one of the few functional indices that gives each component variable weight or value. The weighting scheme appears to be based on clinical judgment of the time and amount of actual physical assistance required for a patient who is unable to perform the activity independently. It has been used extensively to study patient care outcomes in institutionalized settings.

Instrumental ADL Scale

Lawton and his colleagues at the Philadelphia Geriatric Center (PGC) were among the first to develop standardized measures of instrumental ADL.[11] They define instrumental ADL as behaviors that are more complex and less directly body-oriented than physical self-maintenance. Their original instrument examines ability to use a telephone, shop, prepare food, keep house, do laundry, use public transportation, take responsibility for one's medications, and to handle finances. Each item is scored on a 3-, 4-, or 5-point scale that reflects the amount of assistance used or limitation in performing the activity. The original instrument is designed to record professional judgment; it has been adapted to be used to record self-report information. The self-report version focuses on the frequency with which meal preparation, shopping, and laundry are performed. Table 5-4 illustrates the eight scale items. Both versions yield coefficients of reproducibility for Guttman scalogram analysis[11] of .9. Evidence of their validity has not been reported.

Table 5-4. Philadelphia Geriatric Center Instrumental ADL Scale Items

A. Ability to use telephone
B. Shopping
C. Food preparation
D. Housekeeping
E. Laundry
F. Public transportation
G. Responsibility for own medications
H. Ability to handle finances

Lawton MP, Assessing the competence of older people. In Kent D, Kastenbaum R, Sherwood S (eds): Research Planning and Action for the Elderly. Behavioral Publications, New York, 1972.

The PGC instrumental ADL scales represent an early attempt to standardize instrumental activity assessment. The authors note that these scales only begin the process of conceptual differentiation and operational definition of instrumental activities. Only a limited number of activities are assessed. The instruments are most relevant to the elderly, particularly older women. Paid employment is not assessed in either version.

Kenny Self-Care Index

The Kenny Self-Care Instrument is a standardized protocol for recording professional judgment of rehabilitation patients' basic physical function.[28] The instrument consists of six major activities (i.e., bed activities, transfers, locomotion, dressing, personal hygiene and feeding) encompassing the 17 individual self-care items illustrated in Table 5-5. Each item is rated on a 5-point scale, where 0 equals completely dependent in performing the item, 1 equals uses extensive assistance, 2 equals moderate assistance, 3 equals minimal assistance and/or supervision, and 4 equals totally independent. A total score is derived by developing an average score for activities within each of the six categories and then adding the category scores to obtain a summary score for

Table 5-5. List of Items in the Kenny Self-Care Index

1. Bed	4. Dressing
a. Move in bed	a. Upper trunk and arms
b. Rise and sit	b. Lower trunk and legs
2. Transfers	c. Feet
a. Sitting	5. Personal hygiene
b. Standing	a. Face, hair, arms
c. Toilet	b. Trunk, perineum
3. Locomotion	c. Lower extremities
a. Walking	d. Bowel program
b. Stairs	e. Bladder program
c. Wheelchair	6. Feeding

Schoening H, et al: Numerical scoring of self-care status of patients. Arch Phys Med Rehabil. Oct 1965:689.

basic physical function. The Kenny Instrument focuses on basic ADL; abilities necessary for life outside of a health care institution are omitted.

There appears to be no formal evidence of the Kenny Self-Care Instrument's reliability; however, there has been some work on its validity. In studies conducted with patients in rehabilitation centers, strong negative correlations were found between the Kenny Instrument's scores and the amount of time spent helping a patient perform a transfer, an indicator of staff workload. In other words, as functional independence increased (as reflected by high scores on the Kenny Instrument) less staff time was required to help a patient perform a transfer.

The Kenny Self-Care Instrument is a frequently used tool for recording health professional judgment of patient's functional capacity. It is especially useful for hospitalized rehabilitation patients. Its emphasis on only basic ADL makes it less appropriate for noninstitutionalized groups. The instrument could be more carefully standardized to improve its reliability in different settings and when used by different professionals. The definition of assistance is unclear; does it include human assistance, equipment, or both? What is the time frame for the assessment? Is it the day of administration, the past week, or what? Ambiguities of this nature could substantially reduce its reliability when used by different therapists or in different settings over time.

Linn Rapid Disability Rating Scale

Linn's Rapid Disability Rating Scale is a short global disability assessment tool developed for gerontological research.[29] This scale is designed to standardize professional judgment about a patient's level of disability based on easily observable data. The Linn Rapid Disability Rating Scale, shown in Table 5-6, contains 16 items that focus on physical function (e.g., eating, walking) as well as a number of other conceptual dimensions (e.g., diet, medication, speech, incontinence, depression). Each item is rated on a 3-point scale that assesses frequency of occurrence, or degree of assistance. A total disability score is obtained by adding scores across the 16 items. The scale has demonstrated significant inter-rater reliability (.913 Kendall's W) in 60 independent ratings of 20 patients in a comparison of hospital nursing personnel ratings with nursing home staff ratings on the same group of elderly patients. It has also achieved substantial test–retest reliability (product moment correlation .831). The Linn Rapid Disability Rating Scores have displayed statistically significant correlations with physician prognostic judgment, number of previous hospitalizations, and length of hospitalization. The magnitude of these correlations has not been reported.[29]

Linn's Rapid Disability Rating Scale is a short efficient approach to documenting disability status that has demonstrated substantial reliability and some evidence of validity. As with other global rating approaches, this scale offers very limited information on physical function. One might also question the arbitrary equal weighting of each component in deriving a summary score. For example, is it appropriate to weight degree of dependence in shaving the same

Table 5-6. Rapid Disability Rating Scale

Patient's Name _____

Rater _____

Date _____

Directions: On the basis of your knowledge about the patient, at the present time, will you please rate the following items:

1. *Eating*

   No assistance | Moderate assistance | Considerable assistance
2. *Diet*

   Regular diet | Modified regular diet | Special diet
3. *Medication*

   Rarely | Occasionally | Every day
4. *Speech*

   Not impaired | Moderately impaired | Unable to be understood
5. *Hearing*

   Normal | Moderately impaired | Deaf
6. *Sight*

   Normal (glasses) | Moderately impaired | Blind
7. *Walking*

   No assistance | Crutches/someone's help | Unable to walk
8. *Bathing*

   No assistance | Moderate assistance | Considerable assistance
9. *Dressing*

   No assistance | Moderate assistance | Considerable assistance
10. *Incontinence*

    Never | Occasionally | All the time
11. *Shaving*

    No assistance | Moderate assistance | Considerable assistance
12. *Safety supervision*

    Never | Sometimes | All the time
13. *Confined to bed*

    Not at all | Part of the day | All the time
14. *Mentally confused*

    Never | Occasionally | All the time
15. *Uncooperative*

    Never | Occasionally | All the time
16. *Depression*

    Never | Occasionally | All the time

Linn MW: A rapid disability rating scale. J Am Gerontol Soc 15:211, 1967.

as frequency of incontinence? One might even question the meaningfulness of adding scores across these 16 conceptual dimensions to derive a total disability score.

Jebsen Hand Function Test

The Jebsen Hand Function Test is a short, easily administered performance test that assesses the amount of time taken to complete a broad range of standardized hand functions commonly used in daily life activities.[30] The instrument is designed as an objective evaluation of several major aspects of hand function and to evaluate the effectiveness of specific treatments applied to patients with hand disabilities. The Jebsen test examines seven hand activities: writing, card turning, picking up small common objects, simulated feeding, stacking check-

Table 5-7. Examples of Jebsen Hand Function Test Items and Testing Protocol

Writing

Procedure—The subject is given a black ball-point pen and four 8-by-11-inch sheets of unruled white paper fastened, one on top of the other, to a clip board. The sentence to be copied has 24 letters and is of third-grade reading difficulty.* The sentence is typed in all capital letters and centered on a 5-by-8-in index card. The card is presented with the typed side face down on a bookstand. After the articles are arranged to the comfort of the subject (see Instructions), the card is turned over by the examiner with an immediate command to begin. The item is timed from the word "go" until the pen is lifted from the page at the end of the sentence. The item is repeated with the dominant hand, using a new sentence.

Instructions—"Do you require glasses for reading? If so, put them on. Take this pen in your left hand and arrange everything so that it is comfortable for you to write with your left hand. On the other side of this card (indicate) is a sentence. When I turn the card over, and say 'Go,' write the sentence as quickly and as clearly as you can using your left hand. Write, do not print. Do you understand? Ready? Go."

Simulated Feeding

Procedure—Five kidney beans of approximately ⅜-in length are placed on a board** clamped to a desk in front of the subject 5 in from the front edge of the desk. The beans are oriented to the left of center, parallel to and touching the upright of the board 2 in apart. An empty 1-lb coffee can is placed centrally in front of the board. A regular teaspoon is provided. Timing is from the word "go" until the last bean is heard hitting the bottom of the can. The item is repeated with the dominant hand, the beans being placed to the right of center.

Instructions—"Take the teaspoon in your left hand please. When I say 'Go,' use your left hand to pick up these beans one at a time with the teaspoon and place them in the can as fast as you can beginning with this one (indicate bean on extreme left). Do you understand? Ready? Go."

* Different sentences were used when subsequent tests were given to a single individual. Available sentences were: (1) The old man seemed to be tired. (2) John saw the red truck coming. (3) Whales live in the blue ocean. (4) Fish take air out of the water.

** A wooden board 41½ in long, 11¼ in wide and ¾-in thick was secured to the desk with a "C" clamp. The front edge (¾-in thickness) of the board was marked at 4-in intervals for easy reference when placing objects. A center piece of plywood, 20 in long, 2 in high, and ½-in thick, was glued to the board 4⅜ in from the right end and 6 in from the front of the board (this is for a secretary-type desk with a right-sided knee hole). The front of the center upright should be marked at 2-in intervals beginning 1-in from each end for convenience in placing objects.

Jebsen RH, et al: An objective and standardized test of hand function. Arch Phys Med Rehabil 50:311, 1967.

ers, picking up large light objects, and picking up large heavy objects. Scores are derived for each standardized task by having trained observers record the time taken to complete the requested task. The authors present very detailed instructions on applying each test in a standardized fashion. Table 5-7 displays the detailed instructions for two of the seven items in the Jebsen instrument.

In a study of 26 patients with stable hand disability, test–retest reliability coefficients ranged from .6 to .9. As a measure of validity, researchers have examined the Jebsen Hand Function Test's ability to discriminate degree of disability in three different patient groups: patients with hemiparesis, rheumatoid arthritis, and quadriplegia. Results indicate a wide distribution of patients' scores within all three patient groups; the instrument was unable to discriminate various degrees of disability represented by patients in these three groups.[30]

In a study with 360 subjects with no known hand disability, Jebsen Test scores varied significantly by age; subjects 60 years and older performed hand tasks significantly more slowly than did younger subjects. Statistically significant sex differences were also observed in this study, but with no observable pattern.[30] Agnew and Mass present additional normative data on the Jebsen Hand Function Test in 382 subjects drawn from a metropolitan area in Australia.[31] They found significant age and sex differences in their study population. Unlike the Jebsen study, these investigators report hand function differences among six age groups: 16 to 25 years, 26 to 35 years, 36 to 45 years, 46 to 55 years, 56 to 65 years, and 66 to 90 years. Men were found to perform significantly better than women on grip strength, moving heavy large objects, and moving large light objects. Women, on the other hand, performed significantly better than men on writing and manipulating small objects.

The Jebsen Hand Function Test is a very practical, standardized approach to examining several major aspects of hand function. Further investigation is needed to determine whether or not the dimension of time required to perform hand tasks will prove to be a valid indicator of hand function.

Patient Classification

The Patient Classification is a multidimensional assessment tool designed to provide a comprehensive assessment of physical health of nursing home patients.[19] The Patient Classification includes checklists that can be used to identify the presence or absence of diagnostically defined conditions, sensory impairment, the presence of risk factors, current care plans, demographic information as well as a section on functional status. The functional status section includes an assessment of 14 different items as illustrated in Figure 5-1. Items range from mobility and other basic ADL, to bowel and bladder function, behavioral pattern, communication of needs, and orientation for time, place, and person.

The Patient Classification is designed as a detailed patient assessment tool. It is a useful approach to standardizing the assessment of a wide range of relevant information. It appears to be most useful for institutionalized populations, and provides a comprehensive patient description that reflects social, psychological, physical, and functional needs. Its architects have published a detailed users' manual that helps standardize the way in which it is used.[32] The Patient Classification has been used in an extensive study of patient status in seven different long-term-care institutions in the metropolitan Boston area. The Patient Classification, when administered by clinicians, demonstrated agreement of 68–98% between different raters.[19]

The Patient Appraisal and Care Evaluation instrument (PACE) is a modification of a Patient Classification form.[33] The PACE assessment, which includes an extensive psychosocial section, is quite similar to the original Patient Classification in most other ways. Reliability and validity have not been reported.

INSTRUCTIONS: CHECK ALL BOXES WHICH APPLY. FILL IN ALL DIAGONALS AS INDICATED. "DESCRIBE HELP" IS TO INCLUDE NUMBER OF HUMAN ASSISTANTS AND/OR TYPE OF MECHANICAL AID.

Patient's Name _____

Patient's Number _____

Name of Facility _____

FUNCTIONING STATUS ITEMS

MOBILITY LEVEL — DATE
- Goes Outside Facility/Home
- Moves About Inside Facility/Home
- Confined to Bed and Chair
- Confined to Bed
- DESCRIBE HELP

WHEELING — DATE
- Does Not Wheel-Walks
- Wheels Self
- Is Wheeled by Others
- Does Not Wheel (Confined to Bed or Bed and Chair)
- DESCRIBE HELP

WALKING
- Walks
- Does Not Walk — (Bed and Chair)
- Confined to Bed
- DESCRIBE HELP

TRANSFERRING
- Transfers Self
- Is Lifted
- Does Not Transfer (Confined to Bed)
- DESCRIBE HELP

BATHING
- Bathes Self
- Is Bathed
- DESCRIBE HELP

STAIRCLIMBING
- Climbs Stairs
- Does Not Climb Stairs
- DESCRIBE HELP

DRESSING
- Dresses Self
- Is Dressed
- Is Not Dressed
- DESCRIBE HELP

EATING/FEEDING
- Feeds Self
- Is Spoon Fed
- Fed via Syringe, Tube, I.V., Clysis
- DESCRIBE HELP

TOILETING
- Uses Toilet Room, Day and Night
- Uses Toilet Room & Bedpan, Urinal and/or Commode
- Does Not Use Toilet Room
- DESCRIBE HELP

BEHAVIOR PATTERN
- Appropriate
- Inappropriate - Once a Week or Less Often
- Inappropriate - More Often Than Once a Week
- DESCRIBE INAPPROPRIATE BEHAVIOR

BOWEL FUNCTION
- Continent
- Incontinent less than once a week
- Incontinent more than once a week
- "Ostomy" or other problem
- TYPE OF OSTOMY CARE OR OTHER PROBLEM

COMMUNICATION OF NEEDS
- Communicates Verbally — English
- Communicates Verbally — Other Language
- Communicates Non Verbally
- Does Not Communicate
- DESCRIBE LANGUAGE BARRIER OR NON-VERBAL COMMUNICATION

BLADDER FUNCTION
- Continent
- Incontinent - less than once a week
- Incontinent more than once a week
- Indwelling Catheter
- "Ostomy" or other problem
- TYPE OF OSTOMY CARE OR OTHER PROBLEM

ORIENTATION: Time, Place and Person
- Oriented
- Disoriented—Some Spheres Some Time
- Disoriented—Some Spheres All Time
- Disoriented—All Spheres Some Time
- Disoriented—All Spheres All Time
- INDICATE SPHERES AFFECTED

HARVARD CENTER FOR COMMUNITY HEALTH AND MEDICAL CARE   JULY, 1975

Fig. 5-1. The Patient Classification. (Denson P, Jones E: An Approach to the Assessment of Long-Term Care: final report of research grant H5-01162. Harvard Center for Community Health and Medical Care, Boston, 1975.)

Table 5-8 PADL Performance Test

Test Items	Props
1. Drink from a cup	Cup
2. Use a tissue to wipe nose	Tissue box
3. Comb hair	Comb
4. File nails	Nail file
5. Shave	Shaver
6. Lift food onto spoon and to mouth	Spoon with candy on it
7. Turn faucet on and off	Faucet
8. Turn light switch on and off	Light switch
9. Put on and remove a jacket with buttons	Jacket
10. Put on and remove a slipper	Slipper
11. Brush teeth, including removing false ones	Toothbrush
12. Make a phone call	Telephone
13. Sign name	Paper and pen
14. Turn key in lock	Keyhole and key
15. Tell time	Clock
16. Stand up and walk a few steps and sit back down	—

Kuriansky J, Gurland B: The Performance Test of Activities of Daily Living. Int J Aging Hum Dev 7:343, 1976.

Performance ADL Test (PADL)

Kuriansky and Gurland developed a test of ADL as part of a cross-national study of geriatric psychiatric patients in the United States and Great Britain.[34] This test (PADL) is designed to generate descriptive estimates of functional capacity in patient populations and to monitor change in function over time. The PADL contains 16 tasks that a patient is asked to demonstrate in a standardized testing situation. The instrument consists primarily of basic ADL; it excludes areas of self-maintenance that can not be easily represented by an activity and reasonably be tested during an interview (e.g., ability to walk a few blocks carrying a package). The PADL utilizes a portable equipment or prop kit, which facilitates standardized administration. The PADL requires a minimum of patient alertness; patients must display a minimal degree of comprehension, attention span, vision, and hearing. Patients need only understand one simple message that asks them to attempt to perform a specific activity. The instrument generates a score for each activity. As a patient attempts to perform each activity, the interviewer scores a 0 if the activity was completed reasonably well on his own without personal assistance, or a 1 if the patient was not able to complete the requested activity on his own. For activities that involve a complex pattern of performance, scores are given for each component of the activity. For example, in the area of "grooming" an independent rating is given for the patient's ability to take a comb into his or her hand, grasp the comb properly, bring the comb up to the hair, and finally, to make combing motions. A list of the 16 items and the accompanying props is included in Table 5-8.

Kuriansky and Gurland reported inter-rater reliability levels of .902 when the PADL was administered to geriatric psychiatric patients by an interviewer and an independent observer. In one formal test of its validity, psychologists administered the PADL to approximately 100 older psychiatric patients from the United States and Great Britain. An overall PADL score was defined as the proportion of tested functions a patient completed correctly.[34] These overall PADL scores correlated as hypothesized with patient physical health, mental status and location at follow-up.[35]

The PADL is a clinically useful standardized approach for assessing basic physical function of patients with a low degree of mental ability. It has demonstrated a high degree of inter-rater reliability and validity when administered by trained professionals; whether or not it would continue to be reliable when administered by nonprofessionals has not been reported. The scoring method does rely on the interviewer's definition of "completes the activity reasonably well." This may reduce its reliability when it is used by paraprofessionals. The PADL limits its scope to observable basic ADL; instrumental ADL are not included. It restricts the definition of dependence to use of human assistance and does not consider the use of adaptive equipment. The use of standardized props and a highly structured testing protocol increases the reliability of the PADL when it is used in different institutions and settings.

Rappaport Disability Rating Scale

The Rappaport Disability Rating Scale is a tool designed for use with head trauma patients.[36,37] It assesses multiple conceptual dimensions (e.g., eye opening, verbalization, motor response); cognitive function (e.g., knowledge of how and when to eat and performance of toileting and grooming); social function (e.g., employability); and physical function. The physical function dimension consists of a 6-point scale that assesses level of global physical functions, where a score of 0 equals completely independent and a score of 5 equals totally dependent. It is a modification of earlier work by Scranton, Fogel, and Erdman.[38] This physical function index is used to evaluate professional judgment of the extent to which a patient requires human assistance to function physically in his or her environment.

The Rappaport Disability Rating Scale is designed to describe overall level of disability as well as to monitor change in disability over time. Inter-rater correlations for the total instrument between pairs of three raters who independently rated 88 head injury patients ranged from .97 to .98. Statistically significant correlations have been reported between the Rappaport Disability Rating Scale and evoked brain potential abnormalities, a proposed measure of severity of the CNS injury. Correlations ranged from .38 to .51; evidence of its construct validity.[36,37]

The Rappaport Disability Rating Scale is a short, clinically feasible approach to quantifying the disability of severe head trauma patients. It provides a useful shorthand global description of the condition of the patient with head injury, is easily learned, is completed quickly, and demonstrates high inter-rater reliability and encouraging validity. As a measure of physical function, however, it has limited utility. The Rappaport Scale provides only a crude global indication of the patient's degree of physical function.

Functional Status Index

The Functional Status Index (FSI), which is derived from the original Katz Index, is a self-report measure of basic and instrumental ADL.[39] It is designed to evaluate functional outcomes in noninstitutionalized chronically disabled populations. The FSI assesses three dimensions of physical function: dependence, pain, and perceived difficulty in the performance of selected daily activities. Functional dependence is assessed on a 5-point scale, where 1 equals completely independent, 2 equals uses equipment, 3 equals uses human assistance, 4 equals uses both equipment and human assistance, and 5 equals completely dependent in performing the activity. The dimensions of pain and difficulty are measured separately on a 7-point ordinal scale, where 1 equals no pain/no difficulty and 7 equals severe pain/severe difficulty in the performance of daily activities. The original instrument assessed 44 different ADL, making it impractical for use in most clinical settings.[17] A more recent version,[40] illustrated in Table 5-9, includes 18 representative activities selected from the original 44.

In a study of elderly, chronically ill patients, the FSI demonstrated interobserver reliabilities in the range of .61 to .78.[17] In a study of adult rheumatoid arthritis patients, the FSI achieved average test–retest and inter-observer reliability values ranging from .65 to .81.[40] Scores derived in each dimension have correlated well with independent measures of function, severity of disease, indicators of its construct validity.[41] In one study, FSI scores did not correlate well with clinical judgment of patient function.[42]

The FSI is most useful for noninstitutionalized populations. It includes a wide range of basic and instrumental ADL. It is unique in its assessment of the dimensions of pain and difficulty. The FSI has been used to monitor physical function in adult rheumatic disease patients.

Modified ADL Index

Sheikh and his colleagues have developed a modified ADL Index that includes 17 items rated on a 3-point scale.[43] The Index includes an assessment of 15 basic ADL and two instrumental ADL. The modified ADL index is designed to assess professional observation of a patient's degree of independence in physical function. This assessment can be completed in a hospital setting using a room equipped with standard domestic appliances or at home where a person's own furnishings are used. Each item is scored on a 3-point scale, where 1 equals the ability to perform the activity without human assistance, 2 equals the ability to perform the greater part of the activity without assistance but with some verbal or physical assistance required, and 3 equals complete inability to contribute in any way to the performance of the activity even with assistance or refusal to perform the activity even though deemed able.

The modified ADL Index is designed as a descriptive tool as well as for use in controlled studies of treatment efficacy following a cerebrovascular ac-

Table 5-9. Functional Status Index

Activity	Assistance (1 → 5)	Pain (0 → 7)	Difficulty (0 → 7)	Comment
Mobility				
Walking inside	____	____	____	
Climbing up stairs	____	____	____	
Transferring to and from toilet	____	____	____	
Getting in and out of bed	____	____	____	
Driving a car	____	____	____	
Personal care				
Combing hair	____	____	____	
Putting on pants	____	____	____	
Buttoning clothes	____	____	____	
Washing all parts of the body	____	____	____	
Putting on shoes/slippers	____	____	____	
Home chores				
Vacuuming a rug	____	____	____	
Reaching into high cupboards	____	____	____	
Doing laundry	____	____	____	
Washing windows	____	____	____	
Doing yardwork	____	____	____	
Hand activities				
Writing	____	____	____	
Opening containers	____	____	____	
Turning faucets	____	____	____	
Cutting food	____	____	____	
Vocational				
Performing all job responsibilities	____	____	____	
Avocational				
Performing hobbies requiring hand work	____	____	____	
Attending church	____	____	____	
Socializing with friends and relatives	____	____	____	

Key: Assistance: 1, independent; 2, uses devices; 3, uses human assistance; 4, uses devices and human assistance; 5, unable to do. Pain: 0 → 7: 0, no pain and 7, extremely severe pain. Difficulty: 0 → 7: 0, not difficult and 7, extremely difficult. Time frame, on the average, during the past seven days.

Jette A: The Functional Status Index: reliability of a chronic disease evaluation instrument. Arch Phys Med Rehab 61:395, 1980.

cident.[44] Table 5-10 illustrates the 17 items along with the distribution of scores in a study of stroke patients.

Inter-observer reliability of the modified ADL Index was assessed with 125 adults undergoing rehabilitation. In over 2,000 simultaneously paired observations made by physical and occupational therapists, there were only 78 (3.7 percent) disagreements; all but two of these disagreements were between adjacent points on the scale. Twenty elderly patients were assessed on each of two consecutive days under similar circumstances to examine the instrument's test–retest reliability. Therapists recorded different scores on 14.4 percent of the 340 paired observations; all but four of these differences were be-

Table 5-10. Modified Index of ADL: Activity Items and Frequency Distribution in 116 Stroke Patients

Items	Percentage of Patients Who Scored		
	1 (%)	2 (%)	3 (%)
Transfer from floor to chair	59	39	2
Transfer from chair to bed	86	14	—
Walking indoors	82	17	1
Walking outdoors	49	41	10
Ascending a flight of stairs	77	18	5
Descending a flight of stairs	76	18	6
Dressing (overgarments)	58	42	—
Washing (simulated)	71	29	—
Bathing (simulated)	58	39	3
Using lavatory (simulated)	78	22	—
Continence (bladder and bowel control)	90	10	—
Grooming (brushing hair or shaving)	96	2	2
Brushing teeth (simulated)	94	3	3
Preparing for making tea	59	28	13
Making tea	78	16	6
Using taps (ordinary sink taps)	98	1	1
Feeding (simulated)	80	19	1

Sheikh K, Smith DS, Meade TW, Goldenberg E, Brennan PJ, Kinsella G: Repeatability and validity of a modified Activities of Daily Living (ADL) index in studies of chronic disability. Int Rehab Med 1:51, 1979.

tween adjacent points on the scale. ADL scores were correlated with the extent of patient's cerebral lesion, in an attempt to judge the instrument's construct validity. A statistically significant correlation of .376 was observed between ADL scores of the stroke patients and extent of cerebral lesion. These investigators also compared observed ADL scores on a subset of 73 patients assessed both in hospital and then at home one week later. Results indicate a slight tendency for scores at home to be higher than those derived in hospital. Almost all discrepancies occurred with ADL activities that involved equipment.[43]

This modified ADL index is a carefully constructed and well-tested, standardized approach to assess accurately the capacity to perform basic ADL. The instrument has achieved high levels of reliability and has demonstrated strong evidence of its validity. This approach has limited its focus to basic ADL presumably because actual testing of instrumental ADL would require extensive equipment and would be difficult to standardize. The instrument only examines use of human assistance and inability to perform an activity; use of adaptive equipment is included in its definition of independence. Thus, a patient who used a walker would be scored as equal in independence in ambulation to a patient who used no device to assist in ambulation. The instrument has proved useful for describing levels of disability in stroke populations and has also demonstrated sufficient precision to monitor changes in patient disability over time.[44,45]

Arm Function Tests

The Arm Function Tests are multidimensional assessment protocols designed to monitor the recovery of arm control in hemiplegic stroke patients.[46] The Arm Function Tests examine 24 different items organized into five di-

Table 5-11. Arm Function Test Dimensions

1. **Passive movement**
   Range of movement more than 50 percent of normal
   a. Wrist
   b. Elbow
   c. Shoulder
2. **Muscle tone**
   a. Spasticity absent
   b. Severy spasticity absent
   c. Flaccidity absent
3. **Pain**
   Free of pain at
       (a) Wrist
       (b) Elbow
       (c) Shoulder
4. **Arm and trunk movement (turning cranked wheel)**
   a. Rotate in both directions in less than 3 seconds
   b. Rotate in both directions in more than 3 seconds
   c. Rotate in clockwise in less than 3 seconds
   d. Rotate in anticlockwise in less than 3 seconds
   e. Rotate in clockwise in more than 3 seconds
   f. Rotate in anticlockwise in more than 3 seconds
   g. Flexion component
   h. Extension component
   i. Exaggerated trunk movement
5. **Hand function**
   a. Open jar
   b. Pick up and place 50-mm cylinder
   c. Pick up and place 16-mm cylinder
   d. Squeeze gauge 100 g and release
   e. Squeeze gauge 50 g and release
   f. Raise glass to mouth
   g. Comb hair

Sheikh K, et al: Repeatability and validity of a modified Activities of Daily Living (ADL) index in studies of chronic disability. Int Rehab Med 1:51, 1979.

mensions: (1) passive ROM, (2) muscle tone, (3) pain, (4) arm and trunk movement, and (5) hand function. Each item is given a binary score relevant to the dimension under study. For example, in the ROM category, a score of 1 equals range of movement greater than 50 percent of the normal range, and 0 equals less than 50 percent of the normal range. This instrument assesses hand function by having patients perform seven specific activities (e.g., open a jar, comb hair) while seated at a table. For each activity, the successful completion of the task scores 1 and failure scores 0. Testing protocols are outlined for each activity shown in Table 5-11.

Inter-observer reliability of the Arm Function Tests was assessed with six observers implementing the total protocol on five patients (a total of 30 observations). Analysis revealed agreement in all but 4 percent of the assessments. Disagreement was greatest for the assessment of pain.[46] Validity was determined by correlating Arm Function Test scores with patients' clinical status and scores from another measure of arm function—pursuit tracking. Pursuit tracking required patients to attempt to track the movement of a randomly moving target symbol on a large cathode-ray display screen with a second symbol under the patients' control. These assessments reveal a highly significant correlation between the Arm Function Test and patients' overall clinical status as well as significant correlation with the pursuit tracking test.[47]

The Arm Function Test is a relatively simple and inexpensive multidimensional protocol that can be used by either health professionals or trained non-health professionals to assess overall upper extremity status. Although its name implies a focus on arm function, its scope is much broader. This procedure provides a relatively crude evaluation of overall upper extremity status that has successfully detected improvement in hemiplegic stroke patients. The Arm Function tests appear to be most relevant for assessing recovery in recent stroke patients in whom a substantial amount of improvement may be expected to occur. It is unclear whether the instrument would be sufficiently precise to detect changes in patients with stroke of long standing.

Activity Pattern Indicators

The Activity Pattern Indicators, a behavioral frequency scale, is part of a set of instruments being developed by the Rehabilitation Indicators Project at New York University Medical Center.[48] It represents an application of the time-budget method to help identify and document the range and scope of change in patient status brought about by rehabilitation efforts. Activity Pattern Indicators are designed to sample and record what people do and how they spend their time. For example, in a recent application of the Activity Pattern Indicators with stroke patients, 14 different basic and instrumental ADL dimensions were recorded, using patient self-report in an open-ended diary format. Examples of the recorded activities include, personal care, home maintenance, housework, child care, social–leisure activities, and social interaction. A wide scope of information can be derived for each ADL dimension from this Activity Pattern approach, including: diversity of activities (i.e., number of different activities performed); frequency of performing each activity; duration of performance; location of activity (i.e., in residence *vs* away); and physical assistance used to perform the activity. A page of an Activity Pattern Indicator diary is illustrated in Figure 5-2.

Limited data are available on the reliability and validity of this approach to functional assessment, in part, because of the complex nature of the data. One study examined the test–retest reliability of the Activity Pattern Indicators by having a sample of patients complete two sets of diaries 1 week apart. Time-use data were reduced to 12 activity categories; of the 12 correlations between sets of data, 10 were found to be statistically significant (M. Brown, personal communication). The magnitude of the correlations were not reported, however, which limits our ability to evaluate the magnitude of agreement achieved. Reliability assessment of time-budget methods of data collection, in general, have been restricted to duration or frequency by activity. The reliability of recording other dimensions of activity has been largely ignored. The Activity Pattern Indicator scores have demonstrated the ability to differentiate between newly impaired persons and those further along in the rehabilitation process,

Timeline Diary for a WEEKEND DAY

Circle one: Saturday Sunday

What did you do all day starting at midnight?

What did you do?	Time began	Time ended	Where were you?	Talk with anyone?	Were you supervised?	Any physical help?	Doing anything else?
	12:00						

GO TO THE NEXT PAGE ▼

Fig. 5-2. Activity pattern indicator diary (Reprinted by permission of the Rehabilitation Indicators Project, New York University Medical Center.)

persons expected to be different with respect to activity participation. No further evidence of the instrument's validity was found.

The Activity Pattern Indicators is a promising attempt to develop measures of physical function beyond the traditional basic ADL. Its developers must address the challenge of demonstrating the reliability and validity of this self-report method if it is to gain widespread acceptance. The Rehabilitation Indicators Project is currently conducting a number of studies that will shed light on these important questions. The Activity Pattern Indicators may prove to be a very useful tool for assessing the impact of rehabilitation efforts on a wide range of important instrumental ADL. A precise assessment of instrumental ADL is beyond the scope of most traditional measures of physical function. This approach, however, is fairly complex, time-consuming, and demands a considerable degree of cognitive ability from a patient. These characteristics of the instrument may limit the type of patient who can use it and restrict its use to large facilities.

Table 5-12 provides a summary of the characteristics of each instrument reviewed. The table displays the conceptual focus, purpose, measurement dimension, and mode of administration for easy reference and review.

Table 5-12. Characteristics of Selected Measures of Physical Function

Instrument	Conceptual Focus	Purpose	Measurement Dimension	Mode of Administration
Katz ADL Index Report	Basic ADL	Description Assessment Monitoring	Assistance	Professional judgment, self
PULSES	Basic ADL Instrumental ADL Impairment	Description Monitoring	Assistance Impairment	Professional judgment
Barthel Index	Basic ADL Impairment	Description Monitoring	Assistance Time	Professional judgement
PGC Instrumental ADL Index	Instrumental ADL	Description	Assistance Frequency	Professional judgement Self report
Kenny Self-Care Index	Basic ADL	Description Assessment Monitoring	Assistance	Professional judgment
Rapid Disability Rating Scale	Global	Description	Frequency Severity	Professional judgement
Jebsen Hand Function Test	Hand function	Description Monitoring	Time	Observation
Patient Classification	Multi-dimensional	Description Assessment Monitoring	Assistance	Professional judgment
Performance ADL	Basic ADL	Description Monitoring	Assistance	Observation
Rappaport Disability Rating Scale	Global	Description Monitoring	Assistance	Professional judgment Observation
Functional Status Index	Basic ADL Instrumental ADL	Description Monitoring	Assistance Pain Difficulty	Self report
Modified ADL Index	Basic ADL	Description Monitoring	Assistance	Observation
Arm Function Test	Upper extremity Basic ADL	Description Monitoring	Performance	Observation
Activity Pattern Indicators	Basic ADL Instrumental ADL	Description Monitoring	Assistance Diversity Frequency Location Duration	Self report

The reader will note that many of these instruments have been developed for disease-specific populations such as patients with stroke or rheumatic disease. A major advantage to this approach is that it allows the investigator to focus on dimensions that are particularly relevant to a specific population. The FSI, for instance, focuses on the dimensions of pain and difficulty in performing daily activities. These dimensions are particularly relevant to patients with rheumatic disease for whom the instrument was designed. The dimensions of pain and difficulty may be less relevant to other populations, for instance, persons with neurologic impairments. Instruments designed for disease-specific populations may limit our ability to draw cross-population comparisons. They also encourage the proliferation of instruments that may be used only by a small group of investigators. Furthermore, we frequently do not know if an instrument that has been developed and shown to reliable and valid on one population will remain so if used in a different group. The shortcomings of disease-specific instruments make necessary the development and use of broader, more generic approaches, with particular emphasis on dimensions of function that are relevant across disease-specific groups. The Patient Classification and PACE instruments represent attempts to do this in the elderly population. Such efforts should be encouraged and expanded into the pediatric population as well as others.

ADVANCING THE STATE OF THE ART IN FUNCTIONAL STATUS ASSESSMENT

One of the attractive features of most formal, standardized approaches to assessing functional status is the ability to summarize detailed information in an overall functional status index. Summary indices facilitate the interpretation of complex data and enable one to draw cross-disease, cross-program, and cross-population comparisons of function. Instruments that lack this feature, such as the Patient Classification and PACE, lose some of their clinical utility and appeal.

Let us consider, for example, a scale that ranges from 0 to 100, where 0 represents complete dependence in physical function and 100 represents complete independence. On such a scale, every individual could be assigned a number from 0 to 100 representing his or her overall functional status. Higher numbers on such a scale would reflect more functional independence. Overall scores would be derived from scores on individual items in the instrument. The fundamental issue is to determine how to develop a value or utility weight for every possible state of function within the overall range. For instance, what score would be given for an individual who was dependent in dressing and bathing *vs* one who was independent in dressing and bathing. Values or utility weights for different functional states can be derived *implicitly* or *explicitly* based on choices or judgments about the desirability of each level of function.

Implicit Utility Weighting

Most functional status instruments that can be reduced to a single summary scale or index rely on implicit judgments about the desirability of each component or level of function.

The Barthel Index, is the clearest example. This instrument assigns a specific weight or value to being dependent in each daily activity. These individual item weights are summed to yield an overall score which ranges from 0 (representing total dependence) to 100 (representing total independence). Inability to transfer from bed to chair without assistance, for instance, receives a score of 10 points, whereas dependence in grooming receives only 5 points. Dependence in transfers is given twice the weight of dependence in grooming. This implicit assignment of values or weights is presumably based on clinical judgment or some other implicit criteria. The problem with such an approach is clear. What is the justification for the weight or value given to a specific activity or level of function? Why is transfer ability weighted twice as much as grooming? Why not three times as much or half as much?

Most instruments (The Katz Index, the FSI, and the Modified ADL) address the problem of utility weighting by giving equal weight or value to each item in an ADL scale. But does this strategy really resolve the issue? One can just as readily question the implicit judgments behind these equal weighting strategies. Should every item be given equal value? Is independence in grooming as important as independence in eating? The problem, therefore, lies in the justification behind these implicit value judgments and not in the specific values or weights themselves.

Explicit Utility Weighting

Problems inherent in almost any implicit weighting scheme have led many methodologic researchers to devise strategies for developing explicit utility or value weighting.

Using three weighting methods—category rating,[49] magnitude estimation,[50] and equivalency,[51] a group of graduate students and health leaders were asked to judge 50 case descriptions representing the 29 function states, 5 age classes and 42 symptom/problem complexes in the Index of Well-Being, a health status indicator.[52] The intent was to develop a reliable and valid summary index of health status. Judges were asked to score their preference for a single day of dysfunction described in each case description. For instance, one subject was described as over 65 years of age, confined to home, moving independently in a wheelchair, able to perform self-care activities, and having one foot or leg missing. In category rating, an equal-interval scaling technique, judges scored the desirability of a day in each case description by circling one number on an 11-point interval scale, where 1 represented least preference and 11 represented maximum preference. For magnitude estimation, a ratio measure, a standard item representing the upper extreme (perfect health) was given a score of 1,000. Judges scored each day in relation to the standard description by selecting any whole and/or fraction >0 and ≤1,000. In the equivalence method, the standard case description was the same, but a decision-making game was used as the scoring method. Judges were told to consider two hypothetical groups of people, both of which would die immediately if not helped. They had the resources to keep one of the groups alive for another year, after which they would also die. The standard group contained 100 people in a state of maximum health. Judges then determined the number of people in each second group (i.e., represented by each case description) that would be equivalent to the 100 people of the same age in the standard group. Explicit utility scores were generated for each possible health state contained in the instrument. The investigators report no significant differences for order of method presentation, interview situation, scaling method, or type of judge.

Explicit weighting schemes of this type have a number of advantages:

1. Explicit schemes enable one to generate reliable and valid estimates of utility weights based on the judgment of a broad base of judges.
2. This approach makes explicit and clear the justification behind the values attributed to certain functional states or activities.
3. Explicit weights enable one to discriminate more precisely among different functional status levels.

Although these approaches are used widely in the development of many global health status indicators, they have not yet been used in the development of functional status instruments. Important work in the area of functional assessments must still be done. The development of reliable and valid weights for a wide range of functional status states will provide a solid foundation on which to advance the study of functional status in population and patient groups.

Summary

In this chapter, I have tried to clarify the conceptual meaning of the term "functional status" as a prerequisite to the scientific study of this important concept. Functional status is one component of the larger concept of health status. It refers to the characteristic performance of the individual. Function reflects one's reaction to a biological condition; it represents the interaction of the individual with his or her environment. Functional status can be further divided into four dimensions: physical, mental, social, and emotional function. I have selected the dimension of physical function as the focus of this chapter. My purpose is to illustrate some of the many physical function assessment tools available to the physical therapist and, even more important, to analyze critically the strengths and weaknesses of each instrument. I have done this by focusing on the criteria of purpose, conceptual focus, measurement dimension, reliability, validity, and mode of administration.

This review points out clearly that there is no one best approach to assessing physical function; nor should there be. A functional status instrument that is useful for one situation may be totally inappropriate for another. This in part reflects the complex nature of the concept as well as its adolescence in the state of the art in this field. In selecting an approach to assessing function, the physical therapist must consider the purpose for which the instrument is being sought, the conceptual focus needed, the measurement dimension sought, and the mode of administration required. A consideration of each of these criteria will lead the therapist to the appropriate instrument. Functional status assessment is in its adolescence. Future methodological work will provide a solid foundation on which to advance the scientific study of functional status.

REFERENCES

1. Baumann G: Diversities in conceptions of health and physical fitness. J Health Hum Behav 3:39, 1961
2. Nagi S: Some conceptual issues in disability and rehabilitation. In Sussman M (ed): Sociology and Rehabilitation, American Sociological Association, Washington, D.C., 1965
3. Haber L: Identifying the disabled: concepts and methods in measurement of disability. Social Security Bulletin 30:17, 1967
4. Koshel J, Granger C: Rehabilitation terminology: who is severely disabled? Rehabil Lit 39:102, 1978
5. Wood P: The language of disablement: a glossary relating to disease and its consequences. Int Rehab Med 2:86, 1980
6. Jette A: Concepts of health and methodological issues in functional assessment. In Granger C, Gresham G (eds): Functional Assessment in Rehabilitation Medicine, Williams & Wilkins, Baltimore, 1984
7. World Health Organization: The First Ten Years of the World Health Organization. Geneva, World Health Organization, 1958
8. Goldsmith S: The status of health status indicators. Health Serv Rep 87:212, 1972
9. American Medical Association Committee on Medical Rating of Physical Impairment: guidelines to the evaluation of permanent impairment. JAMA: 1958
10. Parsons T: Definitions of health and illness in the light of American values and social structure. In Jaco EG (ed): Patients, Physicians and Illness, The Free Press, Glencoe, Illinois, 1958
11. Lawton MP: Assessing the competence of older people. In Kent D, Kastenbaum R, Sherwood S (ed): Research Planning and Action for the Elderly, Behavioral Publications, New York, 1972
12. Kane RA, Kane RL: Assessing the Elderly. Lexington Books, Lexington, Kentucky, 1981
13. Wood P: Appreciating the consequences of disease: the International Classification of Impairments, Disabilities, and Handicaps. WHO Chronicle 34:376, 1980
14. Ruesch J, Brodsky C: The concept of social disability. Arch Gen Psych 19:394, 1968
15. Katz S, Ford A, Maskowitz R, Jackson B, Jaffee M: Studies of illness in the Aged. The Index of ADL: a standardized measure of biological and psychosocial function. JAMA 185:74, 1963
16. Katz S, Downs T, Cash H, Grotz R: Progress in development of the Index of ADL. Gerontologist 10:20, 1970
17. Jette A, Deniston O: Inter-observer reliability of a functional status assessment instrument. J Chron Dis 31:573, 1978
18. Branch L: Understanding the Health and Social Service Needs of People Over Age 65. Boston, Center for Survey Research, University of Massachusetts and the Joint Center for Urban Studies of Harvard University and MIT, 1977
19. Denson P: An Approach to the Assessment of Long-Term Care: Final Report of Research Grant HS-01162. Harvard Center for Community Health and Medical Care, Boston, 1975
20. Sherwood S, Morris J, Mor V, Gutkin C: Compendium of Measures for Describing and Assessing Long Term Care Populations. Hebrew Rehabilitation Center for Aged, Boston, 1977

21. Katz S, Ford A, Downs T, Adams M, Rusby D: Effects of Continued Care: A Study of Chronic Illness in the Home. National Center for Health Services Research and Development, DHEW Publ. No. HSM 73-3010, Washington, D.C., 1972
22. Andrews K, Brocklehurst J, Richards B, Laycock P: The recovery of the severely disabled stroke patient. Rheumatol Rehabil 21:225, 1982
23. Moskowitz E, McCann C: Classification of disability in the chronically ill and aging. J Chron Dis 5:342, 1957
24. Granger C, Greer D: Functional status measurement and medical rehabilitation outcomes. Arch Phys Med Rehabil 57:103, 1976
25. Granger C, Dewis L, Peters N, Sherwood C, Barrett J: Stroke rehabilitation: analysis of repeated Barthel Index Measures. Arch Phys Med Rehabil 60:14, 1979
26. Mahoney F, Barthel D: Functional evaluation: the Barthel Index. Maryland State Med J 14:61, 1965
27. Wylie C: Measuring end results of rehabilitation of patients with stroke. Public Health Rep 82:893, 1967
28. Schoening H, Anderegg L, Bergstrom D, Fonda M, Steinke N, Ulrich P: Numerical scoring of self-care status of patients. Arch Phys Med Rehabil 46:689, 1965
29. Linn M: A rapid disability rating scale. J Am Gerontol Soc 15:211, 1967
30. Jebsen R, Taylor N, Trieschmann R, Trotter M, Howard L: An objective and standardized test of hand function. Arch Phys Med Rehabil 50:311, 1969
31. Agnew P, Maas F: Hand function related to age and sex. Arch Phys Med Rehabil 63:269, 1982
32. Jones E, McNilt B, McKnight E. Patient Classification for Long-Term Care: User's Manual. DHEW Publ. No. HRA 75-3107, U.S. Government Printing Office, Washington, D.C., 1974
33. U.S. Department of Health, Education, and Welfare (DHEW): Working Document on Patient Care Management. Washington, D.C., U.S. Government Printing Office, 1978
34. Kuriansky J, Gurland B: Performance Test of Activities of Daily Living. Int J Aging Hum Dev 7:343, 1976
35. Kuriansky J, Gurland B, Fleiss J, Cowan D, The assessment of self-care capacity in geriatric psychiatric patients. J Clin Psychol 32:95, 1976
36. Rappaport M, Hall K, Hopkins K, Belleza T, Berrol S, Reynolds G: Evoked brain potentials and disability in brain-damaged patients. Arch Phys Med Rehabil, 58:333, 1977
37. Rappaport M, Hall K, Hopkins K, Belleza T, Cope D: Disability rating scale for severe head trauma: coma to community. Arch Phys Med Rehabil 63:118, 1982
38. Scranton J, Fogel M, Erdman W: Evaluation of functional levels of patients during and following rehabilitation. Arch Phys Med Rehabil 51:1, 1970
39. Jette A: Functional capacity evaluation: an empirical approach. Arch Phys Med Rehabil 61:85, 1980
40. Jette A: Functional Status Index: Reliability of a chronic disease evaluation instrument. Arch Phys Med Rehabil 61:395, 1980
41. Shope J, Banwell B, Jette A, Kulik C, Edwards N: Functional status outcome after treatment of rheumatoid arthritis. Rheumatol Practice 1:243, 1983
42. Deniston O, Jette A: Validity of a functional status assessment instrument. Health Serv Res 15:21, 1980
43. Sheikh K, Smith D, Meade T, Goldenberg E, Brennan P, Kinsella G: Repeatability and validity of a modified activities of daily living index in studies of chronic disability. Int Rehab Med 1:51, 1979

44. Smith D, Goldenberg E, Ashburn A, Kinsella G, Sheikh K, Brennan P, Meade T, Zutshi D, Perry J, Reeback J: Remedial therapy after stroke: a randomized controlled trial. Br Med J 282:517, 1981
45. Sheikh K, Smith D, Meade T, Brennan P, Ide L: Assessment of motor function in studies of chronic disability. Rheumatol Rehabil 19:83, 1980
46. DeSouza L, Hewer R, Miller S: Assessment of recovery of arms control in hemiplegic stroke patients. 1. Arm function tests. Int Rehab Med 2:3, 1980
47. DeSouza L, Hewer R, Lynn P, Miller S, Reed G: Assessment of recovery of arm control in hemiplegic stroke patients. 2. Comparison of arm function tests and pursuit tracking in relation to clinical recovery. Int Rehab Med 2:10, 1980
48. Belcher S, Clowers M, Cabanayan A, Fordyce W: Activity patterns of married and single individuals after stroke. Arch Phys Med Rehabil 63:308, 1982
49. Anderson N: Integration theory and attitude change. Psychol Rev 78:171, 1971
50. Sellin T, Wolfgang M: The Measurement of Delinquency. John Wiley, New York, 1964
51. Torgerson W: Theory and Methods of Scaling. John Wiley, New York, 1958
52. Patrick D, Bush P, Chen M: Methods for measuring levels of well-being for a health status index. Health Serv Res 8:228, 1973

6 | Gait Assessment in the Clinic: Issues and Approaches

Rebecca L. Craik
Carol A. Oatis

Locomotion is the act of moving from place to place.[1] Any behavior that results in such movement is a form of locomotion. Locomotion assessment is, therefore, a fundamental element of the physical therapist's functional evaluation. For example, when therapists determine the level of wheelchair independence that a nonambulatory patient has achieved, they have performed a form of locomotion assessment. In ambulatory patients, therapists often describe the patient's walking pattern or ambulatory independence.

Ambulation is the specialized form of locomotion conducted on foot; gait evaluation is the process of describing a person's ambulatory ability. The purpose of this chapter is (1) to discuss the general approaches to gait evaluation, (2) to familiarize the reader with some of the methods currently used clinically, and (3) to discuss some of the limitations of these assessment techniques.

To determine the ambulatory functions that should be assessed for each patient, therapists must be able to identify the information that needs to be sought and analyzed. That is, why is the subject being evaluated? The first section of this chapter reviews the general reasons for gait analysis and why these reasons should guide the evaluation process.

STUDY OF LOCOMOTOR PERFORMANCE

Evaluation Terminology

The terms *measurement, description, analysis,* and *assessment* have, at times, all been used interchangeably to describe the task of examining the movements associated with walking. Winter offers more specific definitions for these terms.[2] According to Winter, *measurement* assigns a numerical value to an observation, e.g., the knee is flexed 25°. *Description* uses several measurements to characterize (or describe) movement. In Winter's terms, a description can be provided from a measurement device when data collected from a marker placed at the center of the knee joint are used to plot the path that the knee center traverses in time and space. The description of a movement can be stated in many forms, e.g., chart recorder curves, oscilloscope traces, or reconstructed stick diagrams. *Analysis* is defined as the mathematical transformation of the data for presentation in another form. Analysis combines the collected data to produce a variable that is not directly measured. For example, measurements can be obtained from a videotape recording and used to provide a description of the movements of the hip, knee, and ankle joints in the sagittal plane. By analysis, joint velocities and accelerations can be derived from this description and used to model the limb movements. Further analysis of the model allows the investigator to predict net forces and muscle moments that caused the observed limb movement. The results of the analysis should, in turn, provide information that allows the examiner to make a judgment about the quality of the movement. *Assessment* is the step in which judgment is introduced so that a statement of "goodness" can be judged.

Assessment can also be made directly from descriptive information without an analytical step. Currently, clinical assessment of ambulatory performance is most commonly derived from descriptive rather than analytical variables. In fact, most of the outcomes of ambulation research have yielded descriptive information. For example, before surgery is performed, a patient with a total knee replacement may demonstrate a shorter stance time and a longer swing time on the involved limb than on the uninvolved limb. Six weeks after surgery, the temporal asymmetry between the limbs diminishes. The clinician then judges the quality and rate of postsurgical locomotor recovery through an assessment of the gait measurements.

Judgment of "goodness" of a gait pattern or the recovery rate is difficult. For example, is locomotor performance improving if the range of knee flexion increases 5° during swing but the average walking velocity simultaneously decreases from 0.7 to 0.4 m/s? Is the patient with a total knee arthroplasty recovering at an appropriate rate if the single support time for the involved limb increases 10 percent in one week? These are difficult questions because of our limited knowledge about the *relationships among gait variables* in normals, let alone in patients. In addition, there is little information that can give an expected *rate* of locomotor recovery regardless of the measured variable or the patient type. Therefore, judgments regarding the quality of gait or of the rate of recovery are now based almost entirely on the clinical experience or therapeutic orientation of the therapist.

Evaluation Goals

Gait evaluations have become widely used because clinical measurements of muscle strength, range of motion (ROM), and postural alignment have not been shown to predict functional, or more specifically, locomotor potential.[3] The goals of gait evaluation usually fall into four broad categories:

1. To describe the degree to which a patient's performance differs from nondisabled performance.
2. To determine whether treatment alters performance.
3. To classify the severity of a walking disability.
4. To identify the mechanisms responsible for producing the abnormal gait.

Perhaps the most common goal of gait analysis is to describe the deviation from the normal gait pattern as demonstrated by an individual patient or patient population. The implications of such data are obvious; therapeutic intervention can, theoretically, be provided or altered in an attempt to reduce or eliminate abnormalities. The classic studies of Eberhart et al were the first performed to describe the differences between normal and abnormal function in selected groups.[4] The biomechanical evaluation of the gait pattern of healthy men provided data that were used by these investigators to assess the performance of subjects with above-knee prostheses. The data provided information that was used to improve designs for prostheses. The improved prostheses better simulated kinetic and kinematic function of the lost limb than did previous versions.

Measures of deviations from the normal gait pattern may be useful. However, they also can confuse the clinician. A recent study which assessed the ability of five knee arthroplasty designs to restore normal function provides an example of how gait evaluation can be used to describe deviations from normal performance.[5] The 26 patients selected for the study were matched based on postoperative pain, passive ROM, and joint stability with normal subjects. All patients were evaluated at least 1 year postoperatively to ensure that optimal recovery had taken place. All patients had an excellent clinical result (i.e., reported little or no pain). Regardless of the prosthetic design, the patients demonstrated abnormal patterns of knee movement during gait when compared with the age-matched healthy subject sample. Therefore, the gait evaluation data indicated that the treatment goal, i.e., recovery of normal performance, had not been achieved. These results appear to suggest that the treatment programs and/or the prosthetic designs must be altered in order to achieve a more "normal" outcome. Yet the clinical results for the subjects were considered excellent. There was no postoperative pain, there were no passive flexion contractures greater than 5°, and the knee joints of patients were stable. Thus, one must ask two questions: Is the description of gait deviations from normal a sensitive measure of clinical outcome? Is the measurement of gait deviations an appropriate measure of clinical success? *Clearly, the most common application of gait analysis, which is to document the amount of deviation from normal, may yield data that are insufficient to assess the subject's gait pattern functionally or meaningfully.* In other words, gait analysis may not yield clinically relevant information, especially when comparisons are made with normal performance.

The utility of an evaluation that discriminates only between what is normal and abnormal may also depend on the patient population that is assessed. Perhaps normal gait should be used as a standard only when the goal of treatment is total recovery to premorbid (normal) function or when there are only subtle differences between the patient and normal performance. For example, Colaso et al used the gait evaluation form developed by Brunnstrom to describe walking performance of patients with hemiparesis.[6,7] Twenty-nine gait patterns were described in a sample of 50 hemiparetic patients. Knowledge that a given patient has five specific gait deviations establishes a baseline that can be used to measure the patient's change. However, a gait evaluation may more effectively assist in planning treatment when ambulatory ability is classified based on meaningful variables. Richards and Knutsson classified the abnormal gait of patients with spastic hemiparesis based on one of three types of electromyography (EMG) patterns produced during walking.[8,9,10] The EMG abnormalities were characterized as: (1) exaggerated stretch responses that disturbed an otherwise well-preserved gait; (2) a lack of or a decrease in the amount of muscle activity during walking; or (3) abnormal coactivation of several muscle groups. In this case, gait evaluation served to classify or categorize three different motor problems in a sample of patients with the same diagnosis, spastic hemiparesis. The description of different types of gait disturbance suggests that therapeutic intervention or treatment goals could be based on the specific type of functional impairment rather than on the clinical diagnosis. Therfore, *use of variables that discriminate performance within a diagnostic category of patients may assist in treatment planning and in documenting of gait deviations.*

Assessing gait helps to describe the mechanisms responsible for producing abnormal gait. Microelectrodes used in animal studies have allowed investigators to describe the activity of neural tracts during locomotion. Gait analyses on these animals have used many of the same approaches used to evaluate human gait.[11,12] However, rather than describing how gait differs from "normal," the questions that are being asked in such animal studies are: (1) How stereotypic is the performance? (2) What aspects of the movement are being controlled? and (3) What aspects of locomotion remain after various central nervous system (CNS) lesions?[13] Although the clinical significance of these kinds of studies is not yet fully evident, the potential relevance of this analytical process has been addressed.[13,14] For example, Grillner has synthesized this research and developed a neural model for locomotion.[14] Included in this model is the suggestion that extension of the hip in terminal stance may initiate flexion for the swing phase. Common problems in the gait of patients with hemiparesis include inadequate flexion of the hip, knee, and ankle during swing. The hip at terminal stance in these patients often exhibits inadequate extension. Based on Grillner's concepts, it can be suggested that hip dysfunction causes the other defects. Although this hypothesis must be tested, this type of approach to gait analysis may not only provide descriptions of aberrant patterns but may provide a method that indicates the cause of the deviations. Thus, in Winter's terms, this application of gait analysis uses measurements and description to isolate more relevant parameters of performance which can be used for assessment and treatment.

In summary, there may be more than one purpose for performing a gait analysis. The purpose should differ with the type of patient being evaluated and the nature of the questions being asked about the patient's condition. In order to know the purpose for gait evaluation or a measurement scheme for a specific type of patient, the therapist must: (1) recognize the goal of treatment, (2) be familiar with the currently available tools, and (3) define the variables that can be measured. This knowledge will also enhance the clinician's ability to analyze the literature, measurement schemes, and the available data bases critically.

PARAMETERS OF GAIT

The biomechanical variables used to describe and analyze movements are kinematic or kinetic. Measurement of physiological performance such as energy costs will not be discusssed here. Winter and Inman et al have defined biomechanical variables and described their uses in assessing functional performance.[2,15] Kinematic variables describe the movement itself. They include displacement, velocity, and acceleration of the moving body or body segments. Kinetic variables describe the internal and external forces that are associated with movement. Analysis using kinetic variables includes determination of the forces applied between the foot and the ground, calculation of resultant forces applied to joints, and the study of power, work, and mechanical energy.

Although muscle contractions contribute to the generation of the internal forces and are, therefore, a kinetic variable, the EMG signal associated with the contraction also contains information that describes the contraction. EMG activity reveals information about the excitation of agonist and antagonist, the onset of the muscle activity following the command to move, and the duration of the contraction.

To date, gait analysis has been carried out in two distinct settings—the clinic and the research laboratory. This has resulted in distinctly different approaches to gait analysis despite apparent similarities in the goals of some of the analyses. Clinicians have relied primarily on the systematic visual inspection of gait to assess function while researchers have commonly employed sophisticated instrumentation. Clinical gait evaluation commonly uses visual assessment to describe deviations in kinematic variables. However, instrumentation that provides a description and analysis of kinematic, kinetic, and EMG variables is being incorporated into many clinical settings. Technological advances have made some of the sophisticated laboratory instruments into clinically feasible tools. The equipment is now smaller in size, sturdier, and easier to operate. Recently developed computer programs for data collection and data analysis can now provide measures at the end of an evaluation session. However, much of the instrumentation was developed to fulfill a research rather than a clinical need; therefore, the rationale and the methodology for clinical use of the instrumentation are not readily available.

Clinicians unfamiliar with current measurement tools may find the plethora of gait variables overwhelming. There are very few guidelines to assist clinicians in selecting the variables to measure during the evaluation. A description of the most common variables is presented in the following section. A discussion of the common methods of data collection and the limitations in our current knowledge are also provided.

Kinematics

A kinematic analysis of movement presents only a detailed description of the movement pattern. For convenience, kinematic variables can be divided into those of joint displacement and those of the spatial and temporal patterns of foot placement.

Joint Displacement.   Displacement patterns are probably the most intensely studied kinematic variables of human locomotion. Although displacement patterns of the body's center of gravity (and of major body segments) have been described, most emphasis has been placed on the relative or absolute displacement patterns of single limb segments. Both translational and rotational movements can be described during locomotion. Motion of the whole body in going from point A to point B is translational, whereas limb segment displacement around a joint axis is rotational. Both translation and rotation occur in all three planes, i.e., sagittal, frontal, and transverse. Therefore, movement in space is said to have six degrees of freedom—three rotational and three translational.

Regardless of the number of planes of motion measured, all kinematic analyses must have a plane of reference. The *absolute spatial reference* system uses the environment as a reference.[2] The *relative reference* system examines the position of one limb segment relative to another limb segment. An *absolute reference* system might tell the examiner that the thigh goes from + 30° to − 10° relative to vertical position during stance. A *relative reference* system might tell the examiner that the hip went through 40° of excursion from relative flexion to relative extension.

Kinematic data has been used to describe abnormal movement patterns associated with many disabilities .[16-19] Individual joint motions are recorded most often. Velocity and accelerations of joint motions have also been examined in subjects with pathologies. In most instances, the kinematic variables have been used to *describe* rather than to *analyze* the locomotor pattern. Studies have identified how several kinematic parameters differed between the subjects with pathology and the normal subjects. Such findings indicate that kinematic variables are sensitive measures that can be used to discriminate between normal performance and performance that is compromised by pathology.

A complete kinematic analysis is complicated, requires sophisticated instrumentation, and generates vast quantities of data. However, a kinematic description can be as simple as a visual inspection of the ROM that occurs in the sagittal plane at the knee. The most common clinical method for the assessment of kinematic variables is direct visual observation.

Observational techniques. Many facilities have developed check lists of kinematic variables. However, despite careful clinical notes, it is often difficult for clinicians to recall accurately the manner in which a patient initially walked. A therapist's approach to gait evaluation apparently depends largely on training, experience, and personality.[20]

Goodkin and Diller used a check list of 17 gait deviations to examine the walking of hemiplegic adults.[20] The form was adapted from a New York University Orthotic Gait Analysis worksheet. Seven physical therapists participated in the study. Patients with hemiplegia (five with left and five with right hemiplegia) were observed. Deviations in joint motion were scored as: 1, acceptable; 2, needs to be minimized; and 3, needs to be encouraged. Only "agreement" statistics were presented. Because each of 10 patients was evaluated by three therapists, a maximum of 30 within-rater agreements could be obtained for each of 17 gait deviations. The highest number of agreements obtained was 28 for four of the deviations, and the lowest number of agreements was 18 for one deviation. The mode was 26.5. A maximum of 51 between-rater agreements could be obtained for a given patient. The highest number of between-rater agreements was 48 for one patient and the lowest was 39 for three patients. The therapists were also asked to name the two major gait deviations observed for each patient. A maximum of six agreements could be obtained for each patient, since three therapists were each required to state the two major deviations. No agreement at all was obtained for three of the 10 patients. Two of the six possible agreements occurred for four of the patients and three of the six possible agreements occurred for two of the patients. There was greatest consensus in four of the six possible agreements for one patient. However, there are limitations in the design of this study: the therapists were not trained to use the form; the same patient was examined at different times by the three therapists so that the patient's performance may have changed between sessions; and within-rater reliability was not assessed. The results stress the need to train evaluators to improve the reliability of observational gait analysis and to make the best possible use of it.

Observational gait analysis forms have been developed to organize systematically the therapist's approach to the patient and to increase the possibility of higher within- and between-rater reliability. Although primary emphasis has been on lower extremity joint rotations in the sagittal and coronal planes, most lists also include observations of the head, trunk, and upper extremities.[7,21,22] An absolute reference is often used to assess the function of the pelvis and hip, whereas relative references are used for the knee and ankle. Investigators at

Rancho Los Amigos and Temple University have developed observational gait analysis forms.

In a presentation in Philadelphia in 1975, describing the Rancho system, Baker stated that a trained observer could reliably detect a change of 5° in joint excursion.[23] However, there is no published report describing the reliability of the Rancho system. Krebs and colleagues examined within-rater and between-rater reliability for three physical therapists trained to use an observational gait analysis form,[24] adapted from those developed at New York University, Rancho Los Amigos, and Temple University. Assessments of three phases of stance were made from video tape recordings of 15 disabled children. Total agreement, both within-raters and between-raters, occurred on approximately two-thirds of the observations. Within-rater Pearson correlations averaged .60 overall. Between-rater intraclass correlations averaged .73. This study suggests that only moderate reliability is present for observational kinematic gait analysis of disabled children. The reliability of observational gait analysis techniques must still be assessed for other populations. Visual analysis can be assisted by the use of video or other recording systems. If the video recording system has a slow play-back or stop-action control, the gait can be examined more easily.

Instrumented techniques.   Other means for the collection of kinematic data include devices such as electrogoniometers and accelerometers and a variety of two-dimensional and three-dimensional imaging systems.[2] Most of these techniques measure displacement. Velocities and accelerations can then be derived from these data. An electrogoniometer is a device similar to a standard goniometer except that the joint angle is converted into an electrical signal, which can then be recorded.[25-28] Electrogoniometers are relatively inexpensive and the data are immediately available on a strip-chart recording, an oscilloscope, or as an input to a computer. There are disadvantages to electrogoniometers, however. The careful application necessary for accurate readings is time-consuming, absolute joint angles must be inferred from the relative excursion of the goniometer's arm, and multiple electrogoniometers also encumber the patient and may distort walking performance.

Figure 6-1 depicts joint excursion of the left hip, knee, and ankle for one subject who walked at a comfortable velocity of 1.3 m/s. The data were collected with electrogoniometers so that only relative excursion can be discussed. Performance of the same subject is depicted on the right side of Figure 6-1. In this case, the subject walked at 0.5 m/s, a velocity that is more consistent with the velocity demonstrated by many patients who are just beginning ambulation training.

An accelerometer is a transducer that measures acceleration. The output signal must be integrated (i.e., area under the curve must be measured) to calculate velocity, and must be integrated twice to calculate displacement. As compared with electrogoniometers, accelerometers are expensive and most of them are fragile.

Imaging methods include cine, video, and multiple exposure photographic techniques.[28,29] The primary constraint of these systems has been that quantification of kinematic variables is very time-consuming and the equipment is

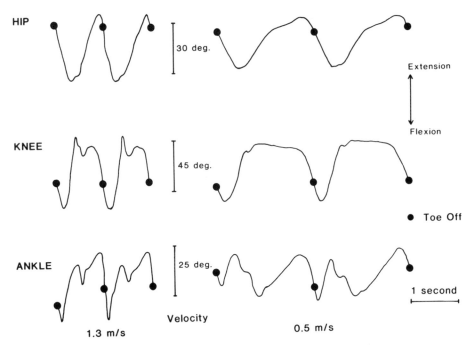

Fig. 6-1. Sagittal plane joint excursion of the hip, knee, and ankle are depicted at two different walking velocities. (Left) sagittal motion that occurred when the subject was walking at a comfortable speed (1.3 m/s); (right) decrease in sagittal plane excursion that accompanies a decrease in walking velocity (0.5 m/s). Two strides at each speed, representing the performance of one subject, are shown (●, toe off)

expensive. For example, a hand-held goniometer or protractor can be used to measure sagittal knee motion, but if ambulation is filmed at 60 frames per second and a cycle lasts 1 second, knee excursion must be measured in each of 60 frames to create an objective measure of sagittal knee displacement for *each stride*. Recent technological advances promise to reduce the time-consuming data reduction process.

There are many commercially available computer-assisted imaging systems but most are of two types. One type requires the subject to wear special lights on each desired site; if the sagittal knee motion is to be measured, lights are placed on the knee, the proximal femur, and the lower leg. The lights are flashed sequentially to denote the location of points of interest and are picked up by a special camera that codes the positions. The other type of system is an optoelectric system, which uses a video system to scan the field for a marker. The markers are placed on anatomical points of interest. If a marker is detected in the video field, *x* and *y* coordinates are determined. A temporal history of the marker is obtained by sequentially scanning the video frames. Optoelectric systems are costly, require engineering and computer support, and their accuracy and reliability have not yet been fully established. However, the advantages of these systems suggest that they will become the preferred method for measuring joint and body translations. Patient encumbrance is minimal and data reduction time is short since computers can collect and analyze the data. In some instances, the data are available by the end of the evaluation session.

The technology of imaging techniques is rapidly advancing; therefore, statements of advantages and disadvantages have temporal limitations. If kinematics are to be observed for more than one joint or more than one plane of motion, data reduction is obtained most efficiently for all of these techniques with the aid of costly computer assistance. Multiple views of the same joint are often required even if only one plane of motion is of interest to insure that joint displacement is not obscured by arm swing or the presence of an assistive device. Multiple views also correct for distortion if the motion is not parallel to or in front of the camera lens. This occurs, for instance, when sagittal knee motion is measured in a patient with internal rotation and adduction of the hip. Multiple views require multiple cameras; this can be costly. Multiple cameras also simultaneously measure more than one side of the body. Movie and video systems often require increased lighting, whereas multiple exposure techniques require diminished lighting or strobe lights to "freeze" motion. Neither of these conditions simulates the natural environment.

Of all of these devices designed to quantify kinematic performance, the electrogoniometer and the video system are the objective measurement instruments most frequently used. The electrogoniometer is commonly used to measure sagittal excursion in one joint, whereas video recordings provide a permanent record of the patient's performance. In this way, the clinician can examine a visual record of ambulation before and after treatment. A systematic visual observation, using one of the check lists, can be performed from the video recording. Viewing a video record repeatedly rather than having the patient walk repeatedly permits the examiner more time to evaluate performance without fatiguing the patient. Video-taping gives the therapist more time to observe the performance. *Variables used to describe the performance still must be carefully selected and the reliability of the selected measures still must be established.*

The primary information derived from kinematic variables has been descriptive. For example, joint displacement data has been used to measure the difference between normal and abnormal performance and to describe the difference that occurs in performance as a result of treatment. There is little information in the clinical literature regarding the neurological or biomechanical mechanisms responsible for the production of abnormal gait patterns. Because the displacement patterns of body segments are interdependent, studies should focus on the compensatory mechanisms used to maintain function rather than on the changes in performance that occur at a single joint.

Spatial and Temporal Patterns of Foot Placement. The spatial patterns of foot placement include step or stride length and base of support. The temporal patterns of foot placement include swing time (single support), stance time, double support, stride time, and step or stride rate (cadence). To standardize the use of temporal foot placement variables, Perry and Southerland

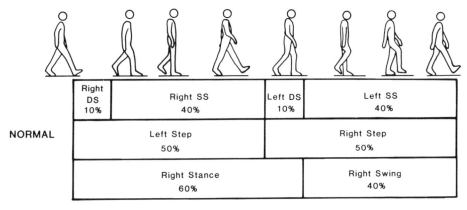

Right DS 10%	Right SS 40%	Left DS 10%	Left SS 40%

NORMAL

Left Step 50%	Right Step 50%

Right Stance 60%	Right Swing 40%

Velocity 1.4 m/s

Fig. 6-2. The pictorial representation characterizes right stride time which in this case encompasses the interval from right heel strike (initial contact) to subsequent right heel-strike (initial contact). The percentages of the stride cycle allotted to the temporal subcomponents at a walking velocity of 1.4 m/s are displayed. This figure represents performance of only one subject; additional data are necessary before the values can be used as a standard data base.

and colleagues recommend that both limbs be referred to throughout the stance and swing phases for the limb of interest.[21,30,31] The stance phase, therefore, becomes subdivided into two double support periods and one single support period; the subsequent swing phase of the limb of interest is the second single support period (Fig. 6-2).

The Functional Ambulation Profile (FAP) is a standardized objective gait evaluation for the clinic. Velocity and cadence measurements are used to assess walking performance. The FAP consists of three phases, progressing from static bilateral stance through independent ambulation. The ambulation test involves asking the patient to walk the length of the parallel bars as quickly as possible. A stopwatch is used to time the task, and the number of steps is counted. Instructions have been carefully prepared for conducting the test to ensure reliability; test–retest reliability for healthy subjects ranged from .90 to .99. Validity and reliability for patient populations has not been documented.

Reports that described the spatial and temporal variables separately for the left and right limbs could not be found in the literature. There are apparently no criteria that can be used to determine whether performance between limbs is symmetrical. In addition, there is a lack of actual step-length measurements, since instrumentation has only recently been developed to measure this variable efficiently. The older reports "derived" stride and step lengths and stride and step times by dividing the total distance walked by the time required to travel that distance and the number of steps or strides taken.

Each investigator in such studies attempts to define and normalize step length uniquely. Step length is dependent upon anthropomorphic characteristics, e.g., a short person usually demonstrates a shorter step length than a tall person.[33,34] Therefore, step length has been divided by the subject's height and has been reported as a percent of that height.[33] Other investigators feel that leg length is a more functional normalization factor than subject height; they report step length as some percent of leg length.[34-36] In addition, there are investigators who have attempted to describe the relationship between weight, height, and step length.[36] No standard method for the measurement leg length has been reported; therefore, the reader is cautioned to examine carefully the methodology of a study before using the results as a normal reference for clinical gait analysis.

The evaluation of the spatial and temporal components of patterns of footfall have gained increased acceptance as a clinical tool. Progress in ambulatory recovery can be objectively measured with these variables. The variables appear sensitive enough to indicate lower extremity disability and to reflect change in the ambulatory pattern that is a result of therapeutic intervention. Because a stride encompasses both a left and right step, any asymmetrical performance, particularly in patients, can be masked by a single stride measurement. Step time and step length rather than stride time and stride length are the variables that should be measured if the degree of asymmetrical performance between limbs is of interest.

Until recently, methods of measuring spatial or temporal data have required a compromise; spatial and temporal data were rarely measured simultaneously. A commonly used clinical method to obtain spatial data involves recording of an imprint of some part of the subject's foot. Such measurement techniques have included inked shoes and paper,[37,38] chalked shoes and a black rubber mat, oiled shoes and absorbent paper,[39,40] walking over thin metal foil that retains the impressions of the feet,[41] and use of a commercially available carbon paper system (Notecare, Inc). Recently, it was suggested that a felt-tipped marker attached to the back of each shoe could mark each foot contact on paper taped to the floor.[42] Data reduction with these techniques involves manual measurement of spatial patterns and tends to be awkward and time-consuming. However, the instrumentation is inexpensive and readily available; the data can be collected in 10 minutes, and can be examined or reduced later.

Temporal measurement schemes often use electrical contact systems to record the contact of the foot with the floor. One such system incorporates a microprocessor to aid in data reduction.[43] Other systems use switches inside the shoes to detect the timing of the foot contact.[44,45] None of these systems provides actual spatial information. Stride length or step lengths are reported as derived values rather than as measured values. Cinematographic, video, and time-lapse photographic methods have also been used because both spatial and temporal gait parameters can be obtained.[46] However, if these are the only variables to be measured, such methods require expensive equipment, substantial time for data reduction and for photographic techniques, and time and expense for film processing. More recent devices provide simultaneous measurement of both temporal and spatial parameters.[47-49] Location and contact pressure sensitive switches can be used to monitor footfall timing. The switches

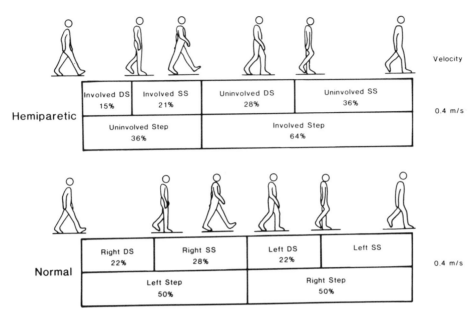

Fig. 6-3. The temporal components of footfall patterns for a patient with hemiparesis and a "normal" subject are illustrated. Please note that these data represent average performance for two subjects. The normal subject walked at the same velocity as the patient. At comfortable walking velocities (1.2 to 1.5 m/s), each swing phase (single support for the other lower extremity) usually requires approximately 40 percent of the stride cycle. At l0.4 m/s, the same temporal component represents only 28 percent of the gait cycle for the normal subject. Comparison of both subject's performance at the slow walking velocity (0.4 m/s) suggests that an inadequate time is spent during involved limb single support and that too much time is spent during uninvolved single support for the patient. Such information would not have been apparent if the patient's performance at 0.4 m/s had been compared to the normal standard (1.2 to 1.5 m/s).

are embedded in the walking surface so that there is minimal or no patient encumbrance. A microprocessor is used to collect and reduce the data so that the spatial and temporal parameters of foot placement are available within a few minutes of data collection.

Optimal performance is commonly assumed to be a symmetrical foot placement pattern within a velocity range of 1.2 to 1.5 m/s and with a step rate of 1.6 to 2.0 steps per second (100 to 120 steps per minute). This is the most energy-efficient range for normals and the most cosmetically pleasing.[15] The length and timing of each step serve as overall indicators of ambulation. Foot placement variables indicate whether change occurs over the course of treatment (Fig. 6-3). The patterns of foot contact are the final outcome of the collective motions of all the major segments contributing to ambulation. Thus, foot placement and temporal factors can indicate overall function including compensatory mechanisms. Kinematic data can then be used to identify the individual contributing factors.

Kinetic Analysis

As was described in the last section, kinematics describe the movements without regard to the forces that produce movement. The kinetic analysis of body motion involves examination of the relationship between displacement, velocity, and acceleration. A gait evaluation that yields only kinematic measurements can be used to classify the degree of locomotor impairment and generate baseline data. A combination of kinematic variables and force measurements provides an assessment of function that can be related to the integrity of the musculoskeletal system.

There are very few gait studies that also describe the clinical characteristics of a sample of patients being studied. Without clinical information, the clinician does not know if the patient who is being observed in the clinic is similar to those described in a study or if the changes being described are characteristic of several types of patient groups.

There have been some attempts to identify correlations between kinematic parameters of gait and the results of standard clinical tests, particularly muscle strength and joint ROM tests. Gyory et al found no correlation between passive range of motion at the knee and the range used during locomotion in subjects with arthritis.[3] However, a correlation between quadriceps strength and sagittal plane knee motion and stride length in patients with rheumatoid arthritis was reported. The correlation was not reported but the significance of the correlation was at a level of $P<.01$. Maximum isometric quadriceps strength was measured by a compression–tension transducer attached to the ankle with subject supine and the knee flexed to 35°. Stauffer et al also suggested that isometric muscle strength might be a major determinant of gait patterns in normals and subjects with arthritic knees.[50]

In an attempt to identify simple clinical tests to predict locomotor function, Oatis has proposed that the knee joint complex behaves as a damped spring during locomotion. This concept led her to suggest clinical parameters that could distinguish functional differences between normal young and old men and could also be used to predict the flexion and extension movements of the knee during normal locomotion.[51] The lower extremity was modeled as a simple mechanical system consisting of two rigid links, one representing the thigh and the other the leg–foot complex. The articulation between the rigid links was modeled as a torsional spring with a viscous damper. Six young men and four older men underwent tests to determine the stiffness and damping coefficients of the knee. The frequency and decay of the oscillations of the knee were monitored with an electrogoniometer when the limb was dropped from full extension and allowed to swing passively. Isometric and isokinetic knee extension torques were measured with a Cybex II dynamometer. The gait patterns were examined with high-speed cinematography and the recorded knee motions were compared with those predicted by the model. Preliminary data show significant stiffness differences between the young and the old subject sample. An inverse correlation was seen between quadriceps torque and stiffness. Last, the model appeared to predict the behavior of the knee during the swing and the early stance phase of gait. If these measures also distinguish between normal and patient performance, a simple clinical test may eventually be developed that can predict walking performance and therefore reduce the need for some sophisticated gait analysis equipment.

Torque Measurement. Until more specific clinical tests such as that proposed by Oatis are developed, the relationship between standard clinical measures of performance and ambulation must be more clearly defined, using kinematic and kinetic variables. Laboratory investigations that have examined kinetic variables support the clinical assumption that assessment of the body under static conditions does not necessarily reflect or predict function under dynamic conditions. Winter and Robertson stress the lack of correlation between the force responsible for production of movement in a controlled experiment, e.g., flexion and extension of the knee, and the forces used during gait.[52] The differences in forces required by the two conditions may be attributed to adjacent limb segments.

In gait, the forces caused by acceleration of limbs, as well as the effects of gravity and muscle force are the forces that influence joint motion. Therefore, an evaluation of the muscle's ability to generate and control joint movement and forward progression may be a more meaningful indicator of that muscle's ability to assist in ambulatory function than are isolated tests of muscle strength and active joint ROM. Perhaps this statement is best illustrated by considering knee extension during terminal swing in the patient with an above-knee amputation. Static testing will demonstrate the patient's inability to extend a prosthesis actively. However, the static evaluation will not assess the patient's ability to control the knee when using hip movement during walking. The dynamic event, therefore, bears little resemblance to the static test.

Kinetic analysis of movement is primarily a research tool because it requires sophisticated and highly technical data analysis. However, recent technological advances in the measurement of displacement and computer-based data processing should make the transfer of this measurement scheme to the clinical setting feasible in the future. Now, however, clinical gait analysis of kinetic variables is primarily limited to a description of ground reaction forces.

Ground Reaction Measurement. The ground reaction force is the resultant force applied by the body to the ground. Thus, it is the sum of the static load or weight and the dynamic load caused by the body's acceleration. Typical force data for a normal subject walking at a comfortable velocity are shown in Figure 6-4. The three coordinates of the ground reaction force indicate the normal progression of the body over the foot at a comfortable velocity. The magnitude of the force component is a function of body weight, the speed of walking, and the nature of the gait itself. The peak values of the force components are usually expressed as a percentage of the person's body weight.

Carlsoo et al examined the ground reaction forces of 10 patients with hemiparesis and seven patients with intermittent claudication.[53] Among the findings that they reported were three distinct types of walking that were distinguished among the patients with hemiparesis by the characteristics of the vertical-force curve. One gait produced a vertical-force curve that was similar to the normal

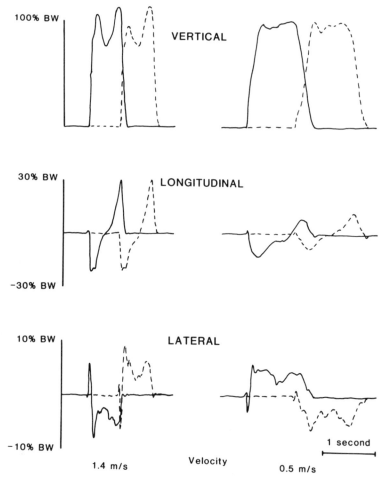

Fig. 6-4. Typical force data for a normal subject walking at a comfortable velocity (1.4 m/s) and at a slow velocity (0.5 m/s) are illustrated. The three coordinates of the ground reaction force have been normalized to the subject's body weight. Note the change in the shape of the force curves and the decrease in the amount of force that accompanies a decrease in walking speed.

gait illustrated for the normal walking velocity depicted in Figure 6-4. A second category of gait produced a force curve that remained relatively constant during the whole support phase without the two crests and intermediate trough. This was similar to the slow velocity curve of the normal subject as depicted in Figure 6-4. The third force pattern increased rapidly towards a maximum force value, and then rapidly decreased back to zero at a rate not consistent with the walking velocity. The peak magnitude of the vertical force was less than body weight for all 10 subjects with hemiparesis. Examining the character of the curve for the involved limb and the uninvolved limb suggested that patients were unable or unwilling to load and unload both limbs at the same rate with the same amount of force for the same duration.

Leiper et al monitored selected kinetic variables and temporal-distance measures of footfall to describe walking performance throughout the time when 14 persons were first learning to use below-knee prostheses.[54] This study was the beginning of an attempt to develop a data base for "typical" acquisition of gait by patients with unilateral below-knee amputations. Among the variables selected to describe the walking pattern were average walking velocity and peak vertical ground reaction force. The force was normalized to each person's body weight. The average walking velocity and the peak vertical force increased over treatment days (Fig. 6-5). The increase in peak force on the prosthetic limb reflected both an increase in walking velocity and an increased confidence in the device. Bilateral step lengths, step times, and single and double support times were also monitored. Statistically significant changes were reported between initial and discharge performance for all variables except peak vertical force on the sound leg, sound leg single support and the involved limb double support time. Evaluation of walking performance throughout the treatment period provides information related to the rate of recovery as well as the quality of recovery. The preliminary study of Leiper described different recovery rates for the 14 patients.[54] If these results continue to be found with large sample sizes, the clinician may have a method to predict total recovery time realistically.

The basic measurement device used to determine the external forces exerted by the body is a force transducer, which provides an electric signal proportional to a force (see Chapter 3). Although there are several kinds of force transducers, most are designed to measure force when a strain is produced within the instrument. Transducers have been developed that can be surgically implanted to measure directly the force borne on a joint surface.[55] However, clinical tools must reflect this force indirectly. A kinematic description of limb displacement and the ability to measure resultant external forces provide the information necessary to calculate joint-reaction forces and to infer muscle moments by applying standard theories of Newtonian mechanics, i.e., writing and solving the equations of motion.

EMG Measurement. There has long been interest in the contributions of specific muscles to physical activity.[56] Some investigators have palpated muscles while subjects walked in order to decipher the phasic activity of muscles during the gait cycle. With the advent of EMG, characterization of muscle activity became more sophisticated. As a result, EMG has become an important tool in studying physical activities.

The phasic activities of the eight major muscle groups of the lower extremity during walking were defined by Eberhart et al.[57] Recently, Hagy et al examined the 30 individual muscles that comprised these groups.[58] General agreement about the timing and levels of activity of these muscles exists among investigators.[59-63] Differences among investigations may result from the use of different data collection systems by the various investigators. The sensitivity

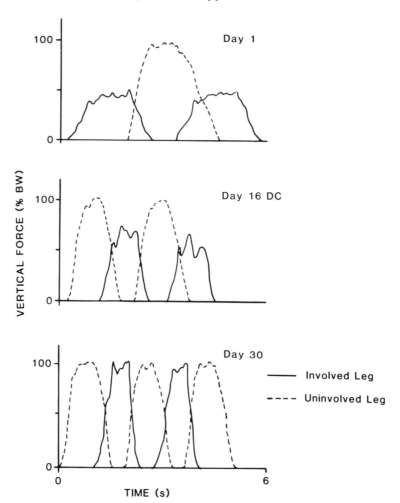

Fig. 6-5. Vertical force data are illustrated for both extremities of a patient with a below-knee amputation.[54] Performance is shown for the first day he walked with his prosthesis, and 16 and 30 days later. Parallel bars were available for assistance as required. Note the increased amount of force and the increased rate of force application that occurred during this time. The shorter time for each stance phase and the increased number of steps reflect an increased walking velocity and cadence, respectively. The involved and uninvolved double support phases also became more symmetrical; double support time is indicated by the intervals of involved and uninvolved limb overlap.

of the instruments can account for reported variations in both the timing and amplitude of the EMG signal.

The descriptions of muscle activity during locomotion remain unchallenged after almost 100 years of investigation. Specifically, *muscles are normally active through very short time periods*—seven-tenths of a second or less. In fact, there are moments in the gait cycle when only minimal muscle activity is observed, implying that much of the motion of the lower extremity is accomplished by inertia or momentum transferred by adjacent limbs. The timing of the muscle activity also leads one to believe that the roles of muscular contraction during walking are primarily those of stabilization and deceleration of the limb. Plantar flexors are primarily responsible for acceleration of the body through activity in midstance and terminal stance. EMG investigation has actually provided the rather startling observation that *muscles are primarily the controlling rather than the propulsive factors in human locomotion.* EMG has been used clinically for defining "out-of-phase" muscle activity in neuropathologies. EMG when used in kinetic analysis, can shed some light on muscle forces.

The reader should be cautioned that data acquisition techniques can influence EMG results (see Ch. 10). There are a wide variety of techniques used in EMG investigations. Electrode type is one source of variation. In kinesiological studies, the choice is essentially between surface and wire electrodes; the literature is replete with examples of occasions in which each type was used.[57,64] It is clear that *the greatest advantage to the surface electrodes is comfort for the subject; it also provides a description of a muscle group's contribution,* e.g., the quadriceps. *The advantage of the wire electrode is greater precision in the ability to monitor a portion of specific muscle,* such as the vastus medialis, but the small area sampled by the wire is a limitation. It is not clear whether data from one type of electrode rather than another are any more clinically valid.

EMG data may also be affected by electrode placement. The amplitude of an EMG signal is influenced by electrode placement[65,66] with a maximum occurring approximately at the center of the muscle belly; few authors precisely describe electrode placement, however. Theoretically, the amplitude of EMG is maximized when the electrode is placed parallel with the muscle fibers and over the bulk of the muscle where there are the largest number of motor units. To insure that the optimal signal is recorded from each subject, electrodes should be similarly placed for all subjects.

After electrode placement, the electrodes are attached in a variety of ways to amplifiers and data collection systems. Because the EMG signal is so small, on the order of 0.5 to 300 mV in kinesiological studies, most investigators have resorted to preamplification to increase the signal-noise ratio. This preamplification may be in each individual electrode[64] or in a central preamplifier for all electrodes. The means of relaying the data between the electrode and the collection system also varies. Hard-wired systems have the disadvantage of requiring encumbering trailing cables, which may interfere with the subject's normal gait pattern.[2] Multichannel biotelemetry systems are being used in several facilities to reduce the constraints applied to the subject by cumbersome apparatus.[2,59,67,68]

Finally, various approaches have been used to quantify the signals obtained in an EMG study. The International Society of Electrophysiological Kinesiology has published a monograph that urges a standard for data collection and reporting of EMG results.[69] The choices range from a subjective analysis of the raw data, to point counting of action potentials, to an analysis of the integrated signal, the last being most frequently used by gait investigators.[2] A variety of low- and high-pass filters are employed to decrease noise. Any of the above techniques have the capacity to demonstrate average amplitude of the signal plotted against time. This is then often compared with the subject's maximal EMG signal elicited by an isometric contraction.[2] Unfortunately, no correlation between EMG amplitude and muscle power has been delineated that is consistent across muscles except for isometric contractions, where $r = .99$ for within-subject correlations.[70] At present, quantification of EMG signals is merely a sophisticated on/off signal. The frequency with which EMG is used in gait laboratories indicates a strong sentiment in favor of its usefulness. Precise definition of abnormal phasic activity in neuropathic disorders has been helpful in prescribing surgical procedures or other therapeutic techniques.[67,68,71,72] EMG data is also essential in a kinetic analysis of gait. Theoretically, by calculating the total force around a joint and the external forces acting on that joint, one can calculate the total muscle force; this can then be related to electromyographic data in an attempt to derive an approximation of the contribution each muscle makes during the gait cycle.[70,73] However, methods for identifying the role played by individual muscles in dynamic tasks such as walking are still being developed. This complicated task requires understanding of each muscle's role in maintaining stability and providing propulsive force.[74]

In summary, insight into the net effect of muscle activity on the production of a movement can be gained with kinetic analysis. A laboratory equipped to provide a kinetic analysis can determine the contribution of the various forces that are acting on the joint to produce movement. These forces include gravitational forces, external (ground reaction) forces, and muscle forces. A kinetic analysis can be used to determine the efficiency of the transfer of potential energy to kinetic energy for a limb or for the whole body.

SELECTION OF ANALYTIC TECHNIQUES

Comprehensive gait analysis requires assessment of kinematic and kinetic variables; however, the equipment necessary to measure ambulatory performance can be extensive. A complete list or description of instruments available to measure ambulation variables is difficult to present because the rapid growth of technology quickly makes any list rapidly obsolete. However, *the clinician interested in developing an objective method for gait evaluation should observe some criteria for the selection of instrumentation.* First and foremost, *the goal of the assessment must be defined.* Only then may more practical issues be addressed. In a presentation at the national meeting of the American Physical Therapy Association in June, 1982, Cook provided questions that clinicians should consider before purchasing equipment to assess ambulatory performance.

1. Is the instrumentation valid and reliable? Does the equipment consistently measure the variable of interest with reasonable accuracy? Is the sampling rate of the recording equipment consistent with sampling theorem? Does the instrumentation superimpose noise on the true signal?

2. Does the instrumentation encumber the patient? Does the weight or bulk of the measurement tool alter the subject's ability to ambulate?

3. What is the equipment application time? Do the donning and calibration processes fatigue the subject before the actual measurement can be taken?

4. What is the space required for the instruments? Because space in most physical therapy departments is usually scarce, where will a measurement system be placed if it requires a 20-m length of uncluttered space or a walkway?

5. What is the cost of the equipment? Equipment and operating costs must be considered. The initial cost of the equipment may be low, but supplies may be expensive and an engineer may be required to maintain the equipment.

6. How are the data recorded? If data are stored on chart recorder paper, is there adequate storage space for the rolls of paper?

7. What is the data reduction time? The initial costs of instrumentation may be low, but 24 hours may be required to reduce the data manually for a single subject. This time requirement limits the number of subjects on whom data can be collected or necessitates a large support staff to keep up with the data reduction.

8. What are staff requirements? Is a computer program required? Is an engineer necessary to maintain the equipment? Can the instrumentation be controlled by one operator or is there a need for more personnel?

These questions should assist individuals interested in purchasing equipment. The questions also should be considered by clinicians who are trying to evaluate conclusions drawn from gait studies. Conclusions cannot be critically examined unless the type of instrumentation is considered. For example, Finley et al reported that the velocity of healthy young women walking at their preferred speed was 0.9 m/s, whereas Murray reported an average walking velocity of 1.3 m/s for women of the same ages.[17,75] Finley et al required subjects to walk on an elevated platform above the level of the floor. Subjects wore electrogoniometers bilaterally to measure sagittal plane motions at the hip, knee, and ankle. Murray's subjects walked on a level surface while wearing black tights that had white strips of material identifying the long bones of the lower extremity. A strobe light was used to freeze many images of the subject on one frame of film. The two situations are so different that it is not surprising that the results differed. Therefore, it is important to recognize the constraints that measurement methods may place on subjects and how this may affect performance.

STANDARDS

If gait evaluations can accomplish all of the purposes outlined and if there are a variety of available measurement tools, why is there a dearth of clinical literature that assesses the quality of a patient's locomotor performance?[76] In

1953, Steindler claimed that gait analysis had become a guide for clinical practice and an "effective adviser" in difficult and controversial situations.[77] There is very little evidence to indicate that gait evaluations have actually achieved this level of sophistication. The bulk of the clinical literature describes some aspect of healthy human walking performance or details an easy-to-use clinical technique for gait evaluation. Perhaps gait evaluations are seldom used in treatment planning because there are inadequate standards, and they are therefore not sensitive for discriminating pathology from normal variations caused by factors such as sex, age, and walking speed. This section will address the use of standards (i.e., criteria) in an attempt to account for the gap between Steindler's dream for the use of gait analysis[77] and the present clinical reality.

Normal Standards

Clearly the most common clinical use of gait analysis is the comparison of patient performance with standards or criteria that have been derived from normal subjects, and classification of patients based on their "gait deviations." This approach was probably inspired by the classic work of Eberhart et al that compared the gait of patients with amputations with that of a matched group of normal subjects.[4] Most advocates of judging patient performance based on normal performance forget, however, that *Eberhart's group had an underlying concept that guided the comparison,* specifically to consider how prosthetic design and management might return those with amputations to normal gait. *Only with a specific concept in mind and only with the use of the appropriate standards can comparisons really be useful.*

If the purpose of the gait evaluation is to describe how a patient's performance differs from "normal," an accurate assessment requires that all differences between the patient's performance and the standard result from the patient's disability. Factors such as height, weight, and shoe type alter the walking performance of healthy subjects.[33,34,75,78] There is also ample evidence to suggest that women demonstrate a higher cadence and shorter single support time than anthropomorphically similar men walking at the same speed.[17,33,75] *Therefore, any standard used to judge a patient's performance must include a description of anthropomorphic characteristics as well as the sex of the subjects examined to generate the standard. Additional factors that should be considered in comparing a normal standard to a patient's performance are age, level of maturation, and walking velocity.*

Clinical observational gait evaluations often use the data from Eberhart et al or Murray et al for use as "normal" standards for the assessment of body translation or joint rotation.[7,21,22,79] However, the original intent of the Eberhart and Murray studies was not to develop a normal data base. The sample sizes were too small, confidence intervals were not developed to predict a range of normal performance, and distributions were never plotted. Ten healthy young men with a mean age of 22 years were evaluated by Eberhart. Although Murray described the kinematics of the lower extremities for subjects of both sexes over a wider age range,[16,46,75,80] the data which are most commonly used clinically were collected from 30 healthy young men ranging in age from 20 to 65 years.[46] Therefore, for example, if a list of gait deviations is developed for an 80-year-old patient using the Murray or Eberhart data, the usefulness of the results would be highly questionable.

Age. Age of subjects must be considered when a data base is selected for use as a standard. Both the aging process and maturation are issues that merit attention. The clinical literature describes a number of age-related gait alterations.[81-84] Murray observed an increased cadence and shortened step length when eight men over the age of 80 years were compared to younger men.[16] Although the majority of quantitative descriptions support an age-related difference in walking,[16,32,19,86-90] a few studies have reported the lack of a relationship.[17,91,91] The disparate findings could result from the fact that in some of the studies the geriatric population may not have been old enough or could have been caused by the inadequacy of the protocols in assessing locomotor capability. Comfortable walking speed was the only walking velocity examined by investigators who reported no age-related differences in walking. Results from a recent study indicate that age-dependent differences in locomotion are minimized when subjects walk at "comfortable" or free walking speed.[93] However, when subjects were asked to demonstrate their range of walking velocities, subjects with a mean age of 70 years were unable to walk as fast (0.3 to 1.6 m/s) as subjects with a mean age of 25 years (0.3 to 2.1 m/s).

Therefore, if the standard selected to compare performance of a 68-year-old, 5 foot tall woman who recovered successfully from a hip fracture and who is walking at 0.7 m/s is derived from a 22-year-old, six-foot-tall man who is walking at 1.2 m/s, then *walking may be erroneously labeled abnormal. Clinicians must select an appropriate data base for comparisons or face the possibility of stating incorrectly that a patient has gait deviations.*

Level of maturation is another variable one must consider when evaluating children. The time frame for the acquisition of the adult walking pattern in children is an area in which normal standards are still being developed.[94-98] Objective gait measurements of children have only recently been attempted, and an adequate sample has not been surveyed. Thus, there is no normative data base. However, research to date has indicated that the gait pattern is age-dependent. This confirms that walking is a behavior that reflects maturation.[96-98] If the quality of walking performance is used as a tool for monitoring treatment progress, as well as an indication of delayed motor development, the following must be considered: (1) gait pattern changes that are dependent on CNS maturation should be distinguished from those that are stature dependent, and (2) gait pattern changes that occur because of therapeutic intervention must be distinguished from those that are dependent on maturation.

The relationship between age and changes in the temporal and distance measurements of foot placement and ground reaction forces in 51 healthy children was described by Beck et al.[98] Children less than 4 years of age demonstrated growth-related gait pattern changes when the test–retest interval was longer than 3 months. The interval between growth related changes is relevant to the clinician who uses gait analysis to assess children before and after treatment. Changes in gait may be inappropriately attributed to treatment when they result, in fact, from maturation. Beck et al reported variations resulting apparently from maturation in velocity, stride length, cadence, stance time, double and single support times, and ground reaction forces. Some of the changes in these variables were also related to changes in stature. For example, when normalized to the child's height, the length of the stride was 76 percent of the child's height regardless of age. In contrast, the peak vertical ground reaction force was 1.37 times body weight for the youngest children and 1.13 times body weight in the 4- to 5-year-old group. Therefore, if normalized to height, stride length can serve as a monitor of treatment progress regardless of maturational level. It appears, however, that the vertical ground reaction force may be a sensitive indicator of CNS maturation for children under the age of 5 years. This study indicates that the effect of maturation on walking performance should be accounted for if pre- and posttreatment gait evaluations are performed. This study also indicates that, depending on the purpose of the evaluation, one gait variable may be more sensitive than another for measuring changes in behavior.

Velocity. The velocity dependence of gait variables is too often neglected in studies that select a data base of healthy subjects to examine the effect of pathology on walking performance. There are many reports in the literature indicating that patients walk more slowly than healthy subjects. For example, Gabel et al reported that preoperative total hip patients walked more slowly, with a slower cadence and a shorter stride length and swing time, than age-matched normals.[80-87] The healthy sample consisted of 140 subjects with 20 subjects in each of 7 age decades. The subjects were instructed to walk at free walking speed. Although this study aids in distinguishing between healthy and abnormal performance, it does not help to determine if hip pathology limits walking speed or if hip pathology reduces speed as well as alters step timing or stepping mechanics. A velocity-matched standard may have provided a more sensitive indication of the effect of hip pathology on walking ability.

The velocity dependence of a variety of gait variables in a "normal" sample has been documented.[4,19,33,35,93,99-102] For example, step length and cadence vary linearly with average walking speed, whereas single and double support times are inversely proportional to walking speed. Average swing phase flexion excursion was 44°, 64°, and 25° at the hip, knee, and ankle, respectively, when five healthy young subjects walked at 1.5 m/s and 26°, 43°, and 17° when the subjects walked at 0.4 m/s.[101] The EMG activity recorded from muscles of the lower extremity also decreases with a decrease in walking speed. The velocity-dependence of joint excursion is supported by numerous investigators.[4,32,34] Ground reaction forces also display velocity dependence. For example, Andriacchi et al reported that one component of the vertical-force curve varied from 90 ± 12.4 percent of body weight at slow gait to 150 ± 12.4 percent of body weight at fast gait.[102]

The problem of comparing a healthy normal person walking at comfortable speed with patients walking more slowly is exemplified by the studies of Knutsson and Richards.[8–10] The ambulatory ability of patients with hemiparesis was assessed by comparing the patients' performances with those of "normal" subjects walking at a free speed. Peat et al used a similar paradigm.[68] Knutsson's and Richards' patients with spastic hemiparesis were subdivided into three categories based on their gait abnormalities. One of the categories was distinguished by an absence or decrease in muscle activity. Similar results were reported by Peat et al. Because EMG amplitude decreases with a reduction in walking speed,[91] it is difficult to determine if the diminished muscle activity reported for the patients was abnormal or merely a speed-dependent observation. The absence of EMG activity may have indicated that patients were unable to develop sufficient muscle activity *or* the diminished muscle activity may have been normal for the patients' velocity. Without the use of a velocity-matched standard, it is impossible to tell which is the case. This has important treatment implications. If a patient is unable to activate muscles, such techniques as EMG biofeedback or functional electrical stimulation may be indicated. However, if the patient is having difficulty changing walking speed, the clinician may elect to work on timing and sequencing instead of just activating isolated muscles.

The velocity dependence of gait variables should be carefully examined when evaluating the integrity of muscles for surgical transfer or release.[63,67,71,72] There is a growing interest in use of EMG analysis as a presurgical tool during the dynamic act of walking instead of during traditional static testing. However, the norms used to judge performance of patients appear to be limited to healthy young subjects walking at free speeds. Perhaps surgical success could be improved through the selection of more appropriate standards.

The results of a study by Smidt and Wadsworth suggest that matching the standard and patient walking speed aids in separating the velocity dependence of the gait variables from other indications of pathology.[103] The performance of 21 patients with hip disease was compared to that of 10 healthy subjects of comparable sex, height, and weight. Unfortunately, there was a disparity in the age of the two samples; the average patient age was 63 years and the average age for the healthy subjects was 32 years. The healthy young sample averaged a free walking speed of 1.28 m/s and a slow speed (e.g., a stroll) of 0.47 m/s. Because the data are limited to mean performance and no inferential statistics were used to compare performance, it is not possible to determine if there were group differences. The trend of the data suggests that, at similar walking velocities, patients took more strides and shorter strides than did subjects in the healthy sample. The rate of vertical force application to the involved extremity also appeared slower and the maximum vertical force applied appeared less than that demonstrated by the healthy subjects walking at comparable speeds.

Figure 6-6 illustrates the need to consider walking velocity when comparing performance of patients and normals. Velocity matching of patients with hemiparesis with normal subjects allows the clinician to separate the effect of a slower speed on gait variables from other indications of pathology. However, identification of the velocity-dependent variables does not leave a residual per-

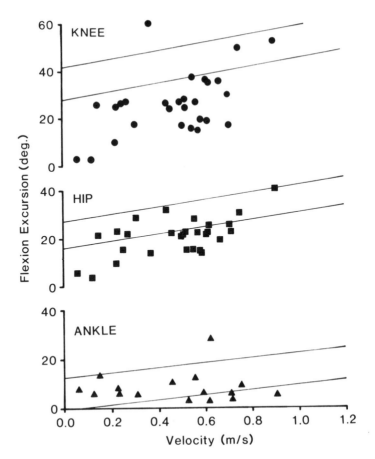

Fig. 6-6. This figure represents the average amount of flexion excursion which occurred during swing and the average walking velocity demonstrated by 28 patients with hemiparesis. The duration of the hemiparesis ranged from 3 months to 9 years. Ankle excursion data was not collected for subjects who wore an ankle–foot orthosis. The area between the two lines on each graph represents one SD for the mean flexion excursion demonstrated by six age- and sex-matched normal volunteers. Velocity-matched comparisons between the normal sample and the patients suggests that the patients demonstrated both inadequate hip knee flexion excursion. These kinds of results should encourage the clinician to focus on the inadequacy of the entire lower extremity rather than limiting focus to the ankle.

formance that can be directly related to pathology. For example, the gait deviations presented in the patients with hip disease in the Smidt and Wadsworth study are not necessarily indicative of hip pathology. The same gait performance deviations may have occurred in any patient who had pain in the lower extremity and walked with an antalgic gait. If the gait assessment is to yield information that guides treatment, the standard must be appropriate, e.g., velocity-matched, and the results of the treatment must be related to the disability.

Attempts to relate walking performance and clinical symptoms assist in addressing the following issues: (1) the specific effect that pathology has on walking ability; (2) the ability to determine the severity of involvement; and (3) the ability to differentiate among types of pathology.

Andriacchi et al examined the effect of pathology on the walking ability of 16 patients who were examined before and after knee surgery. Twenty knees were treated with total joint replacements and three were treated with high tibial osteotomies. Using a velocity-matched standard, it was observed that patients walked with a shorter step length and a higher cadence than did the normal subjects. Among the temporal parameters measured, swing time was the best indicator of gait abnormalities in the patients; 84 percent of the swing-time observations for the patients were "abnormal." Repeated observations of the patients after surgery indicated a shift in the step length and swing time towards normal. The improved gait was related to clinical improvement of the knee joint. The results indicate that controlling extraneous variables such as walking speed and monitoring clinical changes increases the usefulness of the gait evaluation. Clinical observations often consist of lists of gait deviations, which include those that are velocity dependent. By considering the effect of speed, the examiner has measures that can indicate the effect of pathology on performance and that may therefore suggest specific objectives for therapeutic intervention.

The increased sensitivity of the gait evaluation in identification of deviations that relate to clinical pathology when the velocity of the standard is matched has been demonstrated in a study of 22 patients with total knee replacements, 20 patients with total hip replacements, and 14 age-matched healthy subjects.[104] All patients had a successful clinical result after a minimum of 12 months following surgery had elapsed. Deformity, joint stability, passive ROM, and a subjective assessment of pain were used to assess clinical success. The data indicated that the hip patients recovered a more normal gait than did the knee patients. This indication is an assumption because no statistical analysis was performed. The stride length for the hip patients was apparently normal, but the knee patients demonstrated common features that seemed indicative of an abnormal use of the extensor mechanism of the knee: shorter than normal stride length, less than normal knee flexion at midstance, and an abnormal pattern of flexion–extension moments at the knee. Gait abnormalities were also found in hip patients based on the location of the reconstructed joint center. If the distance between the hip joint center and the line of action of the abductor muscles had been shortened during surgery, the gait was normal; if the distance was not surgically shortened, the patients demonstrated a shorter than normal stride length, reduced hip flexion–extension motion, and a higher than normal hip flexion moment. Although the causes of gait abnormalities were not addressed in this study, the results suggest a mechanical cause; thus, a reevaluation of the design and installation criteria for the prostheses seems warranted. If the healthy reference had not been age and velocity-matched, the pathology-specific deviations would not have been detected. Rather, both patient groups would have been reported to walk more slowly than normal.

Although the study just cited evaluated surgical success, a similar approach could be used to examine patients before and after any type of treatment. It is hoped that future studies will describe the variability of performance as well as the mean of performance so that predictors can be developed for normal and abnormal performance.

Assistive Device. What if the patient walks with an assistive device? The normal standard is no longer appropriate because the sequencing of foot placement is different. There have been several attempts to examine the manner in which healthy subjects walk with assistive devices. Smidt and Mommens developed an approach for describing the gait of people using assistive devices and reported data for assisted gait patterns from a sample of 25 young adults.[105] As expected, the healthy subjects walked more slowly when using devices than they did without the devices. The vertical acceleration of the body was greater when subjects used the devices. The increased acceleration suggested an increased vertical loading on some structures of the body as subjects attempted to reduce forces on one lower extremity. These findings demonstrate the differences that occur when a patient is walking with an assistive device and the need to select appropriate standards (criteria) for assessing patient performance.

Another issue raised by the study of Smidt and Mommens deals with the issue of practice. If the gait evaluation is performed to assess the adequacy of performance with an assistive device, then the sample of subjects examined should consist of subjects who are familiar with the use of the device. It is possible that practice with the assistive devices might have increased walking velocity and diminished the increase in vertical acceleration in the naive sample described in this study.

Murray et al assessed veteran cane users to develop reference values for evaluating the use of assistive devices during walking. The forces applied to the canes were examined in 53 disabled men who had predominately unilateral lower extremity problems.[106] Differences in the amplitudes and in the configurations of the force patterns were found among patients with different disabilities. The amplitude and patterns of force application both appeared to relate to the severity of the locomotor disability. For example, a patient with paralysis agitans applied only 1 kg of force to the cane, apparently using the cane as a "feeler." In contrast, a patient with septic arthritis of the knee applied 28 kg of force, apparently in an attempt to reduce weight-bearing on the painful extremity. The cane was used differently depending on the type of disability and severity of involvement. Therefore, *comparison of the way in which healthy subjects walk with assistive devices with the performance of patients may be inappropriate.* Improvement in walking performance could be more appropriately judged if the patient served as his own control or if the patient's performance was compared to a group of patients with a similar disability—or even if performance was evaluated relative to the alterations that were kinesiologically useful.

Standards Derived from Patients

An investigator who is interested in describing the effect of CNS pathology on the control of movement may legitimately select a normal group for comparison. However, the use of a normal standard for clinical gait evaluation may not describe *functional deficits*. For example, the goal of treatment for a patient with rheumatoid arthritis who has just received pharmacologic relief of acute knee pain is often restoration of the function that was lost due to the acute pain. Gait evaluation is one means of evaluating the efficacy of the treatment (restoration of function). The standard used to examine the effect of treatment on managing acute pain should not be derived from an age-matched normal group. Because the patient had rheumatoid arthritis, gait deviations were probably present before the acute episode. If normal performance is the standard, the scale may not be useful for detection of changes in abnormal function. The patient's pretreatment ambulatory status, if known, may be a more useful standard for the evaluation of the treatment's effect. *Changes in the patient's performance may not be noticed when inappropriate standards are used for comparisons.* Appropriate comparisons can be made with data collected from patients with similar disabilities. This could provide a classification of the degree of functional impairment and could establish a realistic goal for functional recovery. There is a need for patient standards that can be used to compare performance; at present, there is a lack of such data.

A study by Takebe and Basmajian demonstrates the potential value of using some types of patients as their own control.[107] Pre- and posttreatment walking performance was measured to evaluate the effect of electrical stimulation (n = 3), intensive conventional therapy (n = 6) or biofeedback and conventional therapy (n = 6) on decreasing foot drop in hemiplegic patients. Joint ROM, single and double support time, and walking velocity were among the variables examined. A case study format rather than a single-case research design was used for reporting results. Therefore, one method of treatment cannot be described as more effective than another in achieving the treatment goal. However, the design of the study provides a useful clinical model, i.e., the comparison of a subject's posttreatment performance with the pretreatment performance.

Use of a normal standard may also be inappropriate if the goal of treatment is a functional gait. *Gait deviations are often adaptive if the goal of treatment is the acquisition of a functional gait. Use of the normal standard may incorrectly label the patient's correct (i.e., adaptive) strategy for improving mobility as a "gait deviation" in need of correction.* The cosmetic appearance of the gait may be irrelevant and the selection of a normal standard will not help in planning a treatment program. In fact, the patient's progress in achieving a functional gait may be hindered if the treatment is directed at making the patient walk "normally" rather than at helping the patient solve a problem in the most efficient manner. For example, is normal ambulation the goal for a person with spastic diplegia or is the goal one of gaining as much independence as possible?

Is the goal for all patients symmetrical, reciprocal, and cosmetically pleasing motions for the lower extremities?

If patient-derived data is selected to aid in evaluating patient performance, descriptors must be detailed so that the therapist can determine if the measured sample matches the characteristics of a specific patient. Ideally, the length and time of therapeutic intervention as well as information such as age, sex, height, weight, and time since onset of injury should be known. Miller conducted a retrospective study of 360 patients with fractures of the hip[108] and determined the outcome in patients with fractures of the hip in terms of survival and ambulation. The assessment scheme defined ambulatory status by describing the patient as: (1) nonambulatory, (2) ambulatory with walker or crutches, or (3) independent. Fifty-one percent of the subjects achieved preinjury ambulatory status 1 year after the injury when classified according to this limited assessment scheme. The authors then identified predictors of ambulatory and nonambulatory performance. These conclusions were based on very limited data, which defined walking ability without any measurement of the performance. The clinical utility of this study would have been markedly enhanced by an objective gait assessment (i.e., something that was reliable) that included descriptions of relevant gait and clinical variables. Such information could then serve as a patient data base and could provide predictors to assist in discriminating among categories of ambulatory performance.

In summary, a major limitation in the current evaluation schemes for gait assessment is the lack of appropriate reference data. There is a lack of standards that can be used to develop realistic goals. Most standards were developed without consideration of such important factors as age, sex, height, weight, and footwear. Current knowledge of "healthy" gait is primarily based on the results of studies on young healthy adults. A comprehensive description of healthy locomotor behavior remains incomplete and unclear. Therefore, a geriatric patient recovering from a hip fracture may not be thought to achieve "optimal" motor performance because performance is compared with a youth-oriented standard rather than because of some pathologic limitation of that patient. Without a velocity-matched data base, the ability to identify the specific effect of a disability on walking performance is limited. Because many gait variables are velocity dependent, comparison of a patient's performance with performance of healthy subjects that are walking faster may only indicate that the patient is walking slowly. If gait assessment is to be a useful clinical tool, the evaluation should not stop with a description of gait deviations. The assessment should proceed to assist in the identification of the causes of gait deviations. This problem-solving process may be enhanced by considering the patient's disability or by comparing the patient's performance with other patients with similar disabilities.

The selection of the appropriate standard is dependent on the purpose of the gait evaluation and the goal of treatment. Presently available standards are sufficient to answer some questions for certain populations. But interpretation of results must proceed cautiously, limited by choice of an appropriate standard.

TESTING CONDITIONS

Traditionally, gait evaluation has implied the assessment of the most common form of ambulation—upright bipedal walking over the level surface. If the purpose of the gait evaluation is to assess the functional limitations in ambulatory ability, perhaps gait should be assessed on other surfaces as well. Andriacchi et al reported that level surface ambulation distinguished age-matched healthy subjects from subjects who had total knee replacements.[5] However, level-surface ambulation did not indicate any difference between patients with five different types of prostheses. When the total knee replacement patients were asked to walk on stairs, the patients who had one type of prosthesis demonstrated more "normal" performance than did patients who had any of the other four prostheses. Apparently, the assessment of ambulation on different surfaces was more sensitive and capable of identifying the differences among the prostheses. This difference would not have been detected if the gait evaluation had been confined to level-surface ambulation.

Reed has suggested that evaluation of ambulation on different surfaces may increase the usefulness of gait assessment.[109] He described the efficacy of a knee orthosis for reducing pain in 10 women subjects with unilateral degenerative joint disease. Ambulation was examined as subjects walked on level surface, up and down standard stairs, and up and down a ramp (with an 8 percent grade). Performance was examined prior to bracing and an average of 3 weeks after bracing. Knee ROM, vertical force and loading rate, swing/stance ratio, and walking velocity were assessed. The variables that demonstrated the most significant improvements were vertical force, loading rate, and velocity. The greatest pre- and post-changes in these variables were seen when ambulation was on the uneven surfaces. The findings of this study indicate that *if the clinician is assessing the ability of a device or treatment to improve function, the evaluation should encompass a variety of ambulatory activities that realistically assess performance.*

The conditions under which gait is assessed determine whether a gait evaluation can describe the patient's functional ability. Does the fact that a patient walks at 0.3 m/s with an asymmetrical step length and inadequate hip, knee, and ankle flexion indicate whether the patient will be able to reach a bus stop before the bus leaves? Nichols pointed out that various assessments such as joint ROM, muscle strength, gait evaluation, and ADL are not clearly related to one another.[110] This is often the case for the gait evaluation. *If the goal of treatment is to restore function, then gait evaluation should afford the clinician an opportunity to assess functional ability.* This suggests more integration of the gait evaluation with ADL assessments. Unfortunately, the literature does not address this issue. Perhaps gait evaluations of the future will incorporate true functional considerations. For example, instead of having the patient walk only in order for gait to be evaluated, the patient could be asked to answer the telephone on the other side of a room before it stops ringing or to catch a bus before it leaves. Certainly, healthy subjects adopt a walking pattern that is goal-dependent, e.g., people stroll when they are window-shopping but rush to get to their car to put money in a parking meter.[17] Perhaps a more appropriate test condition for a gait evaluation is an obstacle course where the patient must walk around objects, over different surfaces, and under various levels of illumination.[111] This kind of assessment may not only be useful in describing performance deficits, but may also be useful in defining the strategies that a patient with CNS pathology (including sensory deficits) has adopted in order to accomplish tasks.

SUMMARY

Smidt reminds us that "to move synchronously, a complex synergy of the nervous system pathways and the muscular system are involved, including 636 muscles, 206 bones, dozens of organs, hundreds of sensing structures, thousands of communication circuits, and gallons of body fluid."[76] Gait measurements are unlikely ever to become the critical element in the medical diagnosis of specific diseases, but evaluation of locomotor performance should gain increased acceptance as a tool to assess treatment. Severity of locomotor pathology can be assessed, the recovery of locomotor function can be documented and correlated with neuromusculoskeletal recovery, and treatment efficacy can be evaluated.

This chapter has attempted to review the purpose of the gait evaluation and to review some of the methods that are currently available to assess locomotor ability. However, the reader is cautioned to avoid getting lost in the details of the gait assessment or the plethora of gait variables. If gait evaluation is to become a useful clinical tool the *purpose* of the assessment, the *goal* of treatment, and the appropriate *standard* must be carefully selected. For some uses, *normal data bases must be developed,* which control for factors such as age, sex, and walking velocity. Gait evaluation measurements in patients must be examined in relation to the pathology and not just stated as deviations from normal. Careful clinical documentation of recovery in a variety of patients is necessary for the development of patient performance norms, and for the description of the deficits common to a given pathology that are not being effectively managed. Last, gait evaluations should truly assess the person's *functional* locomotor ability. The clinical assessment of gait is in its infancy, questions abound, and a vast research effort is needed.

ACKNOWLEDGMENT

The authors would like to acknowledge the technical assistance of Barbara Cozzens, Associate, Gait Analysis Laboratory, Moss Rehabilitation Hospital, Philadelphia, PA

REFERENCES

1. Websters New International Dictionary of the English Language, Ed. Neilson W, Knott TA, Carhart PW. G. and C. Merriman, Springfield, Massachusetts, 1940
2. Winter DA: Biomechanics of Human Movement, John Wiley, New York, 1979

3. Gyory AN, Chao EY, Stauffer RN: Functional evaluation of normal and pathological knee during gait. Arch Phys Med 57:571, 1976
4. Eberhart HD, Inman VT, Saunders JB, et al: Fundamental studies of human locomotion and other information relating to design of artificial limbs, A Report to the National Research Council, Committee on Artificial Limbs, University of California, Berkeley, 1947
5. Andriacchi TP, Galante JO, Fermier RW: The influence of total knee replacement design on walking and stair climbing. J Bone Joint Surg [Am] 64:1328, 1982
6. Colaso M, Joshi J, Singh N: Variation of gait patterns in adult hemiplegia. Neurol India 19:212, 1971
7. Brunnstrom S: Recording gait pattern of adult hemiplegic patients. Phys Ther 44:11, 1964
8. Richards C, Knutsson E: Evaluation of abnormal gait patterns by intermittent light photography and electromyography. Scand J Rehab Med Suppl 3: 61–68, 1974
9. Knutsson E, Richards C: Different types of disturbed motor control in gait of hemiparetic patients. Brain 102:405, 1979
10. Knutsson E: Gait control in hemiparesis. Scand J Rehab Med 13:101, 1981
11. Wetzel MC, Stuart DG: Ensemble characteristics of cat locomotion and its neural control. Prog Neurobiol 7:1, 1976
12. Grillner S: Locomotion in vertebrates: central mechanisms and reflex interaction. Physiol Rev 55:247, 1975
13. Herman R, Wirta R, Bampton S, Finley FR: Human solutions for locomotion: single limb analysis. In: Advances in Behavioral Biology, Vol. 18, p. 13, Plenum Press, New York, 1976
14. Grillner S: Interaction between central and peripheral mechanisms in the control of locomotion. Prog Brain Res 50:227, 1979
15. Inman VT, Ralston HJ, Todd F: Human Walking. Williams & Wilkins, Baltimore, 1981
16. Murray MP, Kory RC, Clarkson BH: Walking patterns in healthy old men. J Gerontol 24:169, 1969
17. Finley FR, Cody KA, Finizie RV: Locomotion patterns in elderly women. Arch Phys Med 50:140, 1969
18. Drillis RJ: The influence of aging on the kinematics of gait. In: Geriatric Amputee. NAS-NRC publication 919, Washington D.C., 1961
19. Crowninshield RC, Brand RA, Johnston RC: The effects of walking velocity and age on hip kinematics. Clin Ortho 132:140, 1978
20. Goodkin R, Diller L: Reliability among physical therapists in diagnosis and treatment of gait deviations in hemiplegics. Percept Mot Skills 37:727, 1973
21. Perry J: The mechanics of walking: a clinical interpretation. Phys Ther 47:778, 1967
22. Bampton S: A guide to the visual examination of pathological gait. Temple University Rehabilitation Research and Training Center No. 8, Philadelphia, 1979
23. Normal and Pathologic Gait Syllabus, Physical Therapy Department, Pathokinesiology Service, Rancho Los Amigos Hospital, Downey, California, 1977
24. Krebs D, Edelstein J, Fishman S: Observational gait analysis reliability in disabled children. Phys Ther 64:741, 1984 (abstr)
25. Tipton CM, Karpovich PV: Electrogoniometric records of knee and ankle movements in pathological gaits. Arch Phys Med 46:267, 1965
26. Johnston RC, Schmidt GL: Measurement of hip-joint motion during walking. J Bone Joint Surg 51-A:1083, 1969

27. Chao EYS, Hoffman RR: Instrumented measurements of human joint motion. ISA Transactions 17:13, 1977
28. Sutherland DH, Hagy JL: Measurement of gait movements from motion picture film. J Bone Joint Surg 54-A:787, 1972
29. Murray MP, Brewer BJ, Gore DR, Zuege RC: Kinesiology after McKee-Farrar total hip replacement. A two year follow-up of one hundred cases. J Bone Joint Surg [Am] 57:337, 1975
30. Sutherland DH, Olshen R, Cooper L, Woo S L-Y: The development of mature gait. J Bone Joint Surg 62-A:236, 1980
31. Sutherland DH, Cooper L, Daniel D: The role of ankle plantar flexors in normal walking. J Bone Joint Surg [Am] 62:354, 1980
32. Nelson AJ: Functional ambulation profile. Phys Ther 54:1059, 1974
33. Molen NH: Problems on the evaluation of gait. Thesis, The Institute of Biomechanics and Experimental Rehabilitation, Free University, Amsterdam, 1973
34. Rosenrot P, Wall JC, Charteris J: The relationship between velocity, stride time, support time and swing time during normal walking. J Hum Movement Stud 6:323, 1980
35. Smidt GL: Hip motion and related factors in walking. Phys Ther 51:9, 1971
36. Wirta RW, Herman R: Some observations of relations among gait variables. Presented at 21st Meeting of Orthopedic Research Society, San Francisco, 1975
37. Ogg HL: Measuring and evaluation of gait patterns of children. Phys Ther 43:717, 1963
38. Boenig D: Evaluation of a clinical method of gait analysis. Phys Ther 57:795, 1977
39. Shirley MM: Development of walking. In: The First Two Years: Study of Twenty-five Babies, Greenwood Press, Connecticut, 1931
40. Clarkson BH: Absorbent paper method for recording foot placement. Phys Ther 63:345, 1983
41. Chodera JD: Analysis of gain from foot prints. Physiotherapy 60:179, 1974
42. Cerny K: A clinical method of quantitative gait analysis. Phys Ther 63:1125, 1983
43. Durie ND, Farley RL: An apparatus for step length measurement. J Biomed Eng 2:38, 1980
44. Bontrager EL: Footswitch Stride Analyzer. In: Annual Report of Progress, p. 45. California, Rancho Los Amigos Engineering Center, 1979
45. Wolf SL, Binder-Macleod SA: Use of the Krusen limb load monitor to quantify temporal and loading measurements of gait. Phys Ther 63:976, 1982
46. Murray MP: Gait as a total pattern of movement including a bibliography on gait. Am J Phys Med 48:290, 1967
47. Gifford GE, Hutton WC: A microprocessor controlled system for evaluating treatments for disabilities affecting the lower limbs. J Biomed Eng 2:45, 1980
48. Taylor DR: An instrumented gait mat. Proceedings of the International Conference on Rehabilitation Engineering, p. 278. Toronto, Canada, 1980
49. Sweeney JK, Smutok MA: Vietnam head injury study: Preliminary analysis of the functional and anatomical sequelae of penetrating head trauma. Phys Ther 63:2018, 1983
50. Stauffer RN, Chao EYS, Gyory AN: Biomechanical gait analysis of diseased knee joints. Clin Orthop 126:246, 1977
51. Oatis C: Functional testing of the knee based on a mechanical model. Phys Ther 62:632, 1982 (abstr)
52. Winter DA, Robertson DGE: Joint torque and energy patterns in normal gait. Biol Cybernet 29:137, 1978

53. Carlsoo S, Dahllof A-G, Holm J: Kinetic analysis of the gait in patients with intermittent claudication. Scand J Rehab Med 6:166, 1974

54. Leiper C, Cozzens BA, Sobel G: Reacquisition of the gait pattern of persons having a below knee amputation, preliminary findings. Arch Phys Med, submitted for publication

55. Carlson CE, Mann RW, Harris WH: A radio telemetry device for monitoring cartilage surface pressure in the human hip. IEEE Trans BME 21:257, 1974

56. Licht S (ed): Electrodiagnosis and Electromyography. Elizabeth Licht, New Haven, Connecticut, 1956

57. Eberhart HD, Inman VT, Bresler B: The principal elements in human locomotion. In: Human Limbs and Their Substitutes, McGraw-Hill, New York, 1954

58. Hagy JL, Mann RA, Keller CW: Normal Electromyographic Data Gait Analysis Laboratory, Shriners Hospital for Crippled Children, San Francisco, 1973

59. Battye CK, Joseph J: Investigation by telemetering of activity of some muscles in walking. Med Biol Eng 4:125, 1966

60. Milner M, Basmajian JV, Quanbury AO: Multifactorial analysis of walking by electromyography and computer. Am J Phys Med 50:235, 1971

61. Dubo HIC, Peat M, Winter DA, et al: Electromyographic temporal analysis of gait: normal human locomotion. Arch Phys Med Rehabil 57:415, 1976

62. Lyons K, Perry J, Gronley JK, et al: Timing and relative intensity of hip extensor and abductor muscle action during level and stair ambulation. Phys Ther 63:1597, 1983

63. Sutherland DH: An electromyographic study of the plantar flexors of the ankle in normal walking on the level. J Bone Joint Surg [Br] 60:533, 1978

64. Basmajian JV: Muscles Alive. 4th Ed. Williams and Wilkins, Baltimore, 1978

65. Inman VT, Ralston HJ, Saunders JB de CM, et al: Relation of human electromyogram to muscular tension. Electroencephalogr Clin Neurophysiol 4:187, 1952

66. Lindstrom L: On the frequency spectrum of EMG signals. Final Report. Laboratory of Medical Electronics, Chalmers University of Technology, Goteborg, Sweden, 1970

67. Perry J, Waters RL, Perrin T: Electromyographic analysis of equinovarus following stroke. Clin Orthop 131:47, 1978

68. Peat M, Dubo HIC, Winter DA, et al: Electromyographic temporal analysis of gait: hemiplegic locomotion. Arch Phys Med Rehabil 57:421, 1976

69. Units, Terms and Standards in the Reporting of EMG Research, International Society of Electrophysiological Kinesiology, August, 1980

70. Woods JJ, Bigland-Ritchie B: Linear and non-linear surface EMG/force relationships in human muscles. Am J Phys Med 62:287, 1983

71. Sutherland DH: An electromyographic study of the ankle in normal walking on the level. J Bone Joint Surg [Am] 48:66, 1966

72. Waters RL, Frazier J, Garland DE, et al: Electromyographic gait analysis before and after treatment for hemiplegic equinus and equinovarus deformity. J Bone Joint Surg [Am] 64:284, 1982

73. Morrison JB: The mechanics of muscle function in locomotion. J Biomech 3:431, 1970

74. Patriarco AG, Mann RW, Simon SR, Mansour JM: An evaluation of the approaches of optimization models in the prediction of muscle forces during human gait. J Biomech 14:513, 1981

75. Murray MP, Kory RC, Sepic SB: Walking patterns of normal woman. Arch Phys Med 51:637, 1979

76. Smidt GL: Methods of studying gait. Phys Ther 54:13, 1974
77. Steindler A: A historical review of the studies and investigations made in relation to human gait. J Bone Joint Surg [Am] 35:540, 728, 1953
78. Schwartz RP, Heath AL, Misick W: The influence of the shoe on the gait. Am J Bone Joint Surg 17:406, 1935
79. Ogg LH: Gait analysis for lower extremity child amputees. Phys Ther 45:940, 1965
80. Murray MP, Frought AB, Kory RC: Walking patterns of normal men. J Bone Joint Surg 46:335, 1964
81. Azar GH, Lawton AH: Gait and stepping as factors in the frequent falls of elderly women. Geront 83, 1964
82. Critchley M: On senile disorders of gait including the so-called "senile paraplegia." Geriatrics 13:364, 1948
83. Steinberg FV: Gait disorders in old age. Geriatrics 21:134, 1966
84. Barron RC: Disorders of gait related to the aging nervous system. Geriatrics 22:113, 1967
85. Masoro EJ, Bertrand H, Leipa G, Yu BP: Analysis and exploration of age-related changes in mammalian structure and function. Fed Proc 38:1956, 1979
86. Drillis RJ: The influence of aging on the kinematics of gait in the geriatric amputee. NAS-NRC Publication 919, Washington D.C., 1961
87. Gabel RH, Johnston RC, Crowninshield RD: A gait analyzer/trainer instrumentation system. J Biomed 12:543, 1979
88. Imms FJ, Edholm OG: The assessment of gait and mobility in the elderly. Age Ageing 8:261, 1979
89. Imms FJ, Edholm OG: Studies of gait and mobility in the elderly. Age Ageing 10:147, 1981
90. Nayak USL, Gabell A, Simons MA, Isaacs B: Measurement of gait and balance in the elderly. J Am Geriatr Soc 30:516, 1981
91. Smith KV, McDermid CD, Shideman FE: Analysis of the temporal components of motion in human gait. Am J Phys Med Rehabil 39:142, 1960
92. Busby C: Gait Pattern of Elderly Men: A Comparative Study in Elderly Women. Master's Thesis, School of Physical Therapy, Duke University, North Carolina, 1981
93. Craik RL, Cozzens BA, Sobel E: The effect of age on walking. Phys Ther, submitted for publication.
94. McGraw MB: Neuromuscular development of the human infant as exemplified in the achievement of erect locomotion. J Pediatr 17:741, 1940
95. Burnett CN, Johnson EW: Development of gait in childhood, part 2. Dev Med Child Neurol 13:207, 1971
96. Stratham L, Murray MP: Early walking patterns of normal children. Clin Orthop 79:8, 1971
97. Sutherland DH, Olshen R, Cooper L, et al: The development of mature gait. J Bone Joint Surg [Am] 62:336, 1980
98. Beck RJ, Andriacchi TP, Kuo KN, et al: Changes in the gait patterns of growing children. J Bone Joint Surg [Am] 63:1452, 1981
99. Grieve DW, Gear RJ: The relationships between length of stride, step frequency, time of swing and speed of walking for children and adults. Ergonomics 8:31, 1966
100. Lamoreux L: Kinematic measurements in the study of human walking. Bull Pros Res 3, 1971
101. Craik R, Cook T, D'Orazio B: Variations in healthy gait with changes in velocity. Phys Ther 60:575, 1980 (abstr)

102. Andriacchi TP, Ogle JA, Galante JO: Walking speed as a basis for normal and abnormal gait measurements. J Biomech 10:261, 1977
103. Smidt GL, Wadsworth JB: Floor reaction forces during gait: comparison of patients with hip disease and normal subjects. Phys Ther 53:1056, 1973
104. Andriacchi TP, Galante JO: The influence of total hip and knee replacement on gait. In: Proceedings of International Conference on Rehabilitation Engineering Toronto, p. 71, 1980
105. Smidt GL, Mommens MA: Systems of reporting and comparing influence of ambulatory aids on gait. Phys Ther 350, 1980
106. Murray MP, Seireg AH, Scholz RC: A survey of the time, magnitude and orientation of forces applied to walking sticks by disabled men. Am J Phys Med 48:1, 1969
107. Takebe K, Basmajian JV: Gait analysis in stroke patients to assess treatments of foot drop. Arch Phys Med 57:305, 1976
108. Miller CW: Survival and ambulation following hip fracture. J Bone Joint Surg [Am] 60:930, 1978
109. Reed B: Evaluation of the CARS-UBC knee orthosis. Orthot Prosthet 33:25, 1979
110. Grieve DW, Leggett D, Wetherstone B: The analysis of stepping movements as a possible basis for locomotor assessment of the lower limbs. J Anat 127:515, 1978
111. Gentile AM: A working model of skill acquisition with application to teaching. Quest 17:3, 1972
112. Craik RL, Leiper CA, Cozzens BA, et al: Comparisons of spatial and temporal patterns. In: Proceedings of IX International Congress of Biomechanics, submitted for publication.

7 Assessment of the Child with CNS Dysfunction

Suzann K. Campbell

The status of measurement by physical therapists of motor development and movement dysfunction in pediatric populations in the 1980s can only be described as in desperate need of improvement. A review of the literature on measurement tools developed by physical or occupational therapists specifically for use in evaluating physically handicapped children with central nervous system (CNS) dysfunction (including cerebral palsy and minor neurologic dysfunction), for example, revealed only a handful of instruments. These identified tools include the following: The Movement Assessment of Infants,[1] the Miller Assessment for Preschoolers,[2] the Southern California Sensory Integration Tests,[3] the Inventory of Developmental Guidelines for Children with Myelodysplasia,[4] the Hughes Basic Gross Motor Assessment,[5] the Test of Sensory Integration,[6] the Motor Age Test,[7] and the Developmental Motor Test.[8] Most of the tests developed by therapists are of recent vintage, and none are yet adequate when compared with the American Psychological Association's standards for test validity and reliability.[9] For example, only a few of these tests have been used in large standardization studies in which norms for performance of children at varying ages are developed, few test developers have documented content validity beyond having selected items from previously available motor development tests, and few have published studies documenting the precision of their instruments for making diagnostic, prognostic, or prescriptive statements based on test results. Nevertheless, the existence of several new tests that are clearly undergoing development in line with accepted psychometric standards is a healthy sign that pediatric therapists recognize and are responding to the need for progress in the ability to measure movement dysfunction in children.

Additional comprehensive tools developed by persons in other professions specifically for assessing pediatric populations with CNS dysfunction include the Bruininks-Oseretsky Tests of Motor Proficiency,[10] the Neurological Examination of the Full Term Newborn Infant,[11,12] the Neurological Assessment of the Preterm and Full-term Newborn Infant,[13] the Test of Motor Impairment,[14] and the Purdue Perceptual-Motor Survey.[15] This list does not intentionally exclude any comprehensive tests of motor dysfunction; rather it includes those familiar to the author. Purposely excluded from this listing, however, were all screening tests, developmental tests designed primarily for normal populations, reflex (only) tests, and tests intended for mentally retarded or learning-disabled populations that omit items for identifying specific sensorimotor handicaps. Readers seeking further information on testing of pediatric populations may wish to consult the *Mental Measurements Yearbook* series,[16] the chapter by Stengel and colleagues in *Pediatric Neurologic Physical Therapy*,[17] the *Tests and Measurements in Child Development* handbooks,[18,19] and reviews of tests published regularly in the journal *Physical and Occupational Therapy in Pediatrics*.

Lack of appropriate tests is not the only problem. Entry-level physical therapy education ill prepares the practitioner for understanding the theory behind valid and reliable measurement and provides inadequate education in child assessment and development (normal *and* abnormal). The clinical specialist in pediatrics gains knowledge and skills primarily from on-the-job experience and in continuing education workshops, which seldom include information on measurement theory (see Ch. 1). This lack of adequate background in measurement results in frequent use of therapist-designed tests compiling original items with selected items excerpted from other tests. Without further psychometric analysis, these tests are of unknown reliability and validity, retard communication among professionals, hinder the development of a unique body of knowledge for physical therapy, and, at worst, may result in inaccurate diagnosis of movement dysfunction. Therapists must also develop more appreciation for the importance, from a humanistic perspective, of accurate testing and measurement. Failure to recognize the need for treatment or inappropriate treatment of a nonexistent condition or one not amenable to correction by physical therapy can result from lack of adequate measurement tools.

Lewko vividly illustrated the sad state of affairs in pediatric therapy in a 1976 survey of tests used in pediatric institutions.[20] Many of the respondents, a large proportion of whom were physical or occupational therapists, reported poor knowledge of sources of information about tests of motor development and inappropriately applied those standardized tests that were in use. Furthermore, large numbers of therapist-designed tests that were not standardized or examined for reliability and validity were in use in preference to the best available tools for assessing motor development.

In summary, few tests are available to assess motor development and coordination in physically handicapped children, therapists are poorly trained in selection or design of proper tools, and continued propagation and use of therapist-designed tests of unknown reliability and validity mitigates against the development of better tools. Last, I believe that the antiquantitative attitudes of some proponents of the major therapeutic approaches to management of children with neurologic dysfunction produce a negative bias against development of formal testing instruments. The unique jargon developed within each approach further hinders communication about exactly what is being assessed and treated.

PROBLEMS WITH CURRENT ASSESSMENTS

The following scenario illustrates today's approach to measurement of the problems of physically handicapped children:

Scenario 1985: Assessment of the Toddler with CNS Dysfunction

The physical therapist performs a Denver Developmental Screening Test (DDST)[21] to verify that the child is delayed in motor development relative to normal age-peers and notes poor quality of movement. These problems of incoordination and abnormal postural tone are assessed by observation and handling and described in extensive anecdotal notes. Passive range of motion (ROM) in areas noted to be restricted on gross assessment is measured with a goniometer. Activities of daily living (ADL) skills are noted from information obtained in a parent interview.
A number of problems exist in this rather typical assessment:

1. The Denver Developmental Screening Test will be useful in verifying that a child with CNS dysfunction is lagging behind age peers, but provides no quantitative information relative to how delayed the child is or what his or her overall age-equivalence is. Furthermore, neither the DDST nor any other motor development test provides norms for performance of children with various types of cerebral palsy. Although development of norms for children with cerebral palsy may represent an unattainable goal given the horrendous nature of the task, availability of the information that, for example, 80 percent of children with spastic diplegia walk independently or with appliances by a certain age would allow: (1) prognostic statements for a given child at a given age; (2) better parent education; and (3) improved assessment of long-term outcome of treatment.
2. Anecdotal notes on problems of incoordination and postural tone are of unknown reliability and provide a poor basis for quantitative assessment of progress during treatment. Moreover, clinical observation methods suffer from lack of validity in that they cannot document adequately the specific problems of abnormal force production, poor timing and isolation of muscular contraction, and inappropriate cocontraction of antagonists and prime movers that are characteristic of the movement patterns of the child with cerebral palsy.[22–25]

3. Only ROM assessments provide a quantitative record of this child's problems. Goniometry, however, has not been adequately studied for its reliability and validity in assessing ROM in children with CNS dysfunction (see Ch. 4). Validity problems are known to exist because of the presence of spasticity and of variation in tone in different positions relative to the force of gravity.[26]

4. The ADL interview and items on the DDST are valuable in providing assessment of the child's actual functional use of movement in purposeful activity. The therapist has only clinical experience and knowledge of normal development to guide judgments regarding the adequacy of the child's performance; however, since no age norms for achievement of skill in ADL activities by children with different types of cerebral palsy are available (see Ch. 5 for a general discussion of problems with standardization of ADL tests).

5. In addition to the problems noted above, the therapist has failed to assess the child's speed or endurance for physical activity, and has failed to document posture or to ascertain whether perceptual problems may be interfering with functional use of movement.

Any attempt to analyze the state of the art in pediatric assessment (or more specifically, assessment of children with CNS dysfunction) must ask the following questions:

1. Does this 1985 scenario represent the best assessment that is currently available? Can assessment of pediatric patients be improved *today*?

2. What is the cost of poor assessment in human terms and in cost to society and the profession of physical therapy in terms of image and effectiveness?

3. What improvements should be made in preparing a tentative scenario for measurement strategies in the year 2000?

In attempting to address these questions, the goals of this chapter are to: (1) discuss the general components of a comprehensive assessment of motor development and movement dysfunction in the pediatric patient; (2) survey and critique tools for assessing these components of motor development and movement dysfunction, specifically in pediatric clients with mild to severe CNS dysfunction; and (3) discuss research on measurement of sensorimotor function in children that gives promise of ultimate translation into useful clinical assessment tools of the future. To make this task manageable, the focus of assessment will be one of the most common of pediatric clients, the child with CNS dysfunction. Some parts of the analysis will be applicable to other pediatric patients, such as the child with myelodysplasia or muscular dystrophy; however, no attempt will be made to discuss the problems of evaluation of other special areas, such as pulmonary dysfunction, orthopedics, or oral motor problems in children.

COMPONENTS OF MOTOR DEVELOPMENT

Therapists describe motor development as consisting of three components: motor milestones, developmental reflexes, and the elusive property, "quality" of movement. From a theoretical perspective, however, research on motor development has resulted in identification of *nine* different aspects of gross and fine motor development of importance in assessment of movement in the age range of 4 to 15 years.[27] These components are the following:

Gross Motor

1. Speed
2. Static body balance
3. Dynamic body balance
4. Coordination
5. Strength

Gross and Fine Motor

6. Visual-motor tracking
7. Response speed to a visual stimulus
8. Visual-motor control of the hand
9. Upper extremity speed and precision in manipulation.

Factor analysis of items designed to test these various components of motor performance in children resulted in summary factors labeled speed, precision, strength, balance, and coordination.[27] Additional factors of special importance in physically handicapped populations include posture, ROM, endurance, and ADL. Problems in these latter areas are the result of abnormal motor control, lack of exercise, and diminished opportunity to practice functional skills; however, they may be the problems most amenable to improvement by therapeutic intervention and thus should be thoroughly documented in initial and repeat evaluations.

Of course, assessment of motor development for infants and toddlers must also include attainment of sequential motor milestones to assess degree of developmental delay, and all children with CNS dysfunction require analysis of postural reflexes, such as righting, protective, and equilibrium reactions. Last, a thorough assessment of the client with abnormal postural tone should include identification of: (1) the presence of abnormal restraint of movement by inappropriate contraction of antagonists to prime movers leading to increased stiffness of limbs; (2) maintained primitive reflexes; (3) abnormally large receptive fields to sensory input, i.e., excessive muscular contraction upon stimulation of peripheral receptors; and (4) inability to perform isolated movements. These abnormalities are the hallmarks of the stereotyped movement characteristic of CNS dysfunction, yet they are only beginning to be described in the scientific literature.[22-26] The work of the future entails study of whether treatment can positively influence these abnormalities of reciprocal innervation, reflex gain, and coordination of muscular synergies.

REVIEW OF AVAILABLE TESTS

In this section, published tests will be analyzed for their ability to assess the components of movement outlined above, as well as on the basis of how well they meet scientific standards for reliability and validity. Table 7-1 summarizes this information for each test. These tools will be discussed in the following three categories:

Tests for Infants at Risk for CNS Dysfunction
Neurological Examination of the Full Term Newborn Infant (NEFTI)
Neurological Assessment of the Preterm and Full-Term Newborn Infant (NAPI)
Movement Assessment of Infants (MAI)
Tests for Children with Mild to Moderate Sensorimotor Dysfunction
Miller Assessment for Preschoolers (MAP)
Hughes Basic Gross Motor Assessment (BGMA)
Bruininks-Oseretsky Test of Motor Proficiency (B-OTMP)
Test of Motor Impairment (TMI)
Southern California Sensory Integration Tests (SCSIT)
Test of Sensory Integration (TSI)
Purdue Perceptual-Motor Survey (PP-MS)
Tests for Children with Cerebral Palsy and Myelodysplasia
Motor Age Test (MAT)
Developmental Motor Test (DMT)
Inventory of Developmental Guidelines for Children with Myelodysplasia (IDG)

Although, out of necessity, brief, each discussion will summarize the purpose of the test, the normative sample, reported reliability data, examples of item content, and validity for diagnostic or prescriptive use, when available.

Tests for Infants at Risk for CNS Dysfunction

NEFTI.[11,12] The NEFTI is intended to provide a comprehensive assessment of neurologic development in the full-term newborn infant. Normative performance for neonates was obtained on a sample of about 1,500 newborns, most of whom were at risk for neurologic dysfunction because of a history of maternal obstetric complications. Test–retest stability (intra-rater reliability) is high after the first three days of life, and inter-rater agreement is reported to be 80 percent or better among highly trained testers.[28,29]

The test is intended only for the assessment of newborns and contains items on reflex development and posture and mobility in several positions. In

Table 7-1. Summary of Movement Components Assessed by Selected Motor Development Tests

						Test							
Component	NEFTI	NAPI	MAI	MAP	BGMA	B-OTMP	TMI	SCSIT	TSI	PP-MS	MAT	DMT	IDG
Speed	No	No	No	Some	No	Yes	Yes	Some	Yes	No	Some	Some	No
Balance	No	No	Yes	Yes	Yes	Yes	Yes	Some	Yes	Yes	Some	Some	No
Coordination	Some	Some	Some	Some	Yes	Some	Some	Yes	Yes	Yes	Some	Some	No
Strength	No	No	No	No	No	Some	No	No	No	Some	No	No	No
Manual dexterity	No	No	Some	Yes	Some	Yes	Yes	Yes	Yes	Yes	Yes	Yes	Yes
Visual motor	Yes	Yes	Yes	Yes	Yes	Yes	No	Yes	Yes	Yes	No	No	No
ADL	No	No	No	No	No	No	No	No	No	No	No	No	Yes
Milestones	Newborn	Newborn	To 1 yr	Above Stand	No	Above Stand	No	No	No	No	Yes	Yes	Yes
Reflexes	Yes	Some	Yes	No	No	No	No	No	Some	Yes	No	No	No
Sensation/ perception	Some	Some	Some	Yes	Some	Some	No	Yes	Some	Yes	No	No	No
Posture/ ROM	Yes	Yes	Yes	No	Yes	No	No	Yes	Some	Some	No	No	No
Endurance	No	No	No	No	No	No	No	No	No	No	No	No	Some
Measurement qualities	Good	Fair	Fair	Good	Good	Good	Good	Fair	Fair	Poor	Poor	Poor	Fair

NEFTI = Neurological Examination for the Full Term Infant
NAPI = Neurological Assessment of the Preterm and Full-Term Newborn Infant
MAI = Movement Assessment of Infants
MAP = Miller Assessment for Preschoolers
BGMA = Hughes Basic Gross Motor Assessment
B-OTMP = Bruininks-Oseretsky Test of Motor Proficiency
TMI = Test of Motor Impairment
SCSIT = Southern California Sensory Integration Tests
TSI = Test of Sensory Integration
PP-MS = Purdue Perceptual-Motor Survey
MAT = Motor Age Test
DMT = Developmental Motor Test
IDG = Inventory of Developmental Guidelines for Children with Myelodysplasia

studies of its validity for predicting long-term neurologic outcome, large numbers of false positives and false negatives are reported; however, the presence in the newborn period of one of a number of syndromes, such as hypotonicity or hyperexcitability, is positively correlated with poor neurologic outcome.[29,30]

NAPI.[13]   The NAPI was designed to provide a brief neurologic assessment covering posture, movement, reflexes, and response to visual and auditory stimulation that could be used to assess preterm or full-term infants, whether sick or well. The purpose of the test is to detect the effects on the neonatal nervous system of drugs, hypoxia, or trauma, and to document the evaluation of neurologic function across time in the neonatal period. Although a formal standardization study has not been reported, the authors state that the test was used over a period of 2 years on more than 500 babies, and only items with very high inter-rater reliability were included.[13]

One of the unique features of this new test is the exceptionally well-designed scoring sheet form, which contains information on testing and scoring each item in highly compact form and provides a graphic visual display of the child's level of performance. Items include limb recoil, traction, reflex, and head control tests; spontaneous posture and movement; irritability; and orientation and response decrement to visual and auditory stimulation. The NAPI does not include assessment of endurance or speed and includes only a few selected reflexes believed to be most discriminating in identifying neurologic dysfunction. Case studies presented in the manual illustrate individual profiles of premature, term, and compromised babies, but no formal validity studies have been reported.

MAI.[1]   The MAI is a new therapist-developed test for children at risk for CNS dysfunction for which normative work is in progress. The purpose of the test is to predict cerebral palsy from assessment of infants at 4 months postterm. The correlation for inter-rater reliability is reported to be .72, and for test–retest reliability .76.[31,32]

The MAI provides for assessment of muscle tone, developmental reflexes, posture and coordination in prone, supine, sitting, and vertical positions at 4 months, but does not include endurance or speed information, and has limited ability to assess perceptual development. Ability to predict cerebral palsy at 2 years of age from these assessments of motor milestones, coordination, and reflex development at 4 months corrected age had 2.4 percent false-negative and 16.7 percent false-positive rates in preliminary study of a high-risk population.[32]

Tests for Children with Mild to Moderate Sensorimotor Dysfunction

MAP.[2]   The MAP is a new test designed and developed by an occupational therapist for the purpose of evaluating the motor development, quality of movement, ocular motor ability, and sensory integrative functions of preschool children between the ages of 2 years, 9 months, and 5 years, 8 months. The original research form of the test was standardized on a nationwide, stratified random sample of 600 normal preschool children and 60 children noted by parents or teachers to have functional delays in behavior, perception or language but who had no specific diagnosis. After revisions, the current version of the MAP was standardized on a new sample of 1,200 preschoolers selected to represent the U.S. population on sex, race, community size, and socioeconomic factors, and 90 children selected because of known functional delays. Inter-rater reliability is .98 for the test as a whole and varies from .84 to .99 for the various subtests.[2] Test–retest reliabilities for the five subtests over 1 to 4 weeks range from 72 percent to 94 percent agreement. Internal consistency coefficient is .79 for the 27 items that make up the core exam.

The 27 items in the basic MAP test the senses of touch, position, and movement; oral, ocular, fine, and gross motor abilities; verbal and nonverbal cognitive skills; and complex activities requiring integration of perception, cognition, and movement, such as writing tasks. This test is unique in being the first comprehensive developmental assessment for the preschool age group that includes, in addition to the core items for diagnosis of moderate to severe delay, supplemental sections intended to describe further the quality of the child's coordination and perceptual functions, with a view toward prescribing remediation strategies to improve the overall level of performance. It does not provide for assessment of strength, endurance, ADL, or early milestones. Only limited aspects of posture are tested.

Although the ultimate level of test development, that of demonstrating validity for predicting school performance problems from preschool MAP results, has not yet been achieved, the MAP is undoubtedly the most well-designed and well-developed test ever constructed by a pediatric therapist. The methodology described in the manual is a useful model for others. Content validity has been studied by factor analysis, and criterion-related validity has been analyzed by comparing MAP scores with scores obtained on four other preschool tests. Correlations with other standardized tests were generally low; thus, it remains for future research to demonstrate whether MAP scores are useful for predicting problems in school and in prescribing remedial strategies. These studies are in progress. The only data on diagnostic accuracy are those indicating that, of the 90 children in the standardization sample selected because their parents or teachers thought they had developmental delays, the MAP classified 75 percent as questionable or abnormal relative to same-age peers.

BGMA.[5]   The BGMA was developed for identification of deviations in gross motor performance in children from 6 to 12 years of age. The test assesses basic gross motor skills that all children over 5 years of age should be able to attain rather than assessing developmental delay in motor performance. The test was normed on 1,260 randomly selected children in Denver, Colorado public schools who had a range of income and racial and ethnic characteristics. Test–retest reliability was .97, and inter-rater reliability was .996.[5]

Test items included in the BGMA are: static balance in standing, stride jump, tandem walking, hopping, skipping, beanbag and yo-yo toss, and ball handling. In addition, the manual describes many clinical observations to be made in assessing quality of performance such as maneuvers used to maintain balance, neurologic signs, spatial orientation problems, delayed responses, and emotional reactions. A factor analysis of the test items supported the theory that motor abilities are specific, rather than general; seven factors were identified.[5] These factors were static balance with eyes open, static balance with eyes closed, ball handling, object control, aiming, dynamic balance, and leg strength and balance. Although postural deviations and neurologic symptoms are to be noted, the test can only be considered a screening device for neurologic dysfunction, and does not attempt to assess fine motor function, motor milestones across the age span, ADL, or other areas. No age equivalencies can be obtained.

Concurrent validity with teacher ratings of motor skill ranges from .22 to .79 for various ages and subtests, with 33 of 36 calculated correlations being significant.[5] The items selected for the test were also tested on a sample of 162 children in special education classes who were classified as educable mentally retarded, learning disabled, or emotionally handicapped; significant differences between the performances of these children and the standardization population were found. The test was found to be at too high a level for the trainable mentally retarded population. Predictive validity studies have not been done.

B-OTMP.[10]   The B-OTMP is a battery of subtests designed to assess the gross and fine motor performance of children between 4.5 and 14.5 years of age. It was specifically designed to provide a range of performance capable of displaying the problems of children with mild to moderate motor disability. Standard scores are obtained for gross motor, fine motor, and a composite of the two. Age equivalencies can also be obtained for each of eight subtests. The test battery was standardized on 765 subjects representative of the 1970 U.S. census according to sex, race, community size, and geographic distribution. Test–retest reliabilities range from .29 to .89 for various ages and subtests.[10] The low reliabilities are exceptional and are found primarily in upper age groups who are performing at the ceiling with little variability. Composite score reliabilities are .68 and greater. Inter-rater reliability for untrained raters on the subtest requiring the most tester judgment was found to be .90 in one study and .98 in another.

Because this test was designed to assess all nine of the major components of motor development listed previously, it purports to cover adequately each of these performance areas in its subtests of running speed and agility, balance, bilateral coordination, strength, visual motor control, and upper limb coordination, response time, and speed and dexterity. The test is not intended for children below school-age nor those who are nonambulatory, although many of the upper extremity tests could be administered to nonwalking children. Posture, ROM, endurance, early developmental milestones, ADL, sensation/perception, and reflexes are not assessed.

Factor analysis and internal consistency studies support the contention that the B-OTMP successfully assesses most of the independent constructs of which motor control is composed, and this test is unique among child development instruments in doing so.[27] Further work on validity has demonstrated that normal children perform better than the mildly-severely retarded and than learning disabled children.[10]

TMI.[14] The TMI was designed for the assessment of children between 5 and 14 years of age with subtle forms of neural dysfunction, such as the clumsy child. The test assesses motor control and balance of the body during static activity, upper extremity coordination, dynamic body control and coordination, and speed and precision of manipulation. Cognitive and perceptual demands were minimized by design. The test was normed on 854 children in 31 schools in an industrial city in Ontario. Reliabilities have been reported to be in the acceptable range, and validity studies have demonstrated correlations between test scores and motor ability ratings of teachers as well as social adjustment scores.[33] Again, motor milestones for young children, reflexes, posture, ROM, ADL, sensation/perception, and endurance are not included in this test.

SCSIT.[3] The SCSIT were designed to evaluate various perceptual abilities and postural and coordination skills that together have come to be defined as "sensory integrative" function. The tests measure form and space perception, postural and bilateral integration, tactile perception, and a variety of motor skills in children from 4 to 10 years of age. The tests were normed on 1,004 children in the area of Los Angeles, California. In addition to geographic restriction, the sample was additionally limited by the gathering of only partial data on 9- and 10-year-olds. Test–retest reliability for various subtests ranges from .01 to .89.[3] Subtests with low reliabilities include those involving localization of tactile stimuli; performance scores on these tests have a small range, which contributes to low reliability. Internal consistency reliability has been calculated only for a motor accuracy subtest and was reported as ranging from .67 for 4-year-olds to .93 for 5-year-olds. Inter-rater reliability is not reported in the manual.

The SCSIT consist of a battery of 17 subtests: space visualization, figure-ground perception, kinesthesia, manual form perception, finger identification, graphesthesia, localization of tactile stimuli, double tactile stimuli perception, motor accuracy, imitation of postures, crossing midline of the body, bilateral motor coordination, right–left discrimination, standing balance with eyes open, standing balance with eyes closed, design copying, and position in space. The SCSIT are intended for children with subtle forms of perceptual and motor dysfunction and do not provide for evaluation of dynamic gross motor function, developmental reflexes, posture, endurance, or ADL.

The SCSIT correlate well with several subtests on the Bender Gestalt, and another validity study reports a positive correlation between SCSIT performance and academic success.[34,35] The tests assess primarily upper extremity functions and perception and are not claimed to be a comprehensive assessment of other areas of motor development. Furthermore, the test is intended for use as a diagnostic tool only. The manual suggests that data from the SCSIT can be used to differentiate four types of sensory integrative disorders. These include dysfunction in form and space perception, praxis, postural and bilateral integration, and tactile processing; however, definitive predictive validity studies have not been published. Additional standardization studies and the development of new subtests are reportedly underway (L. King Thomas, personal communication).

TSI.[6]   The TSI was developed to assess postural control, bilateral motor integration, and reflex integration in preschool children. The test has been normed on 101 normal children and 38 developmentally delayed (not more than moderately mentally retarded) children, primarily from the Washington, D.C. area.[36] The majority of the children were 3 or 4 years old. Test–retest reliability over a 1-week period ranged from .85 to .96 for the three subtests and total test score.[36] Inter-rater reliability was .80 or above for each subtest and total test score except for the reflex integration subtest, which demonstrated unacceptable inter-scorer agreement.

The 36 items on the three TSI subtests were chosen to assess supposedly vestibular-based functions in preschool children that are essential for development of refined gross and fine motor skills, laterality, visual–spatial perception, and motor planning. Predictive validity to test this assumption has not been assessed. The items include measures of ability to assume antigravity flexion and extension postures, diadochokinesis, speed in fine motor activities, bilateral rhythm and coordination activities, and tests of the asymmetrical and symmetrical tonic neck reflexes. The test, therefore, covers certain aspects of posture, speed, strength, and static and dynamic balance as well as coordination and visual motor control. In a study of the ability of the test to classify children correctly as normal or abnormal, total test scores achieved an 81 percent index of accuracy with a sensitivity of 71 percent and a specificity of 85 percent.[36]

PP-MS.[15]   The PP-MS was developed to identify children aged 6 to 10 years who lack the perceptual-motor abilities necessary for academic success. Areas assessed include balance and postural flexibility, eye–hand coordination, ocular control, and form perception. Test–retest reliability over a 1-week period was .95.[37] No norms are available; hence, the test is called a "survey" because it is lacking in technical development.

Items included in the test are those of negotiating a walking board and an obstacle course, jumping, identifying body parts, imitating movements, drawing forms, rhythmic writing, and ocular pursuit tasks. Few validity studies are available, and many of the areas tested have been shown to be unrelated to academic success.[37] The test has been reported to discriminate academic nonachievers from achievers, however, and in a second study of 297 children, test results correlated .65 with teacher ratings.[38]

Tests for Children with Cerebral Palsy and Myelodysplasia

MAT.[7]   The MAT was designed for evaluation of children with cerebral palsy whose motor development level is between 4 months and 6 years. Items were derived largely from the work of Gesell and divided into two separate tests, one for the upper extremities and the other for the trunk and lower extremities, yielding an Upper Motor Quotient and Lower Motor Quotient, respectively. The authors note that test results are reproducible, but no normative studies or formal assessments of reliability and validity have been done. Age placements for items are averages for normal children, not those with cerebral palsy, so one can only note how delayed a child is relative to age peers, not relative to others with physical disabilities.

The items in the lower extremity test are used to evaluate motor milestones and static and dynamic balance in standing, jumping, hopping, and skipping activities. The upper extremity test includes fine motor milestones, manual dexterity items, and speed-tests of reciprocally alternating activity requiring precise finger placement, visual motor tracking, and bilateral coordination activities. Endurance, strength, ADL, and specific patterns of coordination used to accomplish test items are not assessed.

DMT.[8]   The DMT was designed for evaluation of children with cerebral palsy whose motor development level is between 1 month and 6 years. Items were derived from the Gesell and Bayley Scales and divided into upper and lower extremity tests. Items and components of motor development assessed are very similar to those of the MAT, although the latter contains many more manual dexterity items. Again, data on normative performance, reliability, and validity are largely lacking, making the value of the test impossible to determine. In the one reported study using the DMT, months of motor development in 93 children with cerebral palsy at 3 years of age (or predicted for 3 years in younger patients) was used as a severity index to predict each child's potential for walking.[8] An index of 10 (indicating a motor developmental age of 10 months at 3 years of age) was the lowest score compatible with the accomplishment of ambulation without assistive devices.

IDG.[4]   The IDG is a new tool for assessing gross motor activities, personal–social development, and self-help skills in children with myelodysplasia from 3 months to 19 years, 8 months of age. The eventual goal of this work is to provide information on typical rates of development of children with myelodysplasia as a basis for parent education and treatment planning. The inventory was developed based on parent reports of age of attainment of selected developmental skills in 173 children with intelligence or developmental quotients above 70 from the northwestern U.S. Norms for 20 percent, 50 percent, and 80 percent attainment of the skills contained in the inventory are available for children with four different levels of neurologic involvement. In a study of parent report agreement with professional staff raters (including therapists, educators, nurses, and psychologists), 89 percent agreement on ages of attainment of milestones was obtained. Since the initial study was a normative one and was based on parent report, only milestones of development and ADL skills are included in the test, and other areas of motor function not as readily assessed by parents are omitted.

Conclusions

It should be obvious from the preceding review that no one test provides for assessment of all areas of sensorimotor function for all age groups, or even for any one age group, and most of the tests were designed for children with mild to moderate dysfunction or for disorders other than cerebral palsy. No comprehensive assessment for the child with cerebral palsy is available; indeed, no satisfactory test for even *one component* of motor development in children with cerebral palsy is in existence. Yet, the addition of one or more of the reviewed tests to the routine assessment battery for children with cerebral palsy, particularly those with mild to moderate dysfunction, would greatly increase the validity of the evaluation process and broaden the functions assessed (and presumably treated, when appropriate). For example, use of the B-OTMP with a mildly handicapped population might identify subgroups of children with problems on particular subtests but not on others. This finding could result in development of treatment approaches specifically targeted to the needs of each identified subgroup. Even use of some of the individual items from selected tests could be condoned if they were used in repeated assessments across time in order to quantify the rate of achievement of established therapeutic goals. For example, timed items would be useful as an assessment of changes in speed of movement with therapeutic intervention, an area that rarely receives attention in assessment, yet one that may be critical for long-term functional improvement.

The need for improving assessment of moderately to severely involved children with neurologic dysfunction are great. These needs include all of the following:

1. Norms for attainment of motor milestones and self-help skills for children with various types of cerebral palsy.
2. A standardized method of postural assessment (for sitting and standing at a minimum).
3. Standardized methods of gait assessment (see Ch. 6).
4. Standardized assessments of static and dynamic balance, perceptual problems, endurance for physical activity, speed (gross and fine motor), strength, manual dexterity, and visual motor skills.
5. Standardized methods for assessing coordination, including measurement of lack of isolated movement and of degree of restraint of active movement by abnormal conditions, such as ROM limitations, antagonist contraction resisting prime mover function, and degree of spread of sensory input to abnormally enlarged muscular receptive fields.

EXPERIMENTAL LITERATURE

In this section, selected papers from the research literature that will illustrate possible approaches to developing some of the needed assessment tools outlined above are reviewed. None is in itself an attempt to develop a standardized tool, but each report was chosen because the methodology proved valuable in revealing various aspects of movement dysfunction in handicapped children and may eventually prove translatable into clinically useful tools. Such studies have been found in the literature relative to methods of assessing the following components of motor development: speed, balance, coordination (including sensory effects on muscular function), and visual motor control.

Speed

As noted earlier, only one or two items that involve speed of performance have been used in tests for children with cerebral palsy, yet impaired velocity of force development and movement is a major symptom of neurologic dysfunction.[23,24,39] Research investigations provide several examples of problems with reaction time and speed of performance that may give direction for the eventual development of clinical assessment tools. For example, Neilson studied the speed with which spastic or athetoid patients could produce rapidly alternating movements of the elbow.[24,40] Both types of patients were considerably slower than normal subjects and demonstrated movement delays following onset of electromyographic (EMG) activity that were indicative of increased limb stiffness.

Other tasks used in studies of children with Down syndrome and with minimal brain dysfunction are tracing a moving sinusoidal line[39] and reaching for a rapidly moving target,[41] respectively. Both tasks are notable for the requirement that the subject must *predict* the trajectory of the object in order to produce the proper velocity of movement to follow or contact the target. The ability of the nervous system to calculate such predictions is important in functional tasks such as reach and grasp of a proffered object or catching a ball.

In the area of gait analysis, Holt assesses speed of locomotion by timing the child's walk over a standard distance and by observing ability to initiate gait promptly, vary speed, and change direction.[42] Sequential photographs are used as an aid to document initial assessments and are repeated to allow analysis of change over time.

Balance

The methods of Nashner for assessing postural responses to disturbances of static stance equilibrium have been used to evaluate both normal adult subjects and patients with several types of neurologic dysfunction.[43] New studies of children are underway.[44] These methods involve unexpected disturbance of balance in one of several directions while the child is standing on a movable platform while an EMG recording is made of lower extremity muscle responses. From these records, response latency, as well as the pattern of coordination among muscles participating in this functional stretch reflex, can be obtained. With the additional use of conflicting signals, such as visual illusions that appear to contradict the sensations received from somatosensory receptors, information can be obtained regarding patients' ability to substitute use of one sensory input for another and rapidly correct for, or learn to ignore, false impressions while controlling postural sway.

Cinematography provides the ability to capture a record of balance while moving, such as during locomotion, and could easily be used to record standard activities in other positions, such as sitting or quadruped. Although not all clinical settings can be expected to provide this, film records have been used routinely in many orthopedic surgery clinics for years.

Coordination

EMG has been used extensively for research on the timing of muscle activity during locomotion, both for research purposes and for gait analysis prior to surgical intervention.[22,26,45–47] Each of these studies stresses the inadequacy of current clinical tools to distinguish among patients with apparently similar movement dysfunction but with strikingly different patterns of muscle coordination revealed by electromyography. This tool is rapidly being translated into a clinically feasible assessment tool by the use of small computers to integrate and summarize quickly the data obtained.

Chong and colleagues, for example, assessed the electromyographic activity during gait of the hip medial rotators, adductors, and hamstrings in twelve children with abnormal degrees of medial rotation.[45] Three different patterns of muscle activity were identified. In six of the 12 subjects, medial hamstring activity was prolonged beyond its normal period of occurrence during late swing and early stance, while the timing of the other muscles was normal. In two subjects, all of the muscles from which recordings were made cycled on and off at the same time; in the remaining four subjects, activity occurred on and off in the various muscle groups with no predictable relationship to each other or to the gait cycle. Only in the first group of patients, in whom the timing of a single muscle appeared to be responsible for the abnormal degree of medial rotation, was surgical intervention deemed likely to be successful in improving the pattern of locomotion.

Similar studies have been useful in identifying muscle imbalances amenable to surgery at the ankle;[46,47] however, EMG alone remains a crude assessment tool since it reflects primarily the presence or absence of activity in various muscles and does not provide a total picture of the ranges of joint motion and forces produced by muscle activity during locomotion. Nevertheless, EMG clearly can reveal that varying patterns of muscle activity are indicative of clinically similar movement disorders (see Ch. 10). If such analysis can be made feasible for routine use in the clinical setting, it might be beneficial in: (1) classifying patients according to prognosis; (2) documenting treatment effectiveness; and (3) identifying which treatments are most successful for varying patterns of dysfunction.

Sensory Control of Muscle Function

Several interesting experiments in biofeedback suggest the possibility of use of biological feedback systems to assess the patient's ability to use sensory information for learning new or improved skills. For example, a manometric method was used with children with myelodysplasia to assess threshold for subjective appreciation of rectal distention prior to utilization of a 6-hour program of biofeedback training aimed at improving voluntary contraction of the external anal spincter.[48] Although not directly applicable to children with cerebral palsy, this study suggests the possibility of developing methods to evaluate ability to use sensory inputs for other motor control functions, such as postural sway, voluntary isolated muscle contraction or relaxation, or rapid muscle tension development. For example, it is not clear whether children with cerebral palsy have variable ability to improve the isolation of muscle activity with exercise. Assessment of a child's ability to utilize feedback on extent of isolated muscle activity achieved might be used to predict the degree of improvement to be expected from a program of therapeutic exercise.

Consideration of aberrant sensory processing is also important in evaluation of cerebral palsy. Barolat-Romana and David, for example, demonstrated that stimulation of surgically exposed dorsal roots in patients with cerebral palsy produces widespread activation of muscles not normally included in the reflexogenic field of those nerve roots.[25] The degree of such aberrant connections was correlated with level of spasticity and suggests that the initial brain insult results in developmental abnormalities in spinal cord circuits. In a more clinically feasible evaluation system, Mykelbust and colleagues have identified a similar phenomenon in perinatally brain-damaged subjects called reciprocal excitation, in which stretch of the soleus muscle produces an excitatory effect, instead of the normal reciprocal *inhibition* of the motoneurons innervating the anterior tibialis muscle.[49] The investigators have not found this effect in adult injured subjects and, again, suggest that early brain injury is accompanied either by a concomitant lesion of the spinal cord or a secondary developmental abnormality in the establishment of neural connections in afferent somatosensory circuits.

The result of these abnormalities is that incoming information from muscle and other receptors exerts an exceptionally dominating effect on motoneuron output and probably contributes to the frequently observed pattern of co-contraction of all muscles in a limb rather than the normal exquisitely timed interaction of agonists and antagonists during voluntary motion.[22,45] These abnormal patterns of muscle activation can be evaluated with EMG in concert with kinematic information to indicate joint positions during various phases of the movement.

Visual Attention and Motor Control

Two recent studies of visual attention and eye-head coordination, respectively, suggest the need and possibilities for analyzing visual motor control and improving attending behavior.[50,51] Atkin and colleagues studied lateral gaze triggered by a light signal or verbal command in normal and retarded children.[50] For 45° gaze shifts, retarded children showed significantly more head turning than did normal children and a tendency to lead the response with head, rather than eye, movement. Some children demonstrated a "locked eye–head" phenomenon in which head and eye movements could not be dissociated from each other. Because difficulty in performing isolated movements is a hallmark of the neurologic dysfunction in children with cerebral palsy, a movement analysis such as that employed by Atkin and associates might be useful in quantifying aberrant eye–head synergies in the population with cerebral palsy.

Poland and Doebler performed an experiment in which severely retarded, visually impaired children with cerebral palsy were given visual attention training with blacklight conditions under the assumption that ordinary white light might flood the visual field of such children, reducing their ability to use visual cues for learning.[51] The success of their experiment suggests that visually impaired children with cerebral palsy could be evaluated for hypersensitivity to ordinary lighting conditions with a modification of the Poland and Doebler training paradigm.

TASKS FOR THE FUTURE

It is sad that we do not know, in the absence of scientific investigations, whether any of the components of movement can be improved with physical therapy for patients with cerebral palsy. Furthermore, a well-elaborated theory does not exist to suggest which components might be most amenable to exercise-induced change. In many areas of science, however, invention of a new assessment tool has been the key to enhanced understanding of the phenomenon under study. Therapists have barely begun to analyze quantitatively the movement problems of children with cerebral palsy. Indeed, the following statement of Johnson and colleagues[7] made in 1951 is largely true today: "We are unable to describe the patient with cerebral palsy in any way which lends itself to a statistical analysis . . . " The goals of this chapter have been to review the current situation and to suggest some new directions for analysis that might lead to improved understanding of the effects of therapeutic intervention. Should some of the directions outlined prove fruitful, perhaps the scenario for the year 2000 might read as follows:

Scenario 2000: Assessment of the Toddler With CNS Dysfunction

The physical therapist engages the child in performing movement skills in sitting, standing, and walking while a minicomputer automatically calculates errors in force, speed, and timing of movement from information relayed by telemetry from joints and muscles. An electrogoniometer records ROM in key joints during functional activities. Films record postural abnormalities and gait deviations. A developmental assessment is performed, yielding standard scores and age equivalents indicating the degree of lag relative to normal children and those with cerebral palsy. A neuropsychologic test battery reveals sensory, perceptual, motor planning, and visual motor strengths and weaknesses. A questionnaire directed to parents indicates their attitudes and understanding of their child's problems and the child's ADL skills. During instruction in home programming, a checklist of psychomotor skills is performed on the mother to indicate her strengths and weaknesses in performing the motor skills required for the home program.

Improvements in assessment will result not only in more accurate diagnosis, more precise treatment prescriptions, and valid measurement of change produced by therapeutic intervention, but may also lead to the ability to make prognostic statements. Such ability would improve parent and client evaluation, might result in differential treatment approaches to identified subgroups, and allow more efficient use of scarce treatment resources. The fact that prognostic statements regarding locomotion in children with cerebral palsy have been made with some degree of success using our current crude assessment of reflexes and motor milestones suggests that better measurement techniques might yield rich results in improved predictability of ultimate function.[8,42,52]

Evans and Peham, in an assessment of the quality of measurement in occupational therapy, describe the critical need for tests with prognostic capabilities in terms of ethical issues.[53] They note that tests are currently being used to classify and label children, a process that carries implicit prognostic implications. As the review in this chapter shows clearly, most of the tests in use today have not been studied for predictive validity and should be considered to be subject to abuse by users who imply prognostic value in their testing. Invalid labeling has the potential to lower caretaker expectations, impair social–psychological development of children, and result in unnecessary intervention.

In summary, today's methods for measurement of CNS dysfunction in children are rudimentary. New understanding of the neurologic aberrations and movement abnormalities is growing, however, in tandem with expanding technology for quantifying the components of movement. The juxtaposition of rapidly developing theory and new instrumentation promises a bright future for therapeutic intervention with brain-damaged clients. Physical therapists must realize, however, that most the work cited in this paper was *not* done by therapists. Improved education for physical therapy, heightened commitment to research, and interdisciplinary cooperation are necessary to maintain the predominant role of physical therapists in pediatric rehabilitation.

ACKNOWLEDGMENTS

During the period in which this chapter was written, the author was supported by a training grant from the Maternal and Child Health Services, DHHS, USPHS. Valuable assistance in test identification and evaluation was provided by Thomas J. Stengel.

REFERENCES

1. Chandler LS, Andrews MS, Swanson MW: Movement Assessment of Infants—A Manual. Movement Assessment of Infants, Rolling Bay, Washington, 1980
2. Miller LJ: Miller Assessment for Preschoolers. Foundation for Knowledge in Development, Littleton, Colorado, 1982

3. Ayres AJ: Southern California Sensory Integration Tests Manual Revised. Western Psychological Services, Los Angeles, 1980

4. Sousa JC, Telzrow RW, Holm RA, McCartin R, Shurtleff DB: Developmental guidelines for children with myelodysplasia. Phys Ther 63:21, 1983

5. Hughes JE: Manual for the Hughes Basic Gross Motor Assessment. Jeanne E. Hughes, Goldon, Colorado, 1979

6. DeGangi GA: Assessment of Sensorimotor Integration in Preschool Children. Unpublished manuscript, The Johns Hopkins University, Baltimore, 1979

7. Johnson MK, Zuck FN, Wingate K: The Motor Age Test: Measurement of motor handicaps in children with neuromuscular disorders such as cerebral palsy. J Bone Joint Surg [Am] 33:698, 1951

8. Beals RK: Spastic paraplegia and diplegia: An evaluation of non-surgical and surgical factors influencing the prognosis for ambulation. J Bone Joint Surg [Am] 48:827, 1966

9. American Psychological Association: Standards for Educational and Psychological Tests. American Psychological Association, Washington, D.C., 1974

10. Bruininks RH: Bruininks-Oseretsky Test of Motor Proficiency: Examiner's Manual. American Guidance Service, Circle Pines, Minnesota, 1978

11. Prechtl HFR, Beintema D: The Neurological Examination of the Full Term Newborn Infant. Clinics in Developmental Medicine, No. 12. J.B. Lippincott, Philadelphia, 1964

12. Prechtl HFR: The Neurological Examination of the Full Term Newborn Infant. Clinics in Developmental Medicine, No. 63. J.B. Lippincott, Philadelphia, 1977

13. Dubowitz L, Dubowitz V: The Neurological Assessment of the Preterm and Fullterm Newborn Infant. Clinics in Developmental Medicine, No. 79. J.B. Lippincott, Philadelphia, 1981

14. Stott DH, Moyes FA, Henderson SE: Test of Motor Impairment. Brook Educational Publishing, Guelph, Ontario, 1972

15. Roach EG, Kephart NC: The Purdue Perceptual-Motor Survey. Charles E. Merrill, Columbus, Ohio, 1966

16. Buros OK (ed): Mental Measurements Yearbook Series. The Gryphon Press, Highland Park, New Jersey, issued periodically

17. Stengel TJ, Attermeier SM, Bly L, Heriza CB: Evaluation of sensorimotor dysfunction. In Campbell SK (ed): Clinics in Physical Therapy: Pediatric Neurologic Physical Therapy. Churchill Livingstone, New York, 1984

18. Johnson OG: Tests and Measurements in Child Development: A Handbook. Jossey-Bass, San Francisco, 1971

19. Johnson OG: Tests and Measurements in Child Development: Handbook II, Vol. I and II. Jossey-Bass, Washington, D.C., 1976

20. Lewko JO: Current practices in evaluating motor behavior of disabled children. Am J Occup Ther 30:413, 1976

21. Frankenberg WK, Dodds JB, Fandal AW, et al.: Denver Developmental Screening Test Reference Manual, Revised 1975 Edition. LADOCA Project and Publishing Foundation, Denver, 1975

22. Knutsson E: Restraint of spastic muscles in different types of movement. In Feldman RG, Young RR, Koella WP (eds): Spasticity: Disordered Motor Control. Year Book Medical Publishers, Chicago, 1980

23. Milner-Brown HS, Penn RD: Pathophysiological mechanisms in cerebral palsy. J Neurol Neurosurg Psychiatry 42:606, 1979

24. Neilson PD: Voluntary control of arm movement in athetotic patients. J Neurol Neurosurg Psychiatry 37:162, 1974

25. Barolat-Romana G, David R: Neurophysiological mechanisms in abnormal reflex activities in cerebral palsy and spinal spasticity. J Neurol Neurosurg Psychiatry 43:333, 1980

26. Perry J, Hoffer MM, Antonelli D, Plut J, Lewis G, Greenberg, R: Electromyography before and after surgery for hip deformity in children with cerebral palsy: A comparison of clinical and electromyographic findings. J Bone Joint Surg [Am] 58:201, 1976

27. Krus PH, Bruininks RH, Robertson G: Structure of motor abilities in children. Percept Mot Skills 52:119, 1981

28. Beintema DJ: A Neurological Study of a Newborn Infant. Clinics in Developmental Medicine, No. 28. William Heinemann, London, 1968

29. Prechtl HFR: The mother-child interaction in babies with minimal brain damage. In Foss BM (ed): Determinants of Infant Behavior II. John Wiley, New York, 1963

30. Prechtl HFR: Prognostic value of neurological signs in the newborn infant. Proc R Soc Med 58:3, 1965

31. Campbell SK: Movement assessment of infants: an evaluation. Phys Occup Ther Pediatr 1:53, 1981

32. Chandler L, Harris S: Movement Assessment of Infants. Workshop presentation, Northeastern District of the Section on Pediatrics of the American Physical Therapy Association, Amherst, Massachusetts, March 27, 1983

33. Pauker JD: Test of Motor Impairment, Test #881. In Buros OK (ed): The Eighth Mental Measurements Yearbook, Vol. II. The Gryphon Press, Highland Park, New Jersey, 1978

34. Kimball JG: The Southern California Sensory Integration Tests (Ayres) and the Bender Gestalt: A correlative study. Am J Occup Ther 31:294, 1977

35. Punwar A: Spatial visualization, reading, spelling and mathematical abilities in second- and third-grade children. Am J Occup Ther 24:495, 1970

36. DeGangi GA, Berk RA: Psychometric analysis of the Test of Sensory Integration. Phys Occup Ther Pediatr 3:43, 1983

37. Jamison CB: The Purdue Perceptual-Motor Survey, Test #874. In Buros OK (ed): The Seventh Mental Measurements Yearbook, Vol. II. The Gryphon Press, Highland Park, New Jersey, 1972

38. Landis D: The Purdue Perceptual-Motor Survey, Test #874. In Buros OK (ed): The Seventh Mental Measurements Yearbook, Vol. II. The Gryphon Press, Highland Park, New Jersey, 1972

39. Henderson SE, Morris J, Frith U: The motor deficit in Down's Syndrome children: a problem of timing? J Child Psychol Psychiatry 22:223, 1981

40. Neilson PD: Voluntary and reflex control of the biceps brachii muscle in spastic-athetotic patients. J Neurol Neurosurg Psychiatry 35:589, 1972

41. Forsström A, von Hofsten C: Visually directed reaching of children with motor impairments. Dev Med Child Neurol 24:653, 1982

42. Holt KS: Review: The assessment of walking in children with particular reference to cerebral palsy. Child Care Health Dev 7:281, 1981

43. Nashner LM: Analysis of stance posture in humans. In Towe AL, Luschei ES (eds): Handbook of Behavioral Neurobiology, Vol. 5, Motor Coordination. Plenum Press, New York, 1981

44. Nashner LM, Shumway-Cook A, Marin O: Stance posture control in select groups of children with cerebral palsy: deficits in sensory organization and muscular coordination. Exp Brain Res 49:393, 1983

45. Chong KC, Vojnic CD, Quanbury AO, Eng P, Letts RM: The assessment of the internal rotation gait in cerebral palsy—an electromyographic gait analysis. Clin Orthoped 132:145, 1978
46. Perry J, Hoffer MM: Preoperative and postoperative dynamic electromyography as an aid in planning tendon transfers in children with cerebral palsy. J Bone Joint Surg [Am] 59:531, 1977
47. Perry J, Hoffer MM, Giovan P, Antonelli D, Greenberg R: Gait analysis of the triceps surae in cerebral palsy. A preoperative and postoperative clinical and electromyographic study. J Bone Joint Surg [Am] 56:511, 1974
48. Whitehead WE, Parker LH, Masek BJ, Cataldo MF, Freeman JM: Biofeedback treatment of fecal incontinence in patients with myelomeningocele. Dev Med Child Neurol 23:313, 1981
49. Myklebust BM, Gottlieb GL, Penn RD, Agarwal GC: Reciprocal excitation of antagonistic muscles as a differentiating feature in spasticity. Ann Neurol 12:367, 1982
50. Atkin A, Bala S, Herman P, Rogowitz B: Organicity and mental retardation: Analysis of eye and head movements. J Ment Defic Res 25:17, 1981
51. Poland DJ, Doebler LK: Effects of a blacklight visual field on eye-contact training of spastic cerebral palsied children. Percept Mot Skills 51:335, 1980
52. Bleck EE: Locomotor prognosis in cerebral palsy. Dev Med Child Neurol 17:18, 1975
53. Evans PR, Peham MAS: Testing and Measurement in Occupational Therapy: A Review of Current Practice with Special Emphasis on the Southern California Sensory Integration Tests. Institute for Research on Learning Disabilities Monograph No. 15. University of Minnesota, Minneapolis, 1981

8 | Pulmonary Function Testing

Elizabeth J. Protas

Physical therapists utilize information from pulmonary function testing in order to select appropriate treatment, evaluate treatment outcomes, and follow the course of various diseases. Pulmonary testing has become an established part of treatment decisions in patients with respiratory pathology; however, it is often difficult to determine the significance of these test results. For example, it is not uncommon to encounter a patient who would be classified as having moderate to severe pulmonary disease according to pulmonary studies and yet who is still leading an active, functional life. If the physical therapist must rely upon these tests for the evaluation of the patient with pulmonary disease, it is important for the therapist to know the inherent limitations of these measurements and their application to clinical practice.

Pulmonary function testing is not truly diagnostic in the sense of implicating one disease process over another. Pulmonary testing can broadly categorize a variety of disease processes and the physiologic sequelae. Pulmonary studies are used to differentiate obstructive lung pathologies from restrictive lung pathologies. Obstructive diseases increase resistance to airflow by obstructing airways. Narrowing or collapse of the airways generally occurs during expiration, when negative thoracic pressures tend to compress small airways. This leads to a decreased expiratory airflow and a greater volume of air trapped in the lung. Asthma and emphysema are the most prevalent examples of obstructive lung disease. In contrast, restrictive disorders are characterized by decreased expandability of lung tissue or the chest wall and/or a decrease in the amount of functional lung tissue. Restrictive diseases limit to varying degrees the maximum volumes of air that can be inhaled or exhaled. Paralysis of respiratory muscles, bony abnormalities of the chest, lung tumors, and pneumonia are examples of restrictive lung disorders.[1]

Pulmonary function tests, as the name implies, are used to determine the functional characteristics of the lung. A variety of tests are employed to determine: (1) how well air is moved in and out of the lung, (2) how much air the lung contains, and (3) the effectiveness of the lung in oxygenating the blood.

Tests that examine the capacity of the lung to move air are grouped as tests that reflect airflow and resistance to airflow. Airflow and resistance tests include forced vital capacity, forced expiratory volume in one second, flow rates, airway resistance, closing volume, closing capacity, and compliance. Airflow and resistance tests measure dynamic flow rates, volumes, and/or pressures that occur during maximal or quiet breathing.

In addition to airflow capabilities of the lung, it is frequently important to know the total capacity of the lung and how much air is retained following exhalation. The measurement of lung volumes provides this information. Lung volume measures include total lung capacity, functional residual capacity, and residual volume. Obstructive diseases often result in increased lung volumes as a result of air trapping, whereas restrictive pathologies often decrease total lung capacity.

The ability of the lung to oxygenate the blood is determined through tests of gas exchange. Diffusion capacity, the ratio of dead space to tidal volume, the difference between alveolar and arteriolar oxygen, and ventilation–perfusion studies indicate the effectiveness of gas exchange in the lung.

Some tests in the same general functional category provide similar or overlapping information. For example, the forced vital capacity and forced expiratory volume of one second will both indicate impeded airflow resulting from an obstructive condition. The selection of which test or group of tests depends on several factors, such as available equipment and personnel expertise and the nature of the pathology and purpose of the test. Public health screening for the incidence of respiratory disease may involve different tests than those administered to a patient with a long history of chronic lung disease who is hospitalized for adult respiratory distress syndrome.

Often an entire battery of pulmonary function tests is used even if similar information is provided, because of the inherent measurement characteristics of pulmonary function tests. First, pulmonary function is normally variable and highly individualized. This variability is enhanced by lung disease. Second, the ability of these tests to detect abnormalities or changes in status varies greatly between the tests. Thus, a combination of tests with overlapping results may enhance the information provided by any single test. Last, a broad spectrum of pathologies impose the same constraints upon pulmonary function. The etiologies behind muscle paralysis and pneumonia are quite different; yet similar limitations of pulmonary function may result. In fact, categorizing the severity of the limitation may be a more important clinical consideration than indicating the nature of the lung abnormality.

This chapter focuses on the reliability, validity, and methodology of pulmonary measurements, as well as on the clinical significance of pulmonary function testing. In physical therapy, pulmonary testing is valuable in the evaluation and management of patients with acute lung pathologies. Increased understanding of these measures should enhance the therapist's ability to select measurements that will document treatment outcomes.

RELIABILITY, SPECIFICITY, AND SENSITIVITY

Because pulmonary function fluctuates from time to time, it is important to know how repeatable pulmonary testing is. Tests that display less biologic and physiologic variability will produce greater confidence in the test results. Consequently, each test discussed will include a description of test reliability in order to provide the reader with information concerning normal variability and how lung pathology influences that variability. Test reliability is reported as the coefficient of variation. The coefficient of variation (CV) is the variability of the results of repeated tests on the same subject expressed as a percentage of the average of the subject's scores (SD/mean × 100) (see Chapter 1). This measure provides information on the within-subject variability; therefore, it will give the clinician an idea of the variation to expect with repeated testing of the same person.

Another key measurement concept describes how well a test distinguishes between an individual whose pulmonary function is within normal limits and an individual with abnormal pulmonary function. The terms *test specificity* and *test sensitivity* are used to describe these qualities. Test specificity refers to the number of normal individuals identified by a test. Excellent test specificity, however, does not necessarily indicate the ability of a test to identify an individual with an abnormality. For example, broad limits have been established for normal range of motion (ROM). A patient who is being seen for a supraspinatus tendonitis could display shoulder motion of the involved side that is within normal limits, yet when the involved shoulder is compared to the range of the contralateral side, it is considered limited. Test sensitivity is the ability of a test to identify individuals with abnormalities. In the example, ROM testing would have excellent test specificity, but poor test sensitivity when moderate to slight losses of ROM exist. Pulmonary function testing displays various combinations of test specificity and test sensitivity. For example, normal values for forced vital capacity are liberally defined. Therefore, forced vital capacity has excellent test specificity for identifying normal individuals. On the other hand, a considerable decrease in vital capacity is necessary before the test is considered abnormal. Forced vital capacity testing has poor sensitivity in relation to detecting slight to moderate abnormalities.

A discussion of the coefficient of variation, test specificity, and test sensitivity has been included for each test. This will provide the physical therapist with a basis for comparing these tests as well as information for interpreting the results.

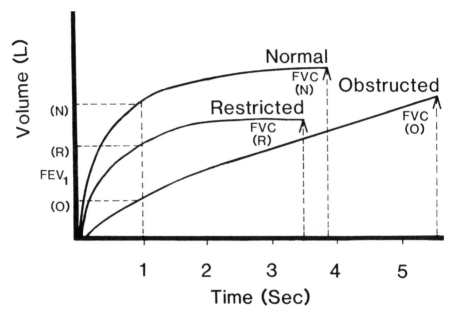

Fig. 8-1. A schematic comparison of the forced vital capacity (FVC) and forced expiratory volume in one second (FEV₁) in normal individuals (N) and in individuals with either obstructed (O) or restricted (R) lung pathology.

PULMONARY FUNCTION TESTS

Airflow and Resistance to Airflow

Forced Vital Capacity. Measurement of the forced vital capacity (FVC) requires complete and rapid exhalation from full inspiration.[1] The expired volume is the maximum amount of air that can voluntarily be moved from the lung. The test is begun at total lung capacity or full inspiration and ends when air can no longer be forced from the lung. Spirometers are used to measure and record the FVC (Fig. 8-1).

The FVC consists of approximately 80 percent of the total lung capacity in healthy, young adults.[2] Normative values for FVC are based upon age, height, and sex.[3–5] Because normative FVC values are based upon large samples, the FVC test specificity is excellent.[6] The FVC, however, is relatively insensitive to the presence of certain types of lung abnormalities.[6–8] In other words, an individual with a positive history of disease and abnormalities on other pulmonary function tests would not necessarily have a reduced FVC. Several factors contribute to this apparent paradox of the FVC having excellent specificity but poor sensitivity. The first is a wide range of values that may be considered normal for a person of a given age, height, and sex, and the second is the type of lung function reflected by the FVC.

When actual values of FVC are compared to predicted values, a wide distribution of values becomes apparent. Parot reviewed data for 822 men and women from several studies.[9] He suggested that 95 percent confidence intervals would result in a range of ± 0.7 L of the predicted value for women and ± 1.0 L for men. This broad range makes it difficult to assess whether any one individual is normal or abnormal. An individual's FVC could be reduced to 4 L from a value of 5 L and would still be considered normal. The reverse is also true. An individual could display 100 percent of a predicted normal value and still be constricted if the individual's FVC is ordinarily much greater than 100 percent of the predicted value. Thus, any one person can be classified as normal in relation to predicted values of FVC, yet still have reduced lung function.

Several authors have suggested that FVC reflects only the function of large airways; changes in the smaller, more peripheral airways of less than 2-mm diameters are not evident in the FVC measure.[10–13] For example, abnormal FVC values were found in only 6 percent of 55 cigarette smokers who were known to have peripheral airway obstruction.[7] Thus, the sensitivity of FVC to small changes in the periphery of the lung is poor, although it can document advanced central airway obstruction.

However, FVC has been shown to be one of the most reliable and repeatable of the standard spirometric measures (Table 8-1). The within-subject coefficients of variation in normals range from 1.9 percent to 4.5 percent when subjects are retested on the same day,[14,15] over several weeks,[16–18] or over several months.[19,20] The within-day variations, however, are generally less than day-to-day and week-to-week variations.[21] Thus, some of the variability reflects changing biological states, whereas a portion is caused by inaccuracies in measuring FVC. The variability is significantly greater in patients with cystic fibrosis[14] and chronic bronchitis.[20]

Forced Expiratory Volume in One Second. The volume of air exhaled in the first second of the FVC is the forced expiratory volume in one second (FEV_1). The measure is taken during the most rapid portion of the FVC test, and normal values of FEV_1 can encompass from 51 percent to 97 percent of the FVC in men and 59 percent to 93 percent in women.[1]

Because FEV_1 is such a large component of FVC, the two measures are highly correlated. Consequently, much of the discussion of FVC applies to FEV_1. FEV_1 has an excellent specificity, but a poor sensitivity.[22] The FEV_1 coefficients of variation of normal individuals are comparable to FVC coefficients, ranging from 3 percent to 5 percent (Table 8-1). McDonald and Cole, using canonical variate analysis on the pulmonary function tests of 25 normal adults, concluded that the FEV_1 contributed almost no unique information when compared with the FVC. They suggested that FEV_1 could be excluded if there is a need to reduce the number of tests, although they do caution that these comments are based upon tests of normal individuals and should not be generalized to patient populations.[6]

Flow Rates. Forced expiratory flow during the middle portion of forced exhalation ($FEF_{25-75\%}$), peak expiratory flow rate (PEFR), and flow rates after 50 percent and 75 percent of the vital capacity have been exhaled ($FEF_{50\%}$ and $FEF_{75\%}$) provide indications of airflow at different points during expiration. $FEF_{25-75\%}$ can be recorded from a spirogram, whereas PEFR and $FEF_{50\%}$ and

Table 8-1. Within-Subject Coefficients of Variations (%) for Expiratory Volumes and Flows

Author	FVC		FEV$_1$		FEF$_{25-75\%}$		FEF$_{50\%}$		FEF$_{75\%}$	
Lebowitz et al[19]	3.5–3.6		3.5–3.6		7.5–8.2		7.5–8.2		12.0–13.4	
Nickerson et al[15]	3.5	(6.0)[a]	3.6	(5.3)	5.5	(9.3)	6.1	(10.1)	8.4	(11.3)
Knudson et al[14]	4.5		4.7		9.2		8.7		13.7	
Cochrane et al[16]	2.0		4.0		—		9.0		14.0	
Love et al[17]										
lab	2.6		3.2		—		5.3		12.1	
field	3.7		5.1		—		15.1		19.3	
Afschrift et al[25]		(11.1)		(14.8)		(13.3)		(8.6)		(11.6)
Mungall and Hainsworth[20]	1.9		2.7		—		—		—	
Jorfeldt and Wranne[18]	—		—		—		7.0		10.3	
Bonsignore et al[24]	—		—		—		7.0	(17, 24)	—	
Stanescu et al[26]	—		—		—		5.4	(7.0)	8.9	(12.8)

[a] Numbers in parentheses are from patients with obstructive or restrictive pathologies.

FVC, forced vital capacity; FEV$_1$, forced expiratory volume in one second; FEF$_{25-75\%}$, forced expiratory flow between 25 percent and 75 percent of FVC; FEF$_{50\%}$, forced expiratory flow after 50 percent of the FVC has been exhaled; FEF$_{75\%}$, forced expiratory flow after 75 percent of the FVC has been exhaled.

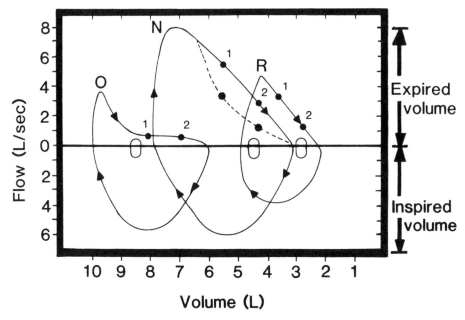

Fig. 8-2. Flow volume loops normally (N) and in obstructed (O) or restricted (R) pathology. The dashed line on the normal flow-volume curve represents a change that may indicate small airway disease. The forced expiratory flow after 50 percent (FEF$_{50\%}$) and 75 percent (FEF$_{75\%}$) of the vital capacity has been exhaled are indicated along the expiratory portion of the loop as 1 and 2, respectively. The peak flow may also be determined from this loop.

FEF$_{75\%}$ are most commonly measured from a maximum expiratory flow-volume curve (MEFV) using a spirometer or a pneumotachygraph with a recording system (Fig. 8-2).[1] PEFR can also be measured using a flow meter.

Flow rates generally have a higher within-subject variability than FVC or FEV$_1$ (Table 8-1). FEF$_{25-75\%}$ and FEF$_{50\%}$ have coefficients of variation ranging from 5.5 percent to 15.1 percent in normals; FEF$_{75\%}$ is highest in this group with values ranging from 8.4 percent to 19.3 percent. In other words, retests of the same subject under the same circumstances can vary by as much as 15 percent for FEF$_{25-75\%}$ and FEF$_{50\%}$ and up to 19 percent for FEF$_{75\%}$. Measurement factors such as the difficulty in isolating a particular volume level on the MEFV curve as well as greater physiological variability associated with lower rates of air flow have been cited as contributing to the within-subject variability.[14,23] Nickerson and associates noted that the coefficients of variation are significantly higher for FEF$_{25-75\%}$, FEF$_{50\%}$ and FEF$_{75\%}$ in patients with cystic fibrosis than in normal subjects.[14] A large variability in flow rates at different volumes has also been observed in asthmatics[24] and in adults with chronic obstructive disease.[25,26] These variations have been attributed to changes in airway mechanics resulting from disease. For example, a redistribution of sputum in the lung during testing contributes to different test results between trials.[14]

The test specificity for normal individuals of the flow measures is not as high as the specificity of FVC and FEV_1; however, the sensitivity of flow rates to small airway disease approaches that of invasive measures, such as radioaerosol lung imaging. In addition, the sensitivity of flow measures is substantially better than that of blood gases in detecting abnormal lung function.[22] The enhanced sensitivity is based on the fact that lower airflow occurs during the later stages of forced exhalation, when the lungs are in a state of low elastic recoil and the small airways are less expanded. If there is a tendency for the small airways to collapse, this occurs when the airways are less expanded. Consequently, $FEF_{50\%}$ and $FEF_{75\%}$ reflect changes in the small airways.[10-13] Tashkin and his colleagues noted that the sensitivity to small airway change of the combined measures derived from the MEFV curve was higher than combined values from spirometry, the closing volume curve, and body plethysmography.[22] In contrast, other researchers have found combined MEFV curve values to be only slightly more sensitive than spirometry in detecting small airway abnormalities, and to be substantially less sensitive than combined measures from closing volume curves of a single breath nitrogen washout test.[7] The question of which test or group of tests is most sensitive to small airway involvement is a subject of current debate, and is, as yet, unresolved.

The combination of the higher variability of flow measures with greater test sensitivity may appear to be inconsistent; however, Sobol et al suggest that a highly variable test may be very sensitive in instances in which the changes induced by pathology are larger than the variability of the measure.[27] Large changes produced by small airway disease were first noted using $FEF_{50\%}$ by McFadden and Linden[28] and using $FEF_{75\%}$ by Mead et al.[29]

Other tests based upon flow-volume curves have been proposed. Dosman suggested the percentage increase in $FEF_{50\%}$ on breathing helium as an index of small airway obstruction.[30] This test, has been shown to be poorly reproducible in normals[6] and less reproducible in asthmatics.[24,31] Similarly, a method proposed by Mead[32] using a computer to calculate slopes along the MEFV curve, (ie, the slope ratios) proved to have coefficients of variation between 50 percent and 80 percent and did not discriminate between normals and patients.[14] On the other hand, a computerized analysis of the MEFV curve, which times airflow at various points in the curve (called mean transit times), has a variability and discrimination comparable to $FEF_{50\%}$ and $FEF_{75\%}$; however, the mean transit time measure does require a sophisticated computer analysis and may not provide any more information than do flow volumes.[14]

Resistance to Airflow.   Although FVC, FEV_1, and flow volumes will provide an indication of resistance to airflow, airway resistance (R_{AW}), closing volume (CV), closing capacity (CC), and lung compliance are also used. The results of R_{AW}, CV, CC, and lung compliance tests will provide other indicators of small airway function and lung elasticity.

R_{AW} is tested with a body plethysmograph to measure pressure, a pneumotachygraph to measure flow, and a recording system (Fig. 8-3). By having

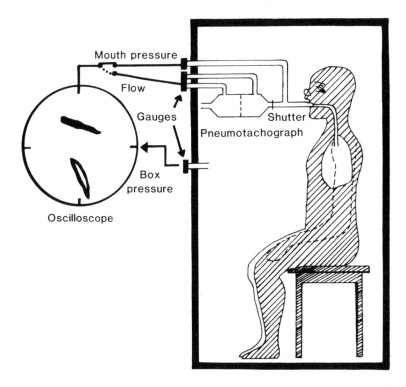

Fig. 8-3. A diagram of the components of a whole body plethysmograph. The mouth pressure is recorded while the subject is panting into an unobstructed airway, i.e., with the shutter open. This produces the lower tracing on the oscilloscope or the pressure loop. The shutter is then closed in order to determine the lung volume at which the pressure is taken. This produces the upper tracing on the oscilloscope. The slopes of these tracings are used to calculate airway resistance (R_{AW}) as changes in pressure (P) over changes in volume (V) ($R_{AW} = \Delta P/\Delta V$). Lung compliance is determined similarly except that a catheter is inserted into the esophagus to record esophageal pressure.

the individual being tested pant rapidly into an open valve, pressure changes (P) in the plethysmograph are recorded (Fig. 8-4). The shutter is then closed in order to record the volume (V) during panting (2 on Fig. 8-4). The slope of these plots are used to calculate R_{AW} as $R_{AW} = \Delta P/\Delta V$.[33] R_{AW} is normally 1.5 to 3.0 cm $H_2O/L/s$ and can increase above 10 cm $H_2O/L/s$ with obstructive disease.[2]

CV and CC are determined by measuring the level of nitrogen or a marker gas during a slow exhalation. This measurement is based upon the fact that the gas concentration is higher in upper zones of the lung, which empty last.[1] When airway closure occurs in the dependent zones of the lung, a sharp increase in marker gas concentration is recorded until residual volume (RV) is reached (Fig. 8-5). The CV is the volume from the onset of airway closure to RV. The CC is CV plus RV. The slope of the longer portion of the recording (phase III

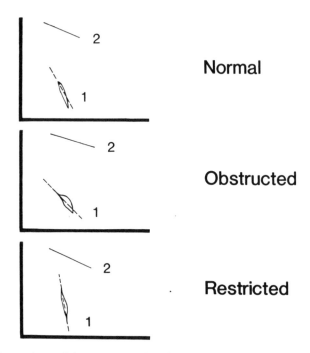

Normal

Obstructed

Restricted

Fig. 8-4.   Illustrations of the pressure (1) and volume (2) tracings recorded from a body plethysmograph in an individual with normal airway resistance (R_{AW}), with increased R_{AW} resulting from obstructed pathology, and with decreased R_{AW} in restricted pathology.

on Fig. 8-5) reflects the degree of homogeneity of inspired gas distribution. Loss of elastic recoil or the patency of the small airways will result in airway closure at higher volumes and poor gas distribution.[2]

Compliance is another measure of the elastic properties or distensibility of the lung. A small balloon catheter is inserted into the esophagus to record changes in esophageal pressure. V and P changes are recorded by a plethysmograph and an integrated pneumotachygraph similar to those described for R_{AW}. Compliance is a ratio of esophageal pressure changes to volume changes (ie, the slope of the curves). Static compliance is measured with an open glottis against an occluded airway at different lung volumes. Static compliance is reduced by changes which increase tissue density such as congestion, atelectasis, and restrictive disease.[2] Dynamic compliance is measured during quiet breathing at generally three to four frequencies from slow to more rapid breathing. A reduction is dynamic compliance as breathing frequency increases is associated with small airway disease.[34]

The specificity of R_{AW} and CV is high and comparable to the specificity of FVC and FEV_1 whereas the test specificity of CC is moderate and approaches that of $FEF_{25-75\%}$. In contrast, the specificity of compliance for detecting normal individuals is relatively low.[22]

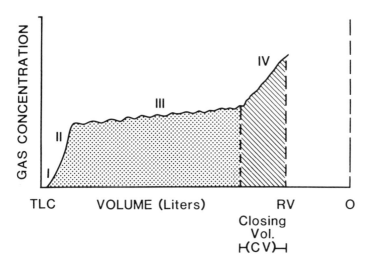

Fig. 8-5. Measuring the concentration of nitrogen or other marker gases exhaled allows the determination of the volume from the point when small airways begin to close to residual volume (RV), or the closing volume (CV). The closing capacity is closing volume plus RV. The slope of the III portion of the graph will indicate gas distribution in the lung.

An almost opposite ordering of test specificity occurs when the test sensitivity of R_{AW}, CV, CC and compliance is examined. In one study, dynamic compliance testing identified 47 percent of the subjects considered abnormal by experienced physicians reviewing the history, physical, and pulmonary testing data, whereas CC testing identified 42 percent. CV results indicated only 26 percent as abnormal, and R_{AW} scores indicated only 5 percent.[22] Thus, the test sensitivity for small airway disease is high in dynamic compliance and CC, moderate in CV and low in R_{AW}.

The sensitivity of the CV curve increases if the results on CV, CC, and the slope of phase III are considered together.[7,22] In other words, an individual who is thought to have small airway disease is more likely to be identified as having an abnormality if all values derived from the CV curve are considered together rather than separately. An analogous example may help to clarify this point. When testing nerve conduction velocities, conduction may be somewhat slowed in a segment. This result alone may be considered normal without additional information; however, when this result is compared to the conduction velocity of other segments of the same nerve and found to be substantially slower, the abnormality becomes more evident. Reports of enhanced sensitivity through examination of all values from the CV curve vary from 53 percent[22] to 90 percent[7] identification of abnormal individuals—substantially better than CV, CC, or phase III slope alone.

Because both flow volume and CV curves are thought to be sensitive to small airway disease, comparisons of the relative sensitivity of the combined measures have been made. The sensitivity of the CV curve values has been reported to be higher than that of the flow volume curve values (90 percent compared to 40 percent)[7] as well as to have a lower sensitivity (53 percent versus 74 percent abnormalities identified).[22] Differences in the population studied and the method for calculating sensitivity contribute to these discrepancies.

Examining the variability of these measures may also help to explain differences in specificity and sensitivity. R_{AW} is poorly reproducible and highly variable within subjects (Table 8-2), a factor that can contribute to its poor sensitivity.[22,33,35] CV as a percent of vital capacity (CV/VC%) is also variable, with retest SDs approaching mean values.[17,22,36] Dynamic compliance measured on eight normal subjects over several breathing frequencies for a 2-year period showed a range of within-subject coefficients of variation of 6 percent to 36 percent, with an average of 17 percent (Table 8-2).[34] MacKenzie and his colleagues, using end inspiratory and end expiratory pressure as a measure of compliance on 42 mechanically ventilated patients, reported a standard deviation of approximately 30 percent of the mean. These investigators used the compliance measure to assess the effects of a single treatment of percussion and postural drainage on patients being ventilated for acute lung pathologies. The compliance increased significantly immediately after and for up to 2 hours following pulmonary physical therapy.[37] This example demonstrates that a variable measure can be used to assess treatment as long as the change produced by the treatment is greater than the variability of the measure.

These measures of airway resistance and elasticity tend to have high within-subject variability. Measurement error and methodology account for part of the variability. For example, computerized analysis decreases the measurement spread when compared with hand calculations,[33,34] and subject training improves reproducibility of test performance.[17]

Lung Volumes

The measurement of static lung volumes is typically more complex than airflow measurement since the methods used are quite involved and the equipment is more complicated. These measures include: total lung capacity (TLC), the volume of gas in the lung with full inspiration; functional residual capacity (FRC), the gas volume in the lung at the end of a normal exhalation; and residual volume (RV), the volume remaining in the lung after complete exhalation.[38] Several methods may be used to measure TLC, FRC, and RV including whole body plethysmography, helium gas dilution methods, or nitrogen washout tests.[1] TLC can also be determined by measuring the area of the lung on a standard chest roentgenogram.[39]

Static lung volumes are used in diagnosing both obstructive and restrictive pathologies.[38] The thoracic gas volume obtained by using body plethysmography in order to derive static volumes has moderate specificity and sensitivity.[22] In one group tested by Marazzini and his co-workers, RV but not TLC

Table 8-2. Within-Subject Coefficients of Variation (%) for Airway Resistance and Gas Exchange Measures

Author	CV%	CC/TLC	R_AW	Compliance	TL-COSB	TL-COSS
Jorfeldt and Wranne[18]	9.5	—	—	—	—	—
Love et al[17]						
lab	20.5	5.8	—	—	7.5	11.0 (50 W)
field	24.6	7.3	—	—	6.6	6.4 (100 W) 22.6 (50 W)
Teculescu et al[35]	—	—	28.0 (13.9)[a]	—	—	—
Douglas et al[34]	—	—	—	6.0—39.0	—	—
Mungall and Hainsworth[20]	—	—	—	—	(15.0)[a]	—

[a] From patients with obstructive pathologies.

CV%, closing volume/vital capacity; CC/TLC, closing capacity/total lung capacity; R_AW, airway resistance; TL-COSB, single-breath carbon monoxide diffusion capacity; TL-COSS, steady-state carbon monoxide diffusion capacity; 50 W, 50 watt bicycle exercise workload; 100 W, 100 watt bicycle exercise workload.

Table 8-3. Within-Subject Coefficients of Variation (%) for Lung Volume Measures

Author	Method	TLC		FRC		RV
Teculescu et al[35]	Plethysmography	4.2	(4.9)[a]	7.5	(7.8)[a]	—
Love et al[17]	Helium dilution					
	lab	2.4		4.9		7.3
	field	3.7		10.4		14.0
Mungall and Hainsworth[20]	Plethysmography		(8.3)[a]	—		—
			(8.8)[a]	—		—
Sterks et al[41]	Closed circuit nitrogen	—		—		7.3

[a] Numbers in parentheses are from patients with obstructive pathologies.
TLC, total lung capacity; FRC, functional residual capacity; RV, residual volume.

or RV/TLC% was significantly increased when smokers were compared to nonsmokers.[36]

The measurement of TLC is as repeatable as FVC and FEV_1 (Table 8-3). Yet, FRC and RV have coefficients of variation in the range of $FEF_{25-75\%}$ and $FEF_{50\%}$.[17,35] Intrasubject variability has also been shown to be greater in obstructive lung disease patients for FRC and RV but not for TLC.[40,41] Wilmore and his colleagues have found the reliability coefficient for normal trained subjects on two closed circuit nitrogen methods for determining RV to be .99.[42] With measures as complex as body plethysmography and gas dilution, the error will not be less than 5 percent unless the correlation coefficients are above .99.[43] In other words, the error becomes exaggerated unless there is a close association between repeated measures.

Static volumes may generally have less applicability in assessing physical therapy outcomes than do functional measures of airflow and airway resistance. This brief discussion of their measurement is presented for comparison with other pulmonary function tests.

Gas Exchange

The most important aspects of lung function are the ability of gas to diffuse through lung tissue and the relationship between ventilation and perfusion. These functions are measured by: diffusion capacity for carbon monoxide either after a single breath (TL_{COSB}) or with steady-state breathing (TL_{COSS}) during rest or exercise, the ratio of physiologic dead space to tidal volume (V_D/V_T), and the gradient between alveolar oxygen tension and arterial oxygen tension $(A-a)DO_2$.[38] Ventilation–perfusion studies can also be performed by following the washout of a radioisotope which has been inhaled (for ventilation) or injected (for perfusion).[44]

Measures of gas exchange are among the few pulmonary function tests that are correlated with exercise tolerance in patients with pulmonary disease.[20,45] Jones points out that some patients with a low arterial partial pressure of oxygen may show an increased arterial oxygen pressure with exercise in instances in which low resting values of ventilation to perfusion improve with exercise.[45] Yet some severely involved chronic pulmonary patients demonstrate a drop in the partial pressure of oxygen with exercise.[46,47] Consequently, resting and exercise gas exchange characteristics may be different. This is clearly important information for the physical therapist. Exercise can be beneficial to the patient who has increased oxygen pressure with activity, but may be detrimental to the patient whose oxygen pressure decreases.

TL_{COSB} is fairly reproducible as a measure of gas diffusion in normal individuals,[17] and slightly less reproducible in patients with chronic obstructive disease (Table 8-2).[20] During steady-state exercise conditions, TL_{COSS} is more reproducible when normal subjects exercise with a 100 W workload on a bicycle ergometer than a lower workload of 50 W.[17] This difference was attributed to the calculation method, which would tend to overestimate TL_{COSS} at lower workloads.

Radioaerosol lung scans are extemely sensitive to abnormalities (84 percent detection) when compared to spirometry, flow volume curves, CV curves, and plethysmographic measures. Radioaerosol scans have also been contrasted with other radionuclide studies (eg, xenon-133) performed on the same population.[22] Xenon-133 ventilation tests and perfusion lung imaging identified only 58 percent and 36 percent, respectively, of those considered to be abnormal by experienced physicians reviewing all of the patient information, whereas $(A - a)DO_2$ calculated from blood samples was only moderately sensitive in showing abnormalities (37 percent).[22] These authors conclude that the addition of more time-consuming and/or invasive tests (such as xenon-133 and drawing of blood samples) did not improve the sensitivity of the battery of tests performed for screening purposes. More pertinent to physical therapy is the potential value of radionuclide studies in relation to evaluating secretion clearance techniques (eg, postural drainage programs). Both the possible applications as well as the problems in using such invasive measures have recently been discussed.[48]

Less cumbersome, noninvasive measures of gas exchange may be of more interest to the physical therapist when evaluating exercise responses of chronic obstructive lung disease patients. Several types of transcutaneous oxygen monitors are available for this purpose.[49-51] One type monitors arterial oxygen when it is attached to the ear lobe and thus is called ear oximetry. Ear oximetry is accurate and reliable when arterial oxygen saturation is above 80 percent, but tends to provide a higher value for arterial saturation when saturation is below 80 percent. Other types of transcutaneous oxygen monitors designed to attach to other skin surface areas have been shown to have poor accuracy with normal arterial partial pressures of oxygen and are even less reliable at reduced oxygen tensions.[50] Ear oximetry is the preferred noninvasive measure of arterial oxygenation at this time.

FACTORS AFFECTING PULMONARY FUNCTION ASSESSMENT

The previous discussion has shown that there is considerable within-subject variability in most pulmonary function tests. This measurement variance reflects not only transient changes in an individual's pulmonary system but also measurement factors. Equipment, measurement error, time, medications, and exercise are frequently cited as influences on the results of testing.

Equipment

Concern that the vast array of devices for measuring pulmonary function were not equivalent led to performance recommendations by the American Thoracic Society.[52] These recommendations require equipment to be accurate within ± 3 percent for FVC and FEV_1, and ± 5 percent for flow values. Several studies using mechanical simulations as testing procedures have indicated that not all equipment can meet these requirements.[53-57] Volume displacement spirometers generally tend to be less variable than flow-sensing devices such as pneumotachygraphs and peak flow meters. In addition, several investigators have indicated that equipment variations may be more pronounced when subject lung volumes are tested than they are in a mechanical simulation.[57-59] Equipment error can be a function of any or several components within a measurement system. Inaccurate sensors, nonlinear responses, leaks, temperature and humidity sensitivity, programming errors in computerized systems, and mechanical problems such as leaky pens, poor seals, and sticky recording paper have all been problematic.[53,54,56,57,60]

Pulmonary testing instruments are complex and sensitive equipment, introducing many possibilities for error. It should also be kept in mind that the technology is changing rapidly, and that new equipment is constantly being introduced into a field with much existing equipment in use. Newer spirometry equipment has been manufactured to meet specific performance standards; however, equipment produced prior to these standards may or may not perform to the same level.[53]

A few general suggestions may help clinicians in making decisions about the quality of the measurement instruments upon which they depend. First, frequent equipment calibration assures that equipment is performing consistently.[54-56,61] Second, patient testing should be conducted on the same type of equipment and, if possible, on the same device.[62] This is particularly important on repeat tests of one patient. Last, because variations occur between equipment of the same model from the same manufacturer,[63] it has been suggested that individual pulmonary function labs should establish reference values for their particular equipment.[14,21] These values can then be used to judge equipment performance and patient evaluation. With these general guidelines in mind, a clinician may feel more confident that the equipment is not contributing significantly to measurement variability.

Measurement Error

The analysis of pulmonary records can be another source of variability. Timed volume, flow volume, pressure volume, or CV values are obtained by finding a particular point on the recorded curve, correcting for barometric pressure and temperature, and frequently, through calculating the final value.

This analysis is completed either by hand or with a computer. All of these manipulations can introduce inaccuracies into the values.[33,56,58,64-66] Furthermore, the variability is greater if several people analyze records than if one person performs the analysis.[35,67,68]

A consistent and well-defined process for analyzing records tends to decrease some of the measurement error. Having technicians who are thoroughly trained in standardized procedures eliminates most errors.[22,52] Multiple observations during testing (eg, three to five) assure that the patient understands the instructions and performs the maneuvers accurately.[47,52,65,69] Peslin and his colleagues concluded that analysis of a composite of five flow volume curves yielded more reproducible results than analysis of only the "best" curve produced.[70] Ideally, when the reproducibility of serial efforts is critical, a single observer should be used to assure greatest consistency in the analysis.

Time

Pulmonary function fluctuates normally throughout the day, from week to week, from month to month, and from year to year. The variation of pulmonary values generally increases as the time between measures increases.[19,21] For this reason, repeated measures should be performed at the same time of day, and when possible, a standard length of time between tests should be established.

Medications and Exercise

Pulmonary function testing before and after provocation tests that induce bronchial spasm is used with asthmatic patients. Bronchial spasm can be provoked by inhaling irritating substances such as histamine,[71] antigens,[72] or water,[73] or following exercise.[74] With these procedures, the tendency for bronchospasm as well as the effectiveness of bronchodilating drugs can be evaluated. Substantial improvements of pulmonary function values have been documented in asthmatics after bronchodilating medications are administered.[75-78]

The effectiveness of bronchodilators and mucolytic agents for secretion clearance in patients with acute lung disease, however, has been questioned.[79] A recent report by Ranchod and his co-workers indicated that β-blocking medications increase airflow obstruction in patients with chronic bronchitis.[80] The influence of medications depends upon the type of medicinal agent and the pathological process.

The patient's medications can be a serious confounding variable and a primary concern of the physical therapist when trying to assess the outcome of the physical therapy treatment regimen. For example, Winning et al reported that the administration of a mucolytic agent lessened the effectiveness of chest physical therapy to increase lung compliance in mechanically ventilated patients.[81] The therapist must identify the type of medication, the time it is administered, and the potential influence the drug may have on pulmonary measures.

Maximal exercise in normal individuals has been shown to increase significantly RV and TLC up to 15 minutes following exercise.[82] A similar phenomenon has been suggested in patients with obstructive lung disease.[83,84] Exercise has also been observed to increase spontaneous coughing in intensive-care patients[85] and in patients with cystic fibrosis.[46] Because activity and exercise are often included with other physical therapy techniques such as secretion clearance and breathing retraining, the differential effects of exercise may have to be distinguished from other treatment approaches.

STANDARDIZED METHODS OF PULMONARY TESTING

Variation in Methodology

The Snowbird Workshop of the American Thoracic Society was an attempt to establish standards for pulmonary testing.[52] During that conference, agreement on recommendations for spirometry and flow volume measures was reached. It is unfortunate that guidelines are not available for all pulmonary function tests. For example, there is no standardization of the measure or the criteria to be used for provocation tests.[75] Considerable disagreement also exists in regard to which test or group of tests is most sensitive to small airway obstruction.

Until there are generally accepted standards, the most pertinent issue for the physical therapist is whether or not there are standardized testing protocols in their facility. The concerns discussed under equipment and measurement error should be addressed in a protocol. Factors such as positioning, timing, repetitions, and methods of analysis for each test should be clearly defined. Well-defined standard procedures can yield more meaningful measures of individual patients while affording therapists the opportunity to categorize responses to treatment more systematically.

Variability in Populations

Interpreting the results of pulmonary function testing may require reference to normative values. In addition to the considerable variations in pulmonary values already discussed, population-specific differences have also been reported. Reference values for healthy white American adults are comparable to caucasian adults in other countries;[86] however, healthy black adults have smaller values for FVC, FEV_1, and $FEF_{25-75\%}$ than do whites of the same age and height.[87] Children tend to display greater variability in lung volumes and flow rates than do adults[88-90]; therefore, separate recommendations for standardization of lung function testing in children have been established.[91] Significant differences in pulmonary volumes and flows have also been observed between boys and girls and between white, black, and Mexican-American children.[92,93] Choosing appropriate normative values for comparison is important in different ethnic groups and children.

CLINICAL SIGNIFICANCE

The effectiveness and outcomes of chest physical therapy have been questioned.[94,95] A recent review of the literature summarizes study results, points out differences in methodology and pathology studied, and identifies areas in which pulmonary physical therapy does or does not have documented benefits.[96] Areas of agreement and controversy have also been well defined.[48] The topic of respiratory care has been the subject of national meetings in 1974 and 1979 by the American Thoracic Society. Both conferences analyzed prior research, generated questions that must be answered, and offered suggestions for research. This is clearly one area of physical therapy in which research studies have been done; however, many questions remain. These studies have led to more careful definitions of the care rendered,[96] and to recognition of problems in using pulmonary function testing to evaluate pulmonary physical therapy.[48,97]

Trying to document change in lungs with chronic, irreversible lung disease is a problem. This group displays more intra-subject variability on most pulmonary function tests[20,24,25] and requires greater change in pulmonary function values before these changes are considered meaningful.[14] For example, in one study concerning cystic fibrosis patients, a 13 percent change in FEV_1 and a 15 percent change in peak flow was needed to produce significant differences in pulmonary functions. Changes of this magnitude do occur if the patient is producing copious sputum.[95,98] Without sputum production, such dramatic changes in pulmonary function do not occur in chronic obstructive lung disease. Other approaches to treatment cannot be expected to produce any change in the status of the abnormal pulmonary function of the patient with obstructive pathology. For example, no change in expiratory flow volume has been observed to follow long-term exercise conditioning in chronic bronchitis and emphysema patients even when substantial cardiovascular conditioning occurs.[99,100]

An important question for the clinician is: How can I determine when a meaningful change in pulmonary function has occurred in the individual patient? Nickerson and his co-workers recommend applying a modification of the sample size formula consisting of:

$$\Delta = \frac{(Z_\alpha + Z_\beta)\sigma}{\sqrt{n}}$$

where Δ is the change required for significance and n is the number of trials per patient. Z_α and Z_β are population values for type I and type II errors of α and β, and σ is population variance. Population values may be estimated from the literature or established from standards developed for a particular facility.

For example, Nickerson established the means, SDs, and confidence intervals for a sample of 15 cystic fibrosis patients tested. These values were then used to determine the percent change within subjects required for significance as follows:

$$\Delta\% = \frac{(t_{0.05,n-1} + t_{0.10,n-1})}{n} \frac{s}{\overline{X}} \cdot 100$$

t values for the sample replaced Z for α and β levels of .05 and .10, respectively, and the sample SD (s) is used as an estimate of the population variance (σ).[14] The change score is then divided by the mean ($\overline{X}$) and multiplied by 100 in order to convert the score to a percentage change. This simple method accounts for error and the variability of the measure in establishing the change required for statistical significance. The clinical significance of a change following treatment depends upon the judgment of the therapist. For example, an increase of FEV_1 from .62 L to .72 L following postural drainage on a child with cystic fibrosis can be statistically significant but may or may not improve the patient's blood gasses.

Another related problem of interest to the physical therapist is the relationship between a patient's ability to perform exercise and pulmonary function. Mungall and Hainsworth tested 13 chronic bronchitis patients six times every two to three weeks for FEV_1, FVC, TL_{CO} and TLC, distance on a 12-minute walking test, and heart rate and ventilation changes on a two-stage treadmill test. They found moderate correlations between TL_{CO} and the ventilation response with the 12 minute walking test ($r = .59$ and $.67$, respectively), but no correlations with other pulmonary function tests. They concluded that submaximal exercise performance is determined more by gas exchange capacity (TL_{CO}) than by airway obstruction. Furthermore, they suggest that the relationship between pulmonary function and exercise performance is poor, and that it decreases with the severity of the condition.[20] Consequently, if enhancing a patient's functional activity tolerance is a treatment goal, the therapist should choose a standard exercise test to objectively assess treatment outcomes in chronic obstructive lung disease rather than pulmonary function measures.

Physical therapists frequently use breathing exercises with both acute and chronic conditions. A recent review suggested that although these procedures have some immediate benefits, there is little evidence of any long-term gains.[101] Long-term goals in chronic obstructive conditions are aimed at promoting relaxation and control during dyspneic attacks.[101,102] However, these goals are difficult to document.

Therapists also think that techniques aimed at enhancing respiratory muscle strength and endurance are important. Leith and Bradley demonstrated different results for a group of normal individuals trained to increase respiratory muscle strength versus a group trained to increase respiratory muscle endurance. The strength group, trained with maximum static inspiration and expiration, significantly increased their maximum inspiratory and expiratory pressure. The endurance group, trained to use rapid breathing to fatigue, significantly increased the fraction of maximum voluntary ventilation (MVV) maintained for 15 minutes, as well as their MVV.[103] Similar changes have been observed following ventilatory muscle strength training in tuberculosis and obstructive lung disease patients,[104] and following ventilatory muscle endurance training in cystic fibrosis patients.[105]

Several measurement problems occur in relation to assessing breathing exercises and ventilatory muscle training. Outcomes such as relaxation, efficiency of breathing, and diaphragmatic excursion can be assessed; however, these assessments are not standardly performed clinically. For example, diaphragmatic excursion can be evaluated by means of roentgenographs or computerized axial tomography, although this evaluation is rarely done. The desired clinical results may require measures which are not pulmonary function tests. The physical therapist may be more interested in improved functional status as a result of breath retraining rather than in the skill the patient displays in performing the maneuvers.

The pulmonary function tests discussed here are more applicable for evaluating acute lung pathologies and secretion clearance. However, other measures may provide more information in relation to the long term management of chronic obstructive conditions. Decisions made by the physical therapist concerning when and how to utilize information generated by pulmonary function tests can shape the practice of pulmonary physical therapy in the future. Factors such as the diagnostic category as well as the severity of the condition, the treatments employed, and the anticipated outcomes of the treatments all have a role in these decisions. This chapter has focused upon the quality of the information provided by pulmonary function tests. An understanding of these tests in combination with the other factors involved will enable the clinician to select appropriate measures for evaluating the patient.

REFERENCES

1. Cotes JE: Lung Function: Assessment and Application in Medicine. Blackwell Scientific Publications, London, 1979
2. Crofton J, Douglas A: Respiratory Diseases. Blackwell Scientific Publications, London, 1981
3. Crapo RO, Morris AH, Gardner RM: Reference spirometric values using techniques and equipment that meet ATS recommendations. Am Rev Respir Dis 123:659, 1981
4. Kory RC, Callahan R, Boren HG, Syner JC: The Veterans Administration—Army cooperative study of pulmonary function. I. Clinical spirometry in normal men. Am J Med 30:243, 1961
5. Morris JF, Koski A, Johnson JC: Spirometric standards for healthy non-smoking adults. Am Rev Respir Dis 103:56, 1971
6. MacDonald JB, Cole TJ: The flow-volume loop: reproducibility of air and helium-based tests in normal subjects. Thorax 35:64, 1980
7. Loss RW, Hall WJ, Speers DM: Evaluation of early airway disease in smokers: cost effectiveness of pulmonary function testing. Am J Med Sci 278:27, 1979

8. Marcq M, Minette A: Lung function changes in smokers with normal conventional spirometry. Am Rev Respir Dis 114:723, 1976

9. Parot S: Some limitations in the use of normal value tables. Respiration 41:188, 1981

10. Cosio M, Ghezzo H, Hobb JC, Corbin R, et al: The relations between structural changes in small airways and pulmonary function tests. N Engl J Med 298:1277, 1978

11. Hogg JC, Macklem PT, Thurlbeck WM: Site and nature of airway obstruction in chronic lung disease. N Engl J Med 278:1355, 1968

12. Knudson RJ, Burrows B: Early detection of obstructive lung disease. Med Clin North Am 3:681, 1973

13. Thurlbeck WM: Small airways: physiology meets pathology. N Engl J Med 298:1310, 1978

14. Knudson RJ, Slatin RC, Lebowitz MD, Burrows B: The maximum expiration flow-volume curve: normal standards, variability, and effects of age. Am Rev Respir Dis 113:587, 1976

15. Nickerson BJ, Lemen RJ, Gerdes CB, et al: Within-subject variability and percent change for significance of spirometry in normal subjects and in patients with cystic fibrosis. Am Rev Respir Dis 122:859, 1980

16. Cochrane GM, Prieto F, Clark TJH: Intrasubject variability of maximum expiratory flow volume curve. Thorax 32:171, 1977

17. Love RG, Attfield MD, Isles KD: Reproducibility of pulmonary function tests under laboratory and field conditions. Br J Ind Med 37:63, 1980

18. Jorfeldt L, Wranne B: Hyperinflation on hyperventilation—a simple test to detect early airway disease. Clin Physiol 2:97, 1982

19. Lebowitz MD, Knudson RJ, et al: Significance of intraindividual changes in maximum expiratory flow volume and peak expiratory flow measurements. Chest 81:566, 1982

20. Mungall IP, Hainsworth R: Assessment of respiratory function in patients with chronic obstructive airways disease. Thorax 34:254, 1979

21. McCarthy DS, Craig DB, Cherniack RM: Intraindividual variability in maximum expiratory flow-volume and closing volume in asymptomatic subjects. Am Rev Resp Dis 112:407, 1975

22. Tashkin DP, Detels R, Coulson AL, et al: The UCLA population studies of chronic obstructive respiratory disease: II. Determination of reliability and estimation of sensitivity and specificity. Environ Res 20:403, 1979

23. Peslin R, Bohadana A, Hannhart B, Jardin P: Comparison of various methods for reading maximal expiratory flow-volume curves. Am Rev Resp Dis 119:271, 1979

24. Bonsignore G, Spina G, Rizzo A, et al: Evaluation of a test of density-dependence of the expiratory flows in the screening of peripheral airways obstruction. Bronchopneumologie 30:457, 1980

25. Afschrift M, Clement J, Peters R, van de Woestyne KP: Maximal expiratory and inspiratory flow in patients with chronic obstructive pulmonary disease: influence of bronchodilation. Am Rev Respir Dis 100:147, 1969

26. Stanescu D, Veriter C, Van Leemputten R, et al: Constancy of effort and variability of maximal expiratory flow rates. Chest 76:59, 1979

27. Sobol BJ, Park SS, Emirgil C: Relative value of early detection of chronic obstructive pulmonary disease. Am Rev Respir Dis 107:753, 1973

28. McFadden ER, Linden DA: A reduction in maximum mid-expiratory flow rate: a spirographic manifestation of small airway disease. Am J Med 52:725, 1972

29. Mead J, Turner JM, Macklem PT, Little JB: Significance of the relationship between lung recoil and maximum expiratory flow. J Appl Physiol 22:95, 1967
30. Dosman J, Bode F, Urbanetti J, Martin R, Macklem PT: The use of helium-oxygen mixture during maximum expiratory flow to demonstrate obstruction in small airways in smokers. J Clin Invest 55:1090, 1975
31. Bonsignore G, Bellia V, Ferrara G, et al: Reproducibility of maximum flows in air and He-O_2 and of ΔV_{max50} in the assessment of the site of airflow limitation. Eur J Respir Dis, suppl., 106:29–34, 1980
32. Mead J: Analysis of the configuration of maximum expiratory flow-volume curves. J Appl Physiol 44:156, 1978
33. Chowienczyk PJ, Rees PJ, Clark THJ: Automated system for the measurement of airways resistance, lung volumes, and flow-volume loops. Thorax 36:944, 1981
34. Douglas NJ, Wraith PK, Brash HM, et al: Computer measurement of dynamic compliance: technique and reproducibility in man. J Appl Physiol 48:903, 1980
35. Teculescu DB, Bohadana AB, Peslin, et al: Variability, reproducibility and observer difference of body plethysmographic measurements. Clin Physiol 2:127, 1982
36. Marazzini L, Vezzoli F, Longhini E: Respiratory function 8 years after a diagnosis of peripheral airways disease. Respiration 42:88, 1981
37. Mackenzie CF, Shin B, Hadi F, Imle PC: Changes in total lung thorax compliance following chest physiotherapy. Anesth Analg (Clev) 59:207, 1980
38. Bokinsky GE, Caldwell EJ: Clinical usefulness of pulmonary function tests. Compr Ther 7:47, 1981
39. Miller RD, Offord KP: Roentgenologic determination of total lung capacity. Mayo Clin Proc 55:694, 1980
40. Cutillo A, Perondi R, Turiel M, et al: Reproducibility of multibreath nitrogen washout measurements. Am Rev Respir Dis 124:505, 1981
41. Sterks PJ, Quanjer PH, van der Maas LLJ, et al: the validity of the single-breath nitrogen determination of residual volume. Bull Eur Physiopathol Resp 16:195, 1980
42. Wilmore JH, Vodak PA, Parr RB, et al: Further simplification of a method for determination of residual lung volume. Med Sci Sports Exerc 12:216, 1980
43. Lorino H, Harf A, Atlan G, et al: Computer determination of thoracic gas volume using plethysmographic "thoracic flow." J Appl Physiol 48:911, 1980
44. Fazio F: Radioisotope imaging. In Clark TJH (ed): Clinical Investigation of Respiratory Disease. Chapman and Hall, London, 1981
45. Jones NL: Exercise tests. In Clark TJH (ed): Clinical Investigation of Respiratory Disease. Chapman and Hall, London, 1981
46. Cerny FJ, Polano J, Cropp G: Adaptations to exercise in children with cystic fibrosis. In Nagel F, Monpoya H (eds): Exercise in Health and Disease, Charles C Thomas, Springfield, 1981
47. Minh VD, Patakas DA, Davies PL, et al: A single-breath method of alveolar O_2 determination. Respiration 37:66, 1979
48. Mackenzie CF: Physiological changes following chest physical therapy. In Mackenzie CF (ed): Chest Physiotherapy in the Intensive Care Unit. Williams & Wilkins, Baltimore, 1981
49. Douglas NJ, Brash HM, Wraith PK, et al: Accuracy and sensitivity to carboxyhemoglobin, and speed of response of the Hewlett-Packard 47201A ear oximeter. Am Rev Respir Dis 119:311, 1979

50. Knill RL, Clement JL, Kieraszewicz ET, et al: Assessment of two noninvasive monitors of arterial oxygenation in anesthetized man. Anesth Analg (Cleve) 61:676, 1982

51. Tremper KK, Shoemaker WC: Transcutaneous oxygen monitoring of critically ill adults, with and without low flow shock. Crit Care Med 9:706, 1981

52. ATS statement: Snowbird workshop on standardization of spirometry. Am Rev Respir Dis 119:831, 1979

53. Gardner RM, Hankinson JL, West BJ: Evaluating Commercially available spirometers. Am Rev Respir Dis 121:73, 1980

54. Petusevsky ML, Lyons LD, Smith AA, et al: Calibration of time derivatives of forced vital capacity by explosive decompression. Am Rev Respir Dis 121:343, 1980

55. Shaw A, Fisher J: Calibration of some instruments for measuring peak expiratory flow. J Med Eng Technol 4:291, 1980

56. Sheen A, Sly RM: Evaluation of calibration of spirometers. Ann Allergy 45:127, 1980

57. Wever AM, Britton MG, Hughes DT, et al: Clinical evaluation of five spirometers. Monaghan M403, Pneumoscreen, Spirotron, Vicatest and Vitalograph. Eur J Respir Dis 62:127, 1981

58. Cissik HJ, Cramer TJ, Shelman LL: Evaluation of the Cavitron Spirometric Computer for accuracy in clinical screening spirometry. Aviat Space Environ Med 52:125, 1981

59. Perks WH, Tams IP, Thompson DA, et al: An evaluation of the miniWright peak flow meter. Thorax 34:79, 1979

60. Petty TL: Spirometric time base considerations. Chest 80:116, 1981

61. Morrill CG, Dickey DW, Weiser, et al: Calibration and stability of standard and mini-Wright peak flow meters. Ann Allergy 46:70, 1981

62. Glindmeyer H: Evaluating commercially avaialble spirometers (letter). Am Rev Res Dis 122:172, 1980

63. Perks WH, Cole M, Steventon RD, et al: An evaluation of the vitalograph pulmonary monitor. Br J Dis Chest 75:161, 1981

64. Knudson RJ, Lebowitz MD, Slatin RC: The timing of the forced vital capacity. Am Rev Respir Dis 119:315, 1979

65. Lisboa C, Ross WR, Jardim J, et al: Pulmonary pressure-flow curves measured by a data-averaging circuit. J Appl Physiol 47:621, 1979

66. Miller A, Chuang MT, Warshaw R, et al: Clinical validation of automated spirometry used in surveys of large occupational groups: comparison with conventional water spirometry. Arch Environ Health 34:266, 1979

67. Li KY, Tan LT, Chong P, et al: Between-technician variation in the measurement of spirometry with air and helium. Am Rev Respir Dis 124:196, 1981

68. Walter S, Nancy NR: Reproducibility of the forced expiratory spirogram. Indian J Med Res 69:319, 1979

69. Sharp JT: Standardization of pulmonary epidemiologic methods. Three blows or five? Chest 76:375, 1979

70. Peslin R, Bohadana A, Hannhart B, et al: Comparison of various methods for reading maximal expiratory flow-volume curves. Am Rev Respir Dis 119:271, 1979

71. Ryan G, Dolovich MB, Roberts RS, et al: Standardization of inhalation provocation tests: two techniques of aerosol generation and inhalation compared. Am Rev Respir Dis 123:195, 1981

72. Hendrick DJ, Marshall R, Faux JA, et al: Positive "alveolar" responses to antigen inhalation provocation tests: their validity and recognition. Thorax 35:415, 1980

73. Lilker ES, Jauregui R: Airway response to water inhalation: a new test for "bronchial reactivity." N Engl J Med 305:702, 1981

74. Johnson JD: Statistical considerations in studies of exercise-induced bronchospasm. J Allerg Clin Immunol 64 (6 pt. 2):634, 1979

75. Avery WG, Maximizing spirometry in reversible airways diseases. Ann Allergy 47 (5 Pt. 2):410, 1981

76. Cole RB, Al-Khader A: Effect of slow-release oral aminophylline on circadian variation in airflow obstruction in asthmatics. J Int Med Res 7:suppl. 1, 40–44, 1979

77. Evans N, Evans PW, Boobis SW: Preliminary experience with controlled-release aminophylline in asthmatic children: salivary levels and peak flow following a single dose. J Int Med Res 7:suppl. 1, 93–97, 1979

78. Thiessen B, Pederson OF: Effect of freon inhalation on maximal expiratory flows and heart rhythm after treatment with salbutamol and ipratropium bromide. Eur J Respir Dis 61:156, 1980

79. Imle PC: Adjuncts to chest physiotherapy. In Mackenzie CF (ed): Chest Physiotherapy in the Intensive Care Unit. Williams & Wilkins, Baltimore, 1980

80. Ranchod A, Keeton GR, Benatar: The effect of beta-blockers on ventilatory function in chronic bronchitis. S Afr Med J 61:423, 1982

81. Winning TJ, Brock-Utner JG, Goodwin NM: A simple clinical method of quantitating the effects of chest physiotherapy in mechanically ventilated patients. Anaesth Intensive Care 3:237, 1975

82. Buono MJ, Constable SH, Morton AR, et al: The effect of an acute bout of exercise on selected pulmonary function measurements. Med Sci Sports Exerc 13:290, 1981

83. Brown HV, Wasserman K, Whipp BJ: Strategies of exercise testing in chronic lung disease. Bull Eur Physiopathol Resp 13:409, 1977

84. Levison H, Cherniak RM: Ventilatory cost of exercise in obstructive lung disease. J Appl Physiol 25:21, 1968

85. Klemic N, Imle PC: Changes with mobility and methods of mobilization. In Mackenzie CF (ed): Chest Physiotherapy in the Intensive Care Unit. Williams & Wilkins, Baltimore, 1981

86. Macfie AE, Harris EA, Whitlock RML: The maximal flow/volume curve in 197 healthy New Zealanders: a comparison with recent American standards. Aust NZJ Med 11:517, 1981

87. Stinson JM, McPherson GL, Hicks, et al: Spirometric standards for healthy black adults. J Natl Med Assoc 73:729, 1981

88. Buist AS, Adams BE, Sexton GJ, et al: Reference values for functional residual capacity and maximal expiratory flow in young children. Am Rev Respir Dis 122:983, 1980

89. Lindemann H: Body plethysmographic measurements in children with an accompanying adult. Respiration 37:278, 1979

90. Wiesemann H, von der Hardt H: Reliability of flow-volume measurements in children. Respiration 41:181, 1981

91. Taussig LM, Chernick V, Wood R, et al: Standardization of lung function testing in children. Proceedings and recommendations of the GAP Conference Committee, Cystic Fibrosis Foundation. J Pediatr 97:668, 1980

92. Boggs PB, Stephens AL, Walker RF, et al: Racially specific reference standards for commonly performed spirometric measurements for black and white children, ages 9–18 years. Ann Allergy 47:273, 1981

93. Hsu KH, Jenkins DE, Hsi BP, et al: Ventilatory functions of normal children and young adults—Mexican-American, white and black. I. Spirometry. J Pediatr 95:119, 1979

94. Anonymous: Chest physiotherapy under scrutiny. (editorial) Lancet 2:1241, 1978

95. Murray JF: The ketchup-bottle method (editorial). N Engl J Med: 300:1155, 1979

96. Mackenzie CF: History and literature review of chest physiotherapy, chest physiotherapy program, patient population and respiratory care of MIEMSS. In MacKenzie CF (ed): Chest Physiotherapy in the Intensive Care Unit. Williams & Wilkins, Baltimore, 1981

97. Peters RM, Turnier E: Physical therapy: indications for and effects in surgical patients. Am Rev Respir Dis:suppl. 5, 122:147–154, 1980

98. Tecklin JS, Holsclaw DS: Evaluation of bronchial drainage in patients with cystic fibrosis. Phys Ther 55:1081, 1975

99. Rochester DF, Goldberg SK: Techniques of respiratory physical therapy. Am Rev Res Dis suppl., 122:133–146, 1980

100. Jankowski LW, Ray LE, Lallee J, et al: Effects of prone immersion physical exercise (PIPE) in patients with chronic obstructive lung disease (COPD). Scand J Rehab Med 8:135, 1976

101. Ciesla N: Postural drainage, positioning and breathing exercises. In Mackenzie CF: Chest Physiotherapy in the Intensive Care Unit. Williams & Wilkins, Baltimore, 1981

102. Frownfelter DL: Breathing exercise and retraining, chest mobilization exercises. In: Chest Physical Therapy, Frownfelter DL (ed):Year book Medical Publishers, Chicago, 1978

103. Leith D, Bradley M: Ventilatory muscle strength and endurance training. J Appl Phys 41:508, 1976

104. Lecoq A, Delkez L, Janssens F, Petit JM: Réentainment de la function motrice ventilatoise chez des insuffisants respiratoires chroniques. Acta Tuberc Pneumol Belg 61:63, 1970

105. Keens TG, Krastens IRB, Wannamaker EM, et al: Ventilatory muscle endurance training in normal subjects and patients with cystic fibrosis. Am Rev Respir Dis 116:853, 1977

9 | Measurements of Cardiovascular Function

David R. Sinacore
Ali A. Ehsani

Many physical therapy departments now offer rehabilitation programs for the patient with cardiovascular disease (postmyocardial infarction, coronary artery disease, and after coronary artery bypass graft surgery). Therefore, physical therapists are not only treating the musculoskeletal complaints of cardiac patients, they are also taking an active role in initiating, prescribing, and supervising exercise programs for such patients. As the involvement of physical therapists with cardiac patients continues to grow, therapists must increase their understanding of cardiovascular physiology and the methods used to assess cardiovascular function.

This chapter reviews the relative quality of the measurements currently used by physical therapists to assess the cardiovascular system. We will also briefly discuss some of the evaluative procedures used by cardiologists. We believe that physical therapists should be aware of the strengths and weaknesses of these methods. This chapter focuses on measurement, and as such, extends some of the practical information presented in the first volume in this series.[1]

The first part of this chapter focuses on the reliability of the cardiovascular measures obtained by physical therapists. These include determination of heart rate (HR), indirect measures of blood pressure (BP) and graded exercise testing (sometimes referred to as stress testing[2] or exercise electrocardiography[3]) and measurements of maximal oxygen uptake capacity. The second part of the chapter briefly discusses selected diagnostic procedures such as radionuclide studies, with comments on their reliability and validity.

HEART RATE

Heart rate is easily and reliably measured by a variety of methods.[4] Clinically, it is the most valuable index of exercise intensity, oxygen consumption, and energy expenditure during dynamic exercise because of the linear relationship between HR and oxygen consumption (i.e., exercise intensity).[4-6] HR is most accurately measured with an electrocardiogram (ECG), but this requires expensive equipment. The HR (or pulse rate) can also be measured by auditory or palpation methods at any number of sites. HR measurements can be made by timing a given number of cardiac cycles (beats) and then determining their frequency per minute by use of a table. A table for determining the HR/minute after timing 30 beats is shown (in Table 9-1). HR is also determined by counting the beats for a short period of time and then multiplying that answer by the appropriate factor to calculate the rate per minute. If HR is to be determined after exercise, the time period during which the pulse is monitored should be short (preferably <15 seconds). The progressive deceleration in HR after cessation of exercise could lead to erroneously low estimates of exercise HR if the time sampled is too long.[7-10]

Recently, Sedlock et al[7] demonstrated in 84 normal subjects that there were no significant differences: (1) between palpated and simultaneously recorded ECG HR determinations during exercise; (2) between carotid and radial palpated pulse rates; and (3) between pulse rates assessed for six- and 10-second periods following cessation of exercise. Immediate postexercise monitoring by palpation yields lower mean heart rates than would be obtained during exercise. However, the difference is modest, less than 4 percent, if HR is monitored within the first 15 seconds after exercise.[7-9] Although immediate postexercise palpated pulse rates (up to 15 seconds postexercise) accurately reflect exercise HR, this relationship has been documented almost exclusively in healthy subjects. It is not known whether patients with various diseases or those on medications can be assessed in this way.

Another important clinical consideration is whether palpation of the carotid artery affects the HR. Considerable controversy exists as to whether palpation of the carotid artery stimulates the carotid sinus reflex, resulting in cardiac deceleration, hypotension and, in some cases, bradyarrhythmias.[7,9,11,12] White reported that 106 of 117 healthy subjects had a lower HR measured by carotid artery palpation than was shown on ECG.[12] This was presumably caused by carotid sinus stimulation during palpation. Oldridge et al, Pollock et al, Gardner et al, and Sedlock et al could not replicate this finding in a variety of patient types, including cardiac patients.[7,9,11,13] They concluded that carotid artery palpation, if properly performed, is a safe and accurate method for determination of postexercise HR.

Table 9-1. Heart Rate Conversion (30 Beats to Rate) Determined by Timing 30 Cardiac Cycles

Time	Rate	Time	Rate	Time	Rate
22.0 sec	82/min	17.3 sec	104/min	12.6 sec	143/min
21.9	82	17.2	105	12.5	144
21.8	83	17.1	105	12.4	145
21.7	83	17.0	106	12.3	146
21.6	83	16.9	107	12.2	148
21.5	84	16.8	107	12.1	149
21.4	84	16.7	108	12.0	150
21.3	85	16.6	108	11.9	151
21.2	85	16.5	109	11.8	153
21.1	85	16.4	110	11.7	154
21.0	86	16.3	110	11.6	155
20.9	86	16.2	111	11.5	157
20.8	87	16.1	112	11.4	158
20.7	87	16.0	113	11.3	159
20.6	87	15.9	113	11.2	161
20.5	88	15.8	114	11.1	162
20.4	88	15.7	115	11.0	164
20.3	89	15.6	115	10.9	165
20.2	89	15.5	116	10.8	167
20.1	90	15.4	117	10.7	168
20.0	90	15.3	118	10.6	170
19.9	90	15.2	118	10.5	171
19.8	91	15.1	119	10.4	173
19.7	91	15.0	120	10.3	175
19.6	92	14.9	121	10.2	176
19.5	92	14.8	122	10.1	178
19.4	93	14.7	122	10.0	180
19.3	93	14.6	123	9.9	182
19.2	94	14.5	124	9.8	184
19.1	94	14.4	125	9.7	186
19.0	95	14.3	126	9.6	188
18.9	95	14.2	127	9.5	189
18.8	96	14.1	128	9.4	191
18.7	96	14.0	129	9.3	194
18.6	97	13.9	129	9.2	196
18.5	97	13.8	130	9.1	198
18.4	98	13.7	131	9.0	200
18.3	98	13.6	132	8.9	202
18.2	99	13.5	133	8.8	205
18.1	99	13.4	134	8.7	207
18.0	100	13.3	135	8.6	209
17.9	101	13.2	136	8.5	212
17.8	101	13.1	137	8.4	214
17.7	102	13.0	138	8.3	217
17.6	102	12.9	140	8.2	220
17.5	103	12.8	141	8.1	222
17.4	103	12.7	142	8.0	225

Time = time for 30 beats; rate = heart rate per minute.

Recent advances in technology are making portable HR monitors available. Most of these use either ECG signals or detect pulse at the earlobe or the finger by optic plethysmographs or photoelectric sensors. The majority of these monitors display HR based on a sample of four beats, but only a few actually display inter-beat-intervals. Aravjo et al evaluated five different monitors and found all to be accurate within ± 4 beats/per minute, 90 percent of the time when subjects were at rest.[14] However, a major limitation of these monitors is that they often become erratic and inaccurate when patients are exercising. Therefore, before using one of these monitors, therapists must determine whether the device will be accurate for the specific type and intensity of exercise to be monitored.

Interpretation of HR responses and the magnitude of the response requires an understanding of nonpathological factors that often influence HR. Some of these will be briefly reviewed.

Maximal HR declines with age and is thought to decrease an average of 10 beats/minute per decade after age 20, although there are variations between individuals. At all exercise intensities (relative and absolute), women tend to have a higher HR than men of the same age.[4,5]

The changes in HR during exercise are mediated primarily by an increase in adrenergic stimulation and by vagal withdrawal.[4] The HR response to exercise is primarily dependent on the intensity of the exercise[4] and the subject's state of training. Endurance-trained athletes have lower resting, submaximal, and—at times—maximal heart rates than do untrained individuals.[5] In addition, for any given level of exercise, HR increases as the ambient temperature, humidity, and altitude increase. HR is also known to vary with the time of day (circadian rhythms), emotional states, nervousness, and apprehension.[4] The magnitudes and types of effects are not known for all factors.

BLOOD PRESSURE

Blood Pressure (BP) measurements have been the topic of extensive review.[16] The ausculatory method of BP measurement, pioneered by Riva-Rocci and described by Korotkoff, is commonly used and widely accepted. However, the origin of the Korotkoff sounds remain incompletely understood[17,18] and sphygmomanometry is known to lack precision and be prone to error.[19–23] There are known physiological variations in BP throughout the day and between days.[24,25] An example of how BP varies within a day is shown in Figure 9-1.[4]

The sources of error in sphygmomanometry are well documented and the reader should consult references 18 through 23 for a review of the subject. In brief, the errors relate to the instrument, the observer, and the interactions of the two. Instrument errors include: improper calibration, inadequate cuff size (length and width), and instrument failure. Observer errors are caused by improper positioning of the patient or of the patient's arm, improper interpretation of Korotkoff sounds, observer bias, and digit preference. Observer bias occurs when the observer reports the BP as lower or higher based on known (i.e.,

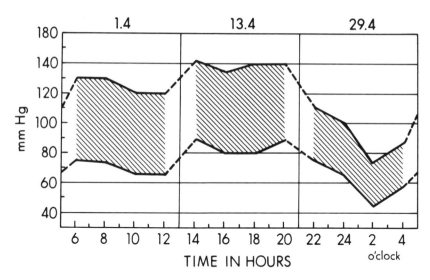

Fig. 9-1. Variation in systolic and diastolic blood pressures within a 24-hour period (Mellerowicz H, Smodlaka VN (eds): Ergometry: Basics of Medical Exercise Testing. Urban & Schwarzenberg, Baltimore, 1981; after W. Menzel).

observer-expected) outcomes or consequences. If, for example, a reading of 140/90 mm Hg is considered the lower boundary between hypertensive and normal BP, an observer might tend to record a more favorable measurement for a young healthy man, but categorize an obese middle-aged man as hypertensive. Digit preference describes a bias for recording a BP ending in zero more often than would be expected. Recently, several instruments have been designed to eliminate observer bias[20,26] and digit preference.[26] Although these devices are not widely used clinically, they have gained acceptance for research purposes. Physiological variables known to influence BP are the ingestion of food, use of tobacco or alcohol, temperature and climactic variations, bladder distention, emotional state, obesity, and exercise. Circadian rhythms also cause variations in BP. Accounting for (i.e., controlling) as many of the aforementioned extrinsic variables as possible is highly recommended.

Indirect methods of measuring resting BP have been compared to direct methods (intraarterial measurements).[16,17,21,27–30] Most investigators report close agreement between direct and indirect measurements for a variety of patient types and for normal subjects of different ages.[27–29] Correlations of the two methods for resting subjects range from .89 to .95 for systolic blood pressure (SBP). Correlations for the fourth Korotkoff sound—diastolic BP$_4$ (DBP$_4$)—range from .83 to .88, and for the fifth Korotkoff sound (cessation of diastolic pressure [DBP$_5$]) from .82 to .93.[28,29] Moss and Adams reported correlations of direct and indirect measurements to be .36 for muffling and .32 for cessation of diastolic pressure.[17] Most investigators agree that indirect methods underestimate direct intraarterial pressures on the average by 3 to 10 mm Hg.[21,27,28] There is still controversy over whether the fourth or fifth Korotkoff sound more accurately reflects the intraarterial diastolic pressure.[17,21,28] However, the American Heart Association recommends recording both pressures (i.e., the pressures at which the muffling sound and cessation of sound occur).[22] In addition, close agreement has been found when the auscultatory method of determining SBP and the palpatory methods (for example, at the radial artery) have been compared.[27]

Devices have been designed to automate BP measurement by controlling the rate of cuff inflation and deflation and by incorporating some form of audiovisual signalling of the endpoints (i.e., SBP, DBP_4 and DBP_5). Nearly all of the designs are based on one of two principles—either detection by the human ear or by microphone of Korotkoff sounds, or the detection of arterial blood flow by Doppler ultrasound.[31] The devices that use auscultation of Korotkoff sounds may reduce observer bias and digit preference by automatic audiovisual signalling but technical difficulties still exist in recognizing and standardizing endpoints. Some of the microphones also have the disadvantage of being sensitive to movement and friction artifacts.

The Doppler ultrasound sphygmomanometers are especially useful when Korotkoff sounds are difficult to detect, as they are in children or in adults in shock or under anesthesia. These devices have been shown to be reasonably reliable and accurate when compared with intraarterial pressures.[23,30] These devices detect variations in frequencies of reflected ultrasonic waves when arteries are occluded and then refilled.[31] They are, however, extremely sensitive and require accurate placement of the crystals over arteries. In addition, they are more costly than standard sphygmomanometers. None of these new devices has been shown to be better than conventional mercury sphygmomanometers if the user has been adequately trained and uses the standard device properly.

Because SBP increases rapidly with HR at the onset of exercise and continues to increase during exercise, progressive indirect measurements of BP are clinically useful. Measurements of SBP are easily obtained during exercise by use of the Korotkoff sounds because they are more distinct than when the subject is at rest. Indirectly obtained diastolic pressures measured during exercise are questionable and may not be reliable.[29] The differences between direct and indirect measures of diastolic pressure increase during and immediately after exercise. Often, DBP_5 remains unaltered down to 0 mm Hg. In these cases, DBP_4 (i.e., muffling) is used as the criterion. With increasing levels of exercise intensity, indirect measures of BP may yield wider variations than would direct measures.[4,29]

EXERCISE TESTING

Use of exercise ("stress") testing has grown enormously over the past 60 years. Although they are used for a variety of purposes, exercise tests are primarily used for (1) the detection, diagnosis, and prognosis of coronary artery disease (CAD), and (2) the assessment of maximal aerobic exercise capacity of normal subjects and patients with cardiac disease who are enrolled in rehabilitation programs. These two indications for stress testing are not mutually exclusive; the same test is often used for both purposes. Many investigators have developed their own exercise tests.[3] These vary according to the purpose, the population being tested, the mode of exercise equipment, and technical and environmental considerations. Exercise tests may differ in the endpoints used to determine when to terminate the test. Endpoints may be classified into four major categories: (1) heart-rate–limited; (2) workload-limited; (3) sign-limited; and (4) symptom-limited.

Heart-Rate–Limited

Heart-rate–limited tests are terminated when a predetermined ("target") HR is reached during exercise testing. A predetermined percentage of the age-predicted maximal HR is often used. Heart rates of 80 percent to 95 percent of the age-predicted maximums are considered more than adequate to induce evidence of myocardial ischemia in most patients.[2,32]

Workload-Limited

Workload-limited tests are concluded when a preselected workload (energy cost) is achieved during exercise. They are not commonly used for the detection of CAD, but they are the most functionally oriented of the tests. They can help determine whether individuals will be capable of performing specific types of jobs or whether they can engage in activities.

Sign-Limited

Sign-limited tests are terminated when signs of myocardial ischemia develop. Classic signs include, (1) the onset of ST segment depression of 0.1 mV or more occurring .08 seconds from the J point; (2) failure of SBP to rise with increasing workload; (3) hypotension; and (4) frequent multifocal premature ventricular contractions (VPC). Results of tests that use sign-limited endpoints appear to correlate more often with coronary angiographic findings than do results of tests that use "target" criteria.[33–39]

Symptom-Limited

Symptom-limited tests continue until symptoms cause termination of exercise, regardless of the HR or the magnitude of the ST segment depression. Symptom-limited tests are thought to have the greatest diagnostic value[40–42] and are used to provide prognostic information, although the validity for long-term prognostication has not been demonstrated.[38,42]

Test Classification

Rather than attempt to review each test protocol (method), we will classify tests according to their purpose and discuss the categories. First, we will consider exercise tests that are used to aid in the diagnosis of CAD.

Exercise testing is widely used for patients with CAD. The most widespread use of exercise testing is for patients who are *symptomatic* from ischemic, valvular, and primary myocardial and congenital heart diseases.[3] Testing is done to determine the existence and extent of the disease and to assess the accompanying functional impairment. Although more controversial, exercise testing is often used in asymptomatic individuals as a screening technique for latent CAD,[43,45] high-risk occupations,[46] and for participation in exercise programs.[3]

Exercise testing, like all "tolerance tests," is based on the assumption that any abnormality (dysfunction) is more likely to become apparent when the organ is subjected to increased demands. Exercise testing can provide information regarding cardiac reserve in patients who do not have anemia or disease of the pulmonary, nervous, or peripheral vascular systems. Exercise is probably the strongest stimulus for the cardiovascular system and especially the heart. Myocardial O_2 demand increases with exercise and, as a result, coronary blood flow must increase proportionally to meet this demand. A defect in blood flow, such as can occur when coronary arteries are stenosed, may result in an inability to meet myocardial O_2 demand during exercise. This can lead to myocardial ischemia, which is often accompanied by the classic symptom of angina pectoris.

In the United States, approximately 1 to 2 million people are affected annually by CAD. Detection of CAD, particularly in the early stages before the disease becomes symptomatic, is highly desirable. Coronary angiography is still the definitive method for detection and assessment of the severity of coronary atherosclerosis. However, it is an expensive and invasive procedure that carries a small but definite risk. Repeated angiography to determine disease progression is impractical in most cases. Because of the inherent risks, coronary angiography is not recommended for asymptomatic subjects, except under unusual circumstances. Therefore, exercise tests and other noninvasive procedures are normally used to detect and predict the presence of significant CAD. The criterion or "gold standard" that is used to evaluate exercise tests is coronary angiography, i.e., how well do they detect CAD demonstrated by angiography. Other noninvasive procedures, such as detecting myocardial perfusion abnormalities with thallium (^{201}Tl) scans or localizing myocardial contraction abnormalities with gated blood pool imaging (radionuclide ventriculography), can be used like exercise ECG to assess myocardial ischemia. These noninvasive measures attempt to assess the physiologic abnormality of myocardial ischemia, whereas coronary artery stenosis is an anatomic measure. Although there may be a high correlation between results of noninvasive tests and invasive tests, none of the noninvasive procedures definitively demonstrate whether an individual has CAD.

Reproducibility of Exercise Tests Used to Detect CAD

The reproducibility of exercise test results is essential for accurate assessment of patient performance and for the evaluation of the results of therapeutic interventions. Stress test reliability has been the subject of many studies.[33,46-49]

Mason and colleagues studied the reproducibility of sign-limited exercise tests by evaluating 15 subjects on three different days and 10 subjects on two different days.[33] Bicycle and escalator ergometers were used with a positive endpoint criterion of 1.0 mm or more of ischemic ST segment depression. They reported that 80 percent of the subjects had reproducible results. Four of the five subjects who did not reproduce their signs underwent a third test, and all had two of three results that agreed.

Smokler et al, using a symptom-limited endpoint (moderately severe angina pectoris), reported similarly high reproducibility for treadmill testing. Average differences of 5.4 percent for total walking time in 40 patients between duplicate tests no more than 6 months apart were reported.[48]

Ellestad et al, using a treadmill test with a combination of endpoints, reported that 92 percent of 25 subjects retested within 90 days performed to an endpoint within 1 minute of the previous test.[49] A majority (60 percent) performed for identical times, and 68 percent developed ischemic ST segment changes at the same time.

Fabian et al investigated the reliability of bicycle ergometer exercise tests using a variety of endpoints in 50 patients.[47] They reported a "reliability coefficient" of .97 for total work performed when the test–retest interval was 3 months. Identical ECG abnormalities were found on both tests in 86 percent of the patients, and 94 percent of the patients were limited because of identical symptoms.

The reliability of exercise testing for the purpose of identifying CAD appears to be reasonably good over various time intervals (several days to 6 months). Numerous authors have reported reproducible results *within* modes of exercise (bicycle,[51] treadmill,[52] arm cranking,[53] and step testing[54]). Similarly, high reliability indices have been reported for varied populations (healthy and patient) and among protocols that use a given mode of exercise (e.g., multistage treadmill tests). However, the investigators did not use the same indices of reliability; therefore, it is difficult to compare the studies.

Variability in results from repeated exercise tests have been reported to be as high as 20 percent.[49] Variations in methods and a lack of standardization in protocols and endpoints may be the cause of this variability. If these factors are controlled, the variability may be greatly reduced. Quantifiable endpoints, such as unequivocal ST segment depression (2 mm or greater) are reproducible and limit variability.

Predictive and Concurrent Validity of Exercise ECG

The clinical usefulness of exercise testing for CAD is not only determined by the *sensitivity* and *specificity* of the test but also by the *prevalence of CAD* in the type of patient (i.e., the population from which they come) being tested.

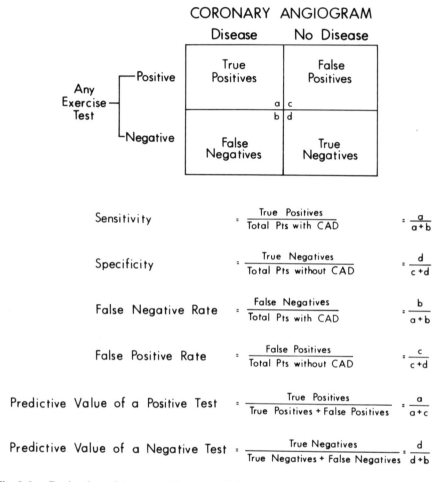

Fig. 9-2. Derivation of the sensitivity, specificity, and predictive values of any exercise test used to screen for coronary artery disease.

Sensitivity is the ratio formed by dividing the number of patients with true-positive responses by the number of those who have the disease.[3] Specificity is the ratio formed by dividing the number of those with true-negative results by the number of patients who do not have the disease.[3] Sensitivity can also be described as the percentage of patients with the disease who exhibit positive findings on exercise testing, whereas specificity is the percentage of those without disease who exhibit negative results (Fig. 9-2). Although sensitivity and specificity are important, they do not necessarily indicate whether exercise tests results provide meaningful clinical and diagnostic information.

The clinician must know the probability that a positive or negative test has in documenting the presence or absence of disease. In other words, the key clinical issue is the *predictive value* of the test, not the specificity or sensitivity. The predictive value of a positive test is the ratio formed by dividing the number of patients with positive results who have the disease (i.e., true positives) by the total number of patients with positive results (both true and false positives).[3] The predictive value of a negative test is the ratio formed by dividing the number of patients without disease who have negative results (i.e., true negatives) by the total number of patients with negative results (both true and false negatives) (See Figure 9-2).

Baye's theorem states that the validity of a diagnostic test is influenced by the prevalence of the disease in the population (to which the patient being examined belongs).[55] For example, the predictive value of a positive exercise (ECG) test in a population with a very low incidence of CAD is small. On the other hand, the predictive value of the same test (exercise ECG) for a patient drawn from a population with a very high incidence of CAD is much greater.[35,37,38,40,56] The following hypothetical examples demonstrate the importance of understanding sensitivity, specificity and predictive value, when characterized according to Baye's theorem, in three distinct populations (patients who are asymptomatic, those who have atypical chest pain, and those with angina pectoris) with different incidences of CAD (see Figs. 9-3 through 9-5).

Most studies indicate that the sensitivity of exercise ECG testing ranges from 47 percent to 80 percent, with an average of 64 percent.[55] If we use the average figure in our example, it would mean that 64 percent of patients with angiographically documented CAD would have positive exercise tests (true positives), whereas 36 percent (the remainder) would have negative tests (false negatives). The specificity of exercise tests vary, with estimates ranging from 65 percent to 95 percent, the average being 90 percent.[55] Therefore, 90 percent of patients with angiographically documented normal coronary artery anatomy would have negative exercise tests (true negatives) and 10 percent (the remainder) would have positive exercise tests (false positives).

Asymptomatic Population. If the prevalence of CAD in an asymptomatic population is 5 percent[35,37,38,40,56] 5 of 100 asymptomatic people will show the presence of CAD and 95 will be normal if an angiogram is performed. Because average sensitivity for this test is 64 percent, three of the five with CAD will have positive stress ECG results, while the other two will have negative (i.e., false negative) results. With the average specificity of 90 percent, 86 of the 95 normal subjects will have negative (i.e., true negative) ECG stress test results while the remaining nine will have positive (i.e., false positive) results. Thus, the predictive value of a positive result will be 25 percent (3/[3 + 9]). The probability that an exercise ECG will identify CAD in a member of this population is only 25 percent and is therefore not sufficiently powerful for a definitive diagnosis. On the other hand, the predictive value of a negative test in the same population is 98 percent. Therefore, when there is a low incidence of CAD in the population (5 percent in our example), a negative stress ECG provides strong clinical evidence to confirm the absence of CAD (Fig. 9-3).

Population with Atypical Chest Pain. The incidence of CAD in patients with atypical chest pain, i.e., chest pain not characteristic of angina pectoris,

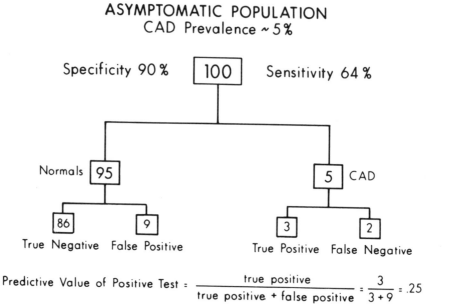

ASYMPTOMATIC POPULATION
CAD Prevalence ~ 5%

Specificity 90 % | 100 | Sensitivity 64 %

Normals | 95 | | 5 | CAD

| 86 | | 9 | | 3 | | 2 |
True Negative   False Positive   True Positive   False Negative

Predictive Value of Positive Test = $\dfrac{\text{true positive}}{\text{true positive + false positive}} = \dfrac{3}{3+9} = .25$

Predictive Value of Negative Test = $\dfrac{\text{true negative}}{\text{true negative + false negative}} = \dfrac{86}{86+2} = .98$

Fig. 9-3. Hypothetical example of the usefulness of any exercise test when the prevalence of coronary artery disease (CAD) is low (5 percent) and the population is asymptomatic.

is ~50 percent;[35,37,38,40,56] that is, 50 of 100 patients will have angiographically documented CAD. Based on the average sensitivity of 64 percent, 32 of the 50 patients with CAD will have positive (true positive) findings from exercise ECG. The remaining 18 with CAD will have negative results (false negatives). The average specificity of 90 percent means that 45 of the 50 patients without CAD will have negative (true negative) results from exercise ECG. Five of those without CAD will have positive ECG tests (false positives). Thus, the predictive value of a positive test for a member of this population is 86 percent, while the predictive value for a negative test is 71 percent. This indicates that for this population (i.e, atypical chest pain patients) exercise ECG tests can predict CAD in 86 percent of those with the disease and predict the absence of the disease 71 percent of the time in persons without CAD (Fig. 9-4).

Patients with Angina Pectoris. In patients with angina, the incidence of CAD is high, on the order of 90 percent, i.e., 90 of 100 patients will have CAD.[35,37,38,40,56] With the average sensitivity and specificity of 64 percent and 90 percent, respectively, we would expect 58 of 90 patients with CAD to have positive (true positive) exercise tests and 32 to have negative (false negative) results. Nine of the 10 without CAD will have negative tests (true negative),

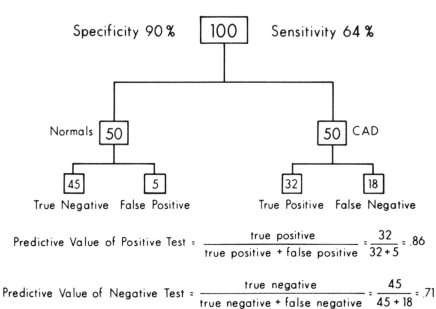

ATYPICAL CHEST PAIN
CAD Prevalence ~ 50%

Specificity 90 % |100| Sensitivity 64 %

Normals |50| |50| CAD

|45| |5| |32| |18|
True Negative False Positive   True Positive False Negative

$$\text{Predictive Value of Positive Test} = \frac{\text{true positive}}{\text{true positive} + \text{false positive}} = \frac{32}{32+5} = .86$$

$$\text{Predictive Value of Negative Test} = \frac{\text{true negative}}{\text{true negative} + \text{false negative}} = \frac{45}{45+18} = .71$$

Fig. 9-4. Hypothetical example of the usefulness of any exercise test when the prevalence of CAD is 50 percent in a population with atypical chest pain.

and one will have a positive test (false positive). The predictive value for a positive test in a member of this population (i.e., those with angina pectoris) is 98 percent. The predictive value of a negative test for this population is 22 percent. Thus, in patients with typical angina pectoris, a negative exercise ECG does not necessarily preclude the presence of CAD, but a positive result provides strong confirmation of the diagnosis (Fig. 9-5).

The following conclusions can be made about the interpretation of ischemic exercise ECG responses, (0.1 mV horizontal or downsloping ST segment depression):

1. The predictive value of a test is more important than sensitivity and specificity.

2. The prevalence of disease in the population from which the patient comes must affect the interpretation of results.

3. Exercise (stress) ECG has limited diagnostic value for patients from populations with very low or very high incidences of CAD. In our examples, it had limited diagnostic value in asymptomatic subjects and greater value for patients with typical angina. In the asymptomatic patient, a positive test is not very useful because of the high false positive rate, whereas a negative test is

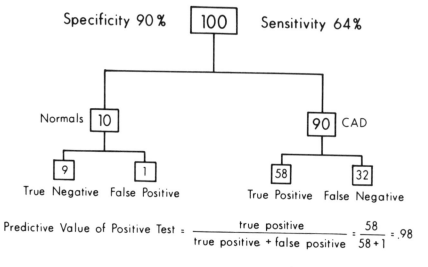

Fig. 9-5. Hypothetical example of the usefulness of any exercise test when the prevalence of CAD is high (90 percent) in a population with angina pectoris.

merely confirmatory. In patients with classic angina pectoris, a normal exercise ECG does not necessarily exclude the presence of CAD and a positive result (i.e., ischemic ST segment changes) only confirms the diagnosis. In patients with unexpected exercise ECG results (based on the predictive values for their populations), either a second noninvasive test, or, in certain circumstances, coronary angiography is recommended.

4. Exercise ECG testing is of most use in patients with atypical chest pain.

5. Sensitivity of stress ECG is lowest in patients with single-vessel CAD.

6. The intensity of exercise should be maximum or near maximum (at least 85 percent of age-predicted HR). If the patient is taking propranolol, there may be a false negative result because it may induce an abnormal chronotropic response.[3]

False-Positive Ischemic ECG Changes. False ischemic changes may be caused by drugs such as digitalis, or by left ventricular hypertrophy, hypokalemia, preexcitation syndrome, hyperventilation, left bundle branch block, cardiomyopathy, mitral valve prolapse, or vasoregulatory asthenia.[3,57]

Interpretation of Exercise Tests

Although exercise tests can provide useful clinical information, detection of CAD by analysis of ST segment response to exercise is limited. Interpretation of exercise test results should not be confined solely to changes seen in the ST segment. Important variables are maximal exercise capacity (i.e., endurance time or $\dot{V}O_{2\,max}$), BP response to exercise, chronotropic response, exercise-induced arrhythmias, and the extent of ST segment depression and whether or not it occurs during the early stages of an exercise test. Exercise capacity provides important prognostic information. Patients with coronary artery disease whose maximal exercise capacity is limited, i.e., those with endurance times of less than 6 minutes when the Bruce protocol is used, have a poor prognosis.[3] Furthermore, patients whose systolic BP falls during exercise are likely to have multivessel CAD with depressed left ventricular function and thus a poor prognosis.[3] ST segment depression of >0.2 mV or the appearance of ST segment depression at low levels of exercise are also suggestive of multivessel CAD.

Although the correlation between exercise-induced ischemic ST segment changes and evidence of CAD obtained from angiography is not always very strong, exercise ECG correlates better with natural history, particularly if other variables such as maximal exercise capacity are taken into consideration.[3] Abnormal exercise ECG tests in asymptomatic individuals should be considered indicative of a risk factor for CAD rather than dignositic of CAD, since evidence suggests an abnormal ECG response may be predictive of future coronary events.[40–42,45,56]

Exercise Tests Used to Assess Maximal Aerobic Capacity

Exercise tests are also routinely used to assess the physiologic limit of the ability to take up, transport, give off and utilize oxygen. This maximal exercise capacity (aerobic capacity) is dependent on a variety of interrelated functions, but is thought to be primarily indicative of the functional capacity of the respiratory, circulatory, and metabolic systems.[4]

Maximal oxygen uptake capacity ($\dot{V}O_{2\,max}$), or maximal aerobic power (MAP) as it is often called, has been shown to relate closely to the intensity of work performance and cardiac output.[58] A variety of tests are used to measure $\dot{V}O_{2\,max}$ and each has its theoretical basis. These tests vary as to the mode of exercise, protocol, method of gas collection, operational definitions of $\dot{V}O_{2\,max}$, and the physiologic response imposed. Therefore, their reliability and validity also vary.

The International Council for Sports Medicine and Physical Education (ICSPE) has adopted standards for ergometry. In order to achieve comparability of data, standardization of methods is essential. The suggested standards attempt to define and control many of the variables previously discussed. Although not all of the criteria for ergometry have been adopted in the United

Table 9.2. Reproducibility of Exercise Tests Used to Assess Maximal Aerobic Capacity Using "Leveling Off" as Criteria

Reference	Mode of Exercise	Correlation Coefficient	Coefficient of Variation (%)	Test Interval
(84) Thompson, 1977	Tm	.98	5.0	Same day
(59) Taylor et al, 1955	Tm	.95	2.4	3–5 days
(66) Mitchell, Sproule and Chapman, 1958	Tm	.92	3.7	Weeks to months
(85) Skubic and Hodgkins, 1963	step	.82	—	–
(62) Cunningham et al, 1977	Tm	.74	4.6	4–5 months
(76) Klissouras, 1971	Tm	—	1.7	2 weeks
(72) Bar-or and Zwiren, 1975	AC	.94	29.0	2 weeks
(74) Bouchard et al, 1979	Tm	.92	12.2	2 weeks
(71) McArdle et al, 1973	bike	.94	12.2	
	Tm	.96	10.7	2 weeks
		Range: .74–.98	Range: 1.7–29.0	

Tm = treadmill; step = step test; AC = arm cranking; bike = bicycle ergometer.

States, most are in the process of being defined. International adoption of a set of standards seems imminent. Mellerowicz[4] has reviewed the topic. Information can also be obtained from the American College of Sports Medicine.*

Reproducibility of Maximal Aerobic Capacity Tests

The criterion for maximal aerobic capacity can vary. The endpoints most often accepted are one of the two first proposed by Astrand.[5] He judged that maximal oxygen uptakes occurs "when oxygen consumption (does) not increase with further rise in workload." This criteria, though it has been modified at times,[59,60] has been shown to be the most reliable endpoint by a number of investigators and, relative to functional capacity, appears to have the best construct validity.[61] The reliability of exercise tests employing this endpoint can be expected to be very high, regardless of the mode of exercise, the population being tested, protocol, or equipment. The range of "reliability coefficients" is from .74 to .98, with an average coefficient of variation of 9.1 percent (See Table 9-2).

The reproducibility of exercise test results can be diminished when plateauing (leveling off) in oxygen consumption has not been achieved, as was demonstrated by Cunningham et al, who reported a "reliability coefficient" of .27 for tests when no plateau had been achieved.[62]

Other criteria have been suggested such as the achievement of (1) specified blood lactate levels[4], (2) maximal HR, (3) signs of fatigue, or (4) the dropping off of oxyhemoglobin saturation during the last minutes of an exercise test.[58] Although studies had indicated that there may be reliability for tests using these criteria, most exercise physiologists believe that these endpoints may not be valid, i.e., they may not be theoretically sound.

---

* American College of Sports Medicine, P.O. Box 1440, Indianapolis, IN 46206.

Most exercise tests use the "leveling off" of oxygen consumption as the endpoint criterion. However, it should be noted that most of the research to date on use of this criterion has been on apparently healthy individuals or well-motivated subjects. Patients with various acute and chronic diseases[63-65] or who are less motivated[62] (e.g., children) do not necessarily achieve this criterion although maximal exercise tolerance is achieved. The clinician interpreting these results must evaluate clinical significance before inferences can be made.

Many tests that do not employ motorized treadmills will not lead to the achievement of the "leveling off" criterion. There are numerous factors that contribute to this, such as the amount of muscle involved in the exercise, physiologic differences in the types of muscle contractions used, subject familiarity with exercise mode, test positions, and other physiologic effects of the elicited exercise. These factors can threaten the reliability and validity of exercise tests that attempt to assess "true" maximal aerobic capacity.

Validity of Exercise Tests Used to Measure Maximal Aerobic Capacity

The standard used to judge all maximal aerobic testing is the multistage maximal treadmill test because the highest oxygen consumption values (liters per minute or milliliters per kilogram per minute) are obtained with this test in any given individual. The criteria of plateauing (leveling off) is also obtained more often with this mode.

Many progressive multistage maximal treadmill tests have been described. Taylor et al[59] pioneered the use of progressive multistage maximal treadmill tests to determine $\dot{V}O_{2\,max}$. Their protocol consisted of having the subject run at 7 mph for 3 minutes at an initial grade of 5 percent. On successive days, the grade was increased by 2.5 percent up to 12.5 percent. Mitchell et al modified Taylor's protocol by using a speed of 6 mph with a grade of 0 for the initial stage.[66] Successive stages were increased by a grade of 2.5 percent, but the rest interval between stages was 10 minutes. The criteria for achieving $\dot{V}O_{2\,max}$ are virtually the same in both protocols; the obtained values would not be expected to differ.

Balke[67] and Bruce[68] advocated the use of protocols they developed although both use continuous multistage maximal treadmill tests. Their protocols differ in the speed, duration, and grades of successive stages, hence in energy costs. The Balke and Bruce protocols, sometimes with modifications, are the most widely used, possibly because they are less time-consuming to conduct.

Froelicher et al[69] examined the Bruce, Balke, and Taylor protocols by assessing the $\dot{V}O_{2\,max}$ measured in the same 15 subjects. The greatest mean oxygen consumption was obtained with the Taylor protocol. The mean $\dot{V}O_{2\,max}$ obtained with use of the Bruce protocol was 6.5 percent lower, whereas the mean was 9.7 percent lower with use of the Balke protocol. These differences are often considered inconsequential in view of the time-saving advantage of the Balke and Bruce protocols.

Considerations such as convenience, space, and equipment expense have led some investigators to advocate other modes for exercise testing. Bicycle ergometers, step tests, and arm cranking have been the modes most often used. A number of studies have examined the differences in maximal oxygen uptake values obtained with the various modes.[58,70–72,74] The r^2 (coefficient of determination) values reported indicate that from 10 percent to 64 percent of the values obtained by maximal treadmill test can be accounted for by the other test modes. There are numerous explanations for this finding. The difference in oxygen uptake values for untrained individuals tested with treadmill tests and bicycle ergometers range from 10 percent to 15 percent.[51,70,71] These differences may result from differences in the amount of muscle involved in each type of exercise, unfamiliarity with the bicycle mode, and fatigue of the leg muscles at high workloads when using the bicycle.[51,70,71]

Bar-or and Zwiren reported that with arm cranking tests, 60 percent to 70 percent of the maximal oxygen uptake values obtained by treadmill testing can be measured.[72] This observation agrees with the findings of other investigators,[53,73,74] which leads to speculation that the lower values are not caused just by the small mass of muscle involved but also by differences in HR, BP, and ventilation during arm cranking.

Despite those limitations and observations, the other modes of exercise have test–retest reliability coefficients similar to those for the treadmill tests. Use of regression equations can provide fairly reliable estimates of "true" maximal oxygen consumption values from those obtained during nontreadmill tests.

Maximal oxygen consumption and the tests used to measure it, cannot be understood unless measurement variability and the factors that can contribute to measurement error are understood. Variability in maximal oxygen uptake measurements was examined by Katch et al.[75] They attempted to quantify the variability in the measurement that was caused by biological factors versus that caused by measurement problems. Of the 5.6 percent total variation they found between tests, they concluded that 90 percent of the variation represented biological phenomena, while only 10 percent was caused by technical problems.[75] Therefore, if methods are standardized and extrinsic factors are controlled, the measurement error (technical error) is small and can be considered negligible. Because most of the variability between repeated tests represents biological factors, the test can be used to understand the effects of disease processes and aging (i.e., when the variability exceeds the expected ranges).

Klissouras examined the variability in the measurement of maximal aerobic power in 25 pairs of monozygous and dizygous twins.[76] He concluded that 93.4 percent of the variability in maximal oxygen uptake was genetically determined. Although there were large assumptions underlying Klissouras' conclusions, the results are thought-provoking, suggesting one explanation for some of the interindividual variation in $\dot{V}O_{2\,max}$.

Maximal oxygen uptake has also been predicted from data obtained during submaximal tests. This approach is attractive because submaximal tests are easy to perform and *most* of the equipment for the test is already found in *most* physical therapy departments. In contrast, the equipment for max testing is costly, more difficult to use, and subjects must be highly motivated and cooperative in order to assure reliable results.[77] Most of the submaximal tests are based on the documented linear relationship between submaximal exercise heart rates and oxygen uptake. By extrapolation, using the predicted age-based maximal heart rate for the subject, maximal oxygen uptake values can be predicted.[5] This is done, for example, when the bicycle ergometer Astrand-Rhyming test is performed. The heart rates of subjects are measured at regular intervals (at predetermined work rates) once steady-state exercise has been achieved. Normograms have been constructed that demonstrate heart rate–work rate relationships.[5] Corrections for reduced maximal heart rate with age must be used.

Astrand has noted that predicitons of $\dot{V}O_{2\,max}$ from submaximal tests has a standard error of 10 percent to 15 percent because of the variability in the linear relationship between heart rate and work at high work rates.[77] Wyndham[60] has suggested that the following assumptions *must* underlie the Astrand-Rhyming test: (1) maximal heart rate occurs at approximately the same work rate as does maximum oxygen consumption; (2) HR and oxygen consumption are linearly related up to maximal values for each; and (3) individual variation about the mean "population" maximum HR is small.

The Astrand-Rhyming bicycle ergometer test normograms were derived from healthy Scandanavian subjects who were familiar with that mode of exercise. The use of this test and the normograms may be questioned when patients with various acute and chronic diseases are tested. Disease processes are known to alter the relationships on which the test is based.[63–65]

Astrand has noted that the state of physical training can influence test results. Predictions may be too high or too low depending on the state of training; however, the direction and the linearity of the estimations require further investigation.

Some investigators have suggested that $\dot{V}O_{2\,max}$ can be estimated from exercise time determined by use of standardized treadmill protocols.[52,67,68] The major limitation of these predictions is that they are only valid up to oxygen uptake values of 50 ml/kg/per minute.[52]

If a standard method is used, results of exercise tests for the purpose of assessing maximal aerobic capacity can be highly reproducible, irrespective of the mode used. "Leveling off" of oxygen uptake even with increased workload is most often demonstrated by use of multistage maximal treadmill tests. Therefore, this test is considered the most valid. Despite the attractiveness of the indirect methods of determining maximal oxygen consumption, they should be used judiciously.

THALLIUM-201 PERFUSION IMAGING

Thallium-201 (^{201}Tl) is a potassium analogue that is taken up by normal myocardial cells. Uptake is dependent on blood flow as well as on the integrity of the myocytes. Decreased uptake indicates dead myocardial tissue (either an acute myocardial infarction or the presence of scar tissue) or decreased blood flow to the region, or both. During exercise, ^{201}Tl uptake normally increases because of increased coronary blood flow, and probably because of the increased metabolic activity of the myocytes. In patients with CAD, ^{201}Tl uptake increases in the regions of the heart supplied by normal arteries, but uptake remains unchanged or even diminished in segments supplied by narrowed arteries. As a result there is a nonhomogeneous distribution of the radio-tracer, which is seen as perfusion defects or cold spots on the scintigram. A few hours after cessation of exercise, the perfusion defects disappear. Perfusion defects that appear only with exercise are caused by narrowed arteries and myocardial ischemia, whereas those that persist at rest (several hours after exercise) are caused by scarring. Sensitivity of ^{201}Tl perfusion scans is generally higher than that for exercise ECG (about 85 percent) and its specificity is slightly higher than exercise ECG.[78] The ^{201}Tl stress test is, therefore, superior to exercise ECG not only because of its higher sensitivity, but also because the scan can demonstrate defects with exercise even though the HR response may not reach maximum or near maximum levels.[78] Perfusion imaging should be used instead of exercise ECG in situations in which false positive ST segment depression might be expected. The limitations of ^{201}Tl imaging are the same as those present for any single photon radiotracer study and include lack of true tomographic resolution as well as a radiation burden.[78]

Reproducibility of Thallium Imaging

McLaughlin et al examined the reproducibility of the results of thallium imaging in 25 patients with known or suspected CAD.[79] Fourteen of these patients had two perfusion imaging studies during maximum exercise. The two exercise tests were performed 1 week apart. Five segments of the left ventricle were assessed in each patient. The results of thallium studies are qualitative, that is, they are judged to have or not to have abnormalities present. In this study, three independent observers interpreted the scans. For 64 of the 70 segments studied (91 percent), findings were reproducible. Inter-observer differences could have accounted for some of the discrepancies in results in the study.

RADIONUCLIDE VENTRICULOGRAPHY

Radionuclide ventriculography using technetium-99m with in vivo or in vitro labeling to determine left ventricular contractile function (i.e., ejection fraction), and regional wall abnormalities at rest and during exercise is also used for the detection of CAD. The test is usually performed during supine or upright bicycle ergometry exercise. The test is based on the observation that exercise-induced myocardial ischemia results in loss of contraction in the regions of the myocardium (wall motion abnormalities) supplied by stenotic coronary arteries. The global ejection fraction is believed to decline during exercise in patients with CAD. Normally ejection fractions increase with exercise. Thus, ^{99m}Tc ventriculography, unlike exercise ^{201}Tl studies, does not display myocardial ischemia but rather the consequences of ischemia (i.e., abnormal contractile function secondary to myocardial ischemia). Experimental studies have demonstrated that documentation of regional abnormalities of contraction are quite reproducible and that the test is more sensitive than exercise ECG.[80,81]

Upton et al measured left ventricular function in the same 10 normal subjects at rest and during exercise.[80] The test–retest "reliability coefficients" for measurement of left ventricular ejection fraction (LVEF) at rest and during exercise at 85 percent of age-predicted maximal HR were $r = .95$. The average variability in LVEF at rest was 4 ± 3.8 percent, and during exercise it was 3.2 ± 2.5 percent.

The sensitivity and specificity of tests for exercise-induced regional wall disorders is higher than that for exercise ECG, averaging 76 percent and 95 percent respectively.[82,83] Although sensitivity of the global ejection fraction is claimed to be higher than that for exercise ECG (88 percent), it is not specific for CAD and its specificity is less than exercise ECG (70 percent).[82,83] Depression of global left ventricular systolic function (ejection fraction) with exercise is not specific for myocardial ischemia. The depression does not prove the presence of CAD, because other conditions—such as cardiomyopathy and aging—may decrease the global ejection fraction measured during exercise.[83] In addition, very high intensity exercise leading to exhaustion within a short period of time may also result in depression of the ejection fraction even in healthy subjects.[80] On the other hand, β-adrenergic blockade may conceal abnormal global ejection fractions during exercise in patients with CAD.[83]

In summary, use of global ejection fractions as a screening test for CAD has serious limitations. However, regional wall motion abnormalities during exercise are a good indicator of CAD.

SUMMARY

A sound, thorough understanding of the relative quality of the measurements used to assess the cardiovascular system is a prerequisite to establishing and assessing therapeutic interventions for cardiovascular disease. Many of our clinical judgments are based on the results of tests and the obtained measurements. We must understand the reliability and validity of cardiovascular measurements. The clinician must also understand and control the factors that are known to influence the measurements.

The reliability and validity of cardiovascular measurements commonly used by physical therapists are relatively good. Measurements of HR and BP are clinically useful and accurate when attention is paid to technique and standardization.

Exercise testing for the purpose of detecting CAD is useful in members of populations with a high incidence of CAD, but it is less useful for other subjects. Exercise testing for the purpose of assessing maximal oxygen delivery capacity has high reliability when precise criteria are used, but to date it has been used mainly on healthy subjects.

Other exercise tests and measurements, such as thallium imaging and radionuclide ventriculography also appear to be reliable and valid and can offer clinical insights that aid the clinician in planning effective treatment programs.

ACKNOWLEDGMENT

The authors gratefully acknowledge the guidance and editorial assistance of Dr. James M. Hagberg and the secretarial assistance of Ms. Phyllis Anderson.

REFERENCES

1. Amundsen LR: Cardiac Rehabilitation, Vol. 1. In: Clinics in Physical Therapy. Churchill Livingstone, Edinburgh, 1981
2. Sheffield LT, Roitman D: Stress testing methodology. In: Sonnenblick EH, Lesch M (eds) Exercise and Heart Disease. Grune and Stratton, New York, 1977
3. Chung EK (ed): Exercise Electrocardiography: Practical Approach, Baltimore, Williams & Wilkins, 1979
4. Mellerowicz H, Smodlaka VN (eds): Ergometry: Basics of Medical Exercise Testing. Urban and Schwarzenberg, Baltimore, 1981
5. Astrand PO, Rodahl K: Textbook of Work Physiology: Physiological Bases of Exercise, 2nd Ed. McGraw-Hill, New York, 1977
6. Gorman PA, Byers WS, Haider R: Exercise electrocardiography. In Naughton JP, Hellerstein HK (eds): Exercise Testing and Exercise Training in Coronary Heart Disease. Academic Press, New York, 1973
7. Sedlock DA, Knowlton RG, Fitzgerald PI, et al: Accuracy of subject-palpated carotid pulse after exercise. Phys Sports Med 11:106, 1983
8. Cotton FS, Dill DB: On the relation between the heart rate during exercise and that of immediate post-exercise period. Am J Physiol 111:554, 1935
9. Pollock ML, Broida J, Kendrick Z: Validity of the palpation technique of heart rate determination and its estimation of training heart rate. Res Q Am Assoc Health Phys Ed, 43:77, 1972
10. McArdle WD, Zwiren L, Magel JR: Validity of the post exercise heart rate as a means of estimating heart rate during work of varying intensities. Res Q Am Assoc Health Phys Ed, 40:523, 1969
11. Oldridge NB, Haskell WL, Single P: Carotid palpation, coronary heart disease and exercise rehabilitation. Med Sci Sports Exerc 13:6, 1980
12. White JR: EKG changes using carotid artery for heart rate monitoring. Med Sci Sports Exerc 9:88, 1977
13. Gardner GW, Danks DL, Scharfsiein L: Use of carotid pulse for heart rate monitoring. Med Sci Sports Exerc 11:111, 1979
14. Aranjo J, Born DG, Rhomas TR: An evaluation of five portable heart monitors. Med Sci Sports Exerc 13:124, 1981
15. Astrand I, Astrand PO, Hallback, Kilbom A: Reduction in maximal oxygen uptake with age. J Appl Physiol 35:649, 1973

16. London SB, London RE: Comparison of indirect pressure measurements (Korotkoff) with simultaneous direct brachial artery pressure distal to the cuff. Adv Intern Med 13:127, 1967

17. Moss AJ, Admas FH: Index of indirect estimation of diastolic blood pressure. Am J Dis Child 106:364, 1963

18. King GE: Taking the blood pressure. JAMA 209:1902, 1969

19. Mitchell PL, Parlin RW, Blackburn H: Effect of vertical displacement of the arm on indirect blood pressure measurements. N Engl J Med 271:72, 1968

20. Wright BM, Dore CF: A random-zero sphygmomanometer. Lancet 1:337, 1970

21. Karvonen MJ, Telivvo LJ, Jarvinen EJR: Sphygmomanometer cuff size and the accuracy of indirect measurement of blood pressure. Am J Cardiol 13:688, 1964

22. American Heart Association: Recommendations for Human Blood Pressure Determination by Sphygmomanometers, Dallas, 1967

23. O'Brien E, O'Malley K: Essentials of Blood Pressure Measurements. Churchill Livingston, New York, 1981

24. Glock CY, Vought RL, Clark EG, Schweitzer MD: Studies in hypertension II: variability of daily blood pressure measurements in the same individual over a three-week period. J Chron Dis 4:451, 1956

25. Armitage P, Rose GA: The variability of measurements of casual blood pressure I: a laboratory study. Clin Sci 30:325, 1966

26. Rose GA, Holland WW, Crowley EA: A sphygmomanometer of epidemiologists. Lancet 1:296, 1964

27. Van Bergen FH, Weatherhead DS, Treloar AE, Dobkin AB, Buckley JJ: Comparison of indirect and direct methods of measuring arterial blood pressure. Circulation 10:481, 1954

28. Holland WW, Homerfelt S: Measurements of blood pressure: comparison of intra-arterial and cuff values. Br Med J 2:1241, 1964

29. Roberts LN, Smiley JR, Manning GW: A comparison of direct and indirect blood pressure determinations. Circulation 8:232, 1953

30. Stegall HF, Kardon MB, Kemmerer WT: Indirect measurement of arterial blood pressure by doppler ultrasonic sphygmomanometry. J Appl Physiol 25:793, 1968

31. Gruen W: An assessment of present automated methods of indirect blood pressure measurements. Ann NY Acad Sci 147:107, 1968

32. Ellestad MH, Wan MKC: Predictive implications of stress testing: follow-up of 2700 subjects after maximum treadmill stress testing. Circulation 51:363, 1975

33. Mason RE, Likar I, Biern RO, Ross RS: Multiple-lead exercise electrocardiography: experience in 107 normal subjects and 67 patients with angina pectoris and comparison with coronary cinearteriography in 84 patients. Circulation 36:517, 1967

34. Martin CM, McConahay DR: Maximal treadmill exercise electrocardiography: correlations with coronary arteriography and cardiac hemodynamics. Circulation 46:956, 1972

35. Friesinger GC, Smith RF: Correlation of electrocardiographic studies and arteriographic findings with angina pectoris. Circulation 46:1173, 1972

36. Kansal S, Roitman D, Sheffield LT: Stress testing with st-segment depression at rest: an angiographic correlation. Circulation 54:638, 1976

37. Proudfit WL, Shirey EK, Stones FM: Selective cine coronary arteriography: correlation with clinical findings in 1,000 patients. Circulation 33:901, 1966

38. Campeau L, Bourassa MG, Bois MA, Saltiel J, Lesperance J, Rico O, Delcan J, Telleria M: Clinical significance of selective coronary cinearteriography. Can Med Assoc J 99:1063, 1968

39. Sketch MH, Mohiuddin SM, Lynch JD, Zencka AE, Runco V: Significant sex differences in the correlation of electrocardiographic exercise testing and coronary arteriograms. Am J Cardiol 36:169, 1975

40. Weiner DA, Ryan TJ, McCabe CH, et al: Exercise testing: correlations among history of angina, ST segment response and prevalence of coronary artery disease in the coronary artery surgery study. N Engl J Med 301:230, 1979

41. Cummings GR, Samm J, Borysyk L, Kich L: Electrocardiographic changes during exercise in asymptomatic men: 3-year follow-up. Can Med Assoc J 112:578, 1975

42. Aronow WS: Five-year follow-up of double master's test, maximal treadmill stress test, and resting and post exercise in asymptomatic persons. Circulation 52:616, 1975

43. Froelicher VF, Thompson AJ, Longo MR, Jr, et al: Value of exercise testing for screening asymptomatic men for latent coronary artery disease. Prog Cardiovasc Dis 18:265, 1976

44. Bruce RA, McDonough JR: Stress testing in screening for cardiovascular disease. Bull NY Acad Med 45:1288, 1969

45. Allen WH, Aronow WS, DeCristofaro D: Treadmill exercise testing in mass screening for coronary risk factors. Cath Card Diagn 2:39, 1976

46. McHenry PL, Fisch C: Clinical applications of the treadmill exercise test. Mod Concepts Cardiovasc Dis 46:21, 1977

47. Fabian J, Stolz I, Janota M, Rohac J: Reproducibility of exercise tests in patients with symptomatic ischaemic heart disease. Br heart J 37:785, 1975

48. Smokler PE, MacAlpin RN, Alvaro A, Kattus AA: Reproducibility of a multistage near maximal treadmill test for exercise tolerance in angina pectoris. Circulation 48:346, 1973

49. Ellestad MH, Allen W, Wan MCK, Kemp GL: Maximal treadmill stress testing for cardiovascular evaluation. Circulation 39:517, 1979

50. Borg G, Dahlstrom H: The reliability and validity of a physical work test. Acta Physiol Scand 55:353, 1962

51. Shephard RJ: The relative merits of the step test, bicycle ergometer, and treadmill in the assessment of cardio-respiratory fitness. Int Z Angew Physiol Einschl Arbeitphysiol 23:219, 1966

52. Pollock ML, Bohannon RL, Cooper KH, Ayres JJ, Ward A, White SR, Linnerud AC: A comparative analysis of four protocols for maximal treadmill stress testing. Am Heart J 92:39, 1976

53. Bobbert AC: Physiological comparison of three type of ergometry. J Appl Physiol 15:1007, 1960

54. Nagle FJ, Balke B, Naughton JP: Gradational step tests for assessing work capacity. J Appl Physiol 4:745, 1965

55. Gibson RS, Beller GA: Should exercise electrocardiographic testing be replaced by radioisotope methods? In Rahimtoola SH (ed). Controversies in Coronary Artery Disease. Cardiovascular Clinics, Vol. 13, Brest AN (ed-in-chief). F.A. Davis, Philadelphia, 1982

56. McConahay DR, McCallister BD, Smith RE: Post exercise electrocardiography: correlation with coronary arteriography and left ventricular hemodynamics. Am J Cardiol 28:1, 1972

57. Erikssen J, Enge I, Forfang K, Storstein O: False positive diagnostic tests and coronary angiographic findings in 105 presumably healthy males. Circulation 54:371, 1976

58. Kasch FW, Phillips WH, Ross WD, Carter JEL, Boyer JL: A comparison of maximal oxygen uptake by treadmill and step-test procedures. J Appl Physiol 21:1387, 1966

59. Taylor SA, Buskirk E, Henschel A: Maximal oxygen intake as an objective measure of cardio-respiratory performance. J Appl Physiol 8:73, 1955

60. Wyndham CH, Williams CG: Improving the accuracy of prediction of an individual's maximum oxygen intake. Int A Angew Physiol Einschl Arbeitsphysiol 23:354, 1967

61. Michels E: Measurement in physical therapy: on the rules for assigning numerals to observations. Phys Ther 63(2):209, 1983

62. Cunningham DA, MacFarlane van Watershoot B, Paterson DH, Lefcob M, Sangal SP: Reliability and reproducibility of maximal oxygen uptake measurement in children. Med Sci Sports Exerc 9:104, 1977

63. Coyle EF, Martin WH, Ehsani AA, Hagberg JM, Bloomfield SA, Sinacore DR, Holloszy JO: Blood lactate threshold in some well-trained ischemic heart disease patients. J Appl Physiol (Respirat Environ Exerc Physiol): 54(1):18, 1983

64. Hagberg JM, Goldberg AP, Ehsani AA, Heath GW, Delmez JA, Harter HR: Exercise training improves hypertension in hemodialysis patients. Am J Nephrol 3:209, 1983

65. Hagberg JM, Coyle EF, Carroll JE, Miller JM, Martin WH, Brooke MH: Exercise hyperventilation in patients with McArdle's disease. J Appl Physiol: Respirat Environ Exerc Physiol 52(4):991, 1982

66. Mitchell JH, Sproule BJ, Chapman CB: The physiological meaning of the maximal oxygen intake test. J Clin Invest 37:538, 1958

67. Balke B, Ware RW: An experimental study of "physical fitness" of Air Force personnel. US Armed Forces Med J 10(6):675, 1959

68. Bruce RA: Methods of exercise testing: step test, bicycle, treadmill, isometrics. Am J Cardiol 33:715, 1974

69. Froelicher VF, Brammell H, Davis G, Noguera I, Stewart A, Lancaster MC: A comparison of three maximal treadmill exercise protocols. J Appl Physiol 36:720, 1974

70. Glassford RG, Baycroft GHY, Sedgwick AW, MacNab RBJ: Comparison of maximal oxygen uptake values determined by predicted and actual methods. J Appl Physiol 20:509, 1965

71. McArdle WD, Katch FI, Pechar GS: Comparison of continuous and discontinuous treadmill and bicycle tests for max $\dot{V}O_2$. Med Sci Sports Exerc 5:156, 1973

72. Bar-or O, Zwiren LD: Maximal oxygen consumption test during arm exercise-reliability and validity. J Appl Physiol 38:424, 1975

73. Astrand P, Saltin B: Maximal oxygen uptake and heart rate in various types of muscular activity. J Appl Physiol 16:977, 1961

74. Bouchard C, Godbout P, Mondor JC, Leblanc C: Specificity of maximal aerobic power. Eur J Appl Physiol 40:85, 1979

75. Katch VL, Sady SS, Freedson P: Biological variability in maximum aerobic power. Med Sci Sports Exerc 14:21, 1982

76. Klissouras V: Heritability of adaptive variation. J Appl Physiol 31:338, 1971

77. Astrand P: Quantification of exercise capability and evaluation of physical capacity in man. In Sonnenblick EH, Lesch M (eds): Exercise and Heart Disease, Grune & Stratton, New York, 1977

78. Botvinick EH, Glazer HB, Shosa DW: What is the reliability and utility of scintigraphic methods for the assessment of ventricular function? In Rahimtoola SH

(ed): Controversies in Coronary Artery Disease. Cardiovascular Clinics, Vol. 13, Brest AN (ed-in-chief). F.A. Davis, Philadelphia, 1982

79. McLaughlin PR, Martin RP, Doherty P, Daspit S, Doris M, Haskell W, Lewis S, Kriss JP, Harrison DC: Reproducibility of thallium-201 myocardial imaging. Circulation 55:497, 1977

80. Upton MT, Rerych SK, Newman GE, Bounous EP, Jones RH: The reproducibility of radionuclide angiographic measurements of left ventricular function in normal subjects at rest and during exercise. Circulation 62:126, 1980

81. Ashburn WL, Schelbert HR, Verba JW: Left ventricular ejection fraction: a review of several radionuclide angiographic approaches using the scintillation camera. Prog Cardiovasc Dis 20:267, 1978

82. Botvinick EH, Shames DM, Gershengorn KM, Carlsson E, Rathsin RA, Parmley WW: Myocardial stress perfusion scintigraphy with rubidium-81 versus stress electrocardiography. Am J Cardiol 39:364, 1977

83. McGowan RL, Martin ND, Zaret BL, Hall RR, Bryson AL, Strauss HW, Flamm MD: Diagnostic accuracy of noninvasive myocardial imaging for coronary artery disease: an electrocardiographic and angiographic correlation. Am J Cardiol 40:6, 1977

84. Thompson, J: The repeatability of the measurement of aerobic power in man and factors affecting it. Q J Exp Physiol 62:83, 1977

85. Skubic V, Hodgkins J: Cardiovascular efficiency tests for girls and women. Res Quart. 34:191, 1963

10 | Measurement Issues in Nerve Conduction Velocity and Electromyographic Testing

John L. Echternach

The purpose of this chapter is to examine the measurement issues associated with nerve conduction and electromyographic examinations. After examining the literature related to this area of testing, especially the early literature, we must conclude that many authors have reported results in a very sketchy fashion.[1-4] Reports of latency and distance measurements in papers concerning nerve conduction velocities or of the abnormalities encountered in electrophysiologic testing of particular types of patients have not always been presented. Clinical procedures have been developed that are successful in defining clinical problems of patients, but the measurement issues evidently have not been completely appreciated by some practitioners.

Nerve conduction and electromyographic testing may be good examples of how technology has been applied to clinical problems before we had an understanding of the physiologic process they were designed to measure. This chapter will raise more questions than it answers. For the clinician who has questions there is often no answer available in the literature. It is hoped that clinicians will be able to use this chapter to improve their understanding of the limitations of clinical testing.

The clinical measurement of nerve conduction velocities has become increasingly popular since the late 1940s. A 1948 article by Hodes et al contained the first clinically relevant discussion of conduction velocity testing and created great interest in the subject.[1] As published reports accumulated, understanding of the usefulness of the method developed. Advances in instrumentation increased the ease and reliability of testing. Both of these factors led to increased use of nerve conduction measurement as an aid in clarifying patient problems. Clinical electromyography has followed similar development, i.e., it was first used in the laboratory and later was applied to clinical problems. From the mid 1940s to the present, there has been an expanding use of clinical electromyography.[2,3]

This chapter will deal with some of the issues in measurement in clinical nerve conduction velocity testing (NCV) and electromyography (EMG). There will also be a brief discussion of some of the problems associated with the use of electromyography for kinesiologic research.

The first thing to ask before a quantity is measured is whether it is measurable. Nerve conduction velocities are measureable.[1,3,4] Nerve conduction velocities are derived measurements dependent on the use of other measurements. In addition, there are several different characteristics of a nerve action potential that are quantifiable and that are frequently obtained while conduction velocity testing is being performed. These are: conduction time or latency which is obtained by measuring the time from the stimulus delivery until a response is observed; amplitude of response or the size of the action potential; and wave form, or a description of the wave characteristics, including the number of phases.

MOTOR NERVE CONDUCTION VELOCITY (MNCV)

In testing nerve conduction velocity, there are several factors that can vary. The issue of reliability can be examined at all points in the process. In MNCV testing, there are eight areas in which error can be introduced into the measurement. These are

1. Electrode placement and skin preparation.
2. Distance from the distal point of stimulation to the recording electrode.
3. Measurements between points of stimulation.
4. Position of limbs for measurement.
5. Measurement of the action potential.
6. Position of stimulating electrodes and related problems.
7. Calculation of conduction velocity.
8. Temperature of body parts and the environment.

Each potential source of error will be discussed separately.

ELECTRODE PLACEMENT AND SKIN PREPARATION

Electrodes must be placed over the belly of the muscle from which the recording will be made so that a maximal response can be obtained; in this way the amplitude of the potential represents all the activity possible for the nerve under study.

The first potential source of error is in electrode placement. Some investigators suggest using the stimulating electrode to find the best motor response over the muscle (i.e., the motor point) and then placing the recording electrode over the motor point. The reference electrode should then be placed a minimum of 2.5 to 3 cm distal to the active electrode. Electrode placement becomes more difficult when patients who have lost the ability to voluntarily contract the muscle (e.g., those with peripheral nerve lesions) are examined. Then the examiner must estimate where the muscle belly is.[5,6]

The amplitude of the action potential represents the voltage or potential difference between the active recording electrode and the reference electrode. The placement and distance between these two electrodes determines to large extent the size of the potential if an adequate stimulus is used. The amplitude of the potential is one of the variables. A decreased amplitude represents a reduction in viable nerve fibers conducting in the nerve stimulated.

Questions remain about the effect of varying inter-electrode distance on the action potential.[7] The importance of placing the active electrode in the best position over the muscle belly suggests that it is also important to have the freedom to place the reference electrode at some point distal to the active electrode, depending on the size of the muscle and the configuration of the body area where the electrodes are to be placed.[8] Those who are in favor of the electrodes being a consistent distance apart feel that this offers a standard that can be used for all muscle sites and all nerves. In general, the placement of the electrodes should be similar for each muscle for each examination.

To ensure standardization of technique, and therefore of results, clinicians must also concern themselves with the procedures used to apply the electrodes. The electrodes should be firmly attached to the skin so that no artifact is created by electrode movement.[9] Skin preparation should follow a standard protocol and should include procedures for cleansing the skin of debris and oils with solvents such as alcohol.

Where to place the ground electrode has been debated. Some authors have suggested that, ideally, the ground electrode should be placed in between the active and reference electrodes, equally distant between the two, preferably over a bony area rather than a muscular area.[10] Sometimes this is not possible, depending on the nerve being tested; therefore, the ground electrode tends to be placed in an area that is convenient for the examiner. When ideal placement is not practical, it is logical to get as close to the ideal placement as possible. Standardized placement between examinations of a given patient is essential.

DISTANCE FROM THE DISTAL POINT OF
STIMULATION TO RECORDING ELECTRODES

The distance between the distal site of stimulation and the recording electrodes becomes an important consideration when examining any nerve that
may be entrapped between these two locations,[11-13] as in a patient who has a
carpal tunnel syndrome with compression of the median nerve beneath the
transverse retinaculum at the wrist. The compression is located between the
most distal point of stimulation of the median nerve, and the abductor pollicis
brevis from which the muscle action potential is recorded. Many examiners
measure a standard distance from the recording electrode to the most distal
point of stimulation of the nerve for this type of problem, usually an 8- to 10-
cm distance for the distal segment of the ulnar or median nerves.[13] This technique also applies to the tibial nerve in the lower extremity.[14] Using a standard
length for a segment in this instance permits comparison of latencies between
two nerves in the same extremity (a common environment) over the same
distance in order to determine if slowing of conduction is occurring, and is
preferable to using an arbitrary upper limit for normal, such as 4 ms. Suppose
that 4 ms was used as a criterion for normal distal motor latency. What does
it mean if a patient has latencies of 4.4 ms for the median nerve and 4.3 ms
for the ulnar nerve, and no ulnar nerve symptoms? Does this patient have
slowing of the distal latency in the median nerve, indicating compression at
the carpal tunnel? Most likely, the patient has no slowing. The larger-than-
expected latency, if measured over equally distant segments of both nerves,
may be normal for this individual (as might occur in the elderly), or may represent neuropathic changes in both nerves. Use of arbitrary criteria for normal
distal latencies may seem to be useful for the clinician, but can lead to faulty
judgments when those criteria are based on isolated measures. This problem
can be avoided by considering as many factors as is reasonable. In our example,
this would include consideration of velocities of both ulnar and median nerves
and of sensory conduction factors, and an electromyographic sample of a few
muscles supplied by these nerves.

Often it is not reasonable to standardize distances between sites of stimulation along the course of nerves because of wide anthropomorphic variations
between patients. Imagine the difficulty in determining the optimal distance
between stimulation sites for the nerve in the forearm (elbow to wrist) in a
person who is 6 feet, 7 inches tall as compared with a person who is a 5 feet
tall. It is obvious that the length of the forearm nerve segment would not be
the same. Should the distances between stimulation sites then be the same?

Conduction time or latency is determined by measuring on the oscilloscope
the time from the initial stimulus to the point at which the muscle action potential begins (Fig. 10-1). Maynard and Stolov reported that when a wave form
was stored on the oscilloscope and experienced examiners were asked to read
the latency as determined by the point of take-off of the muscle action potential,
great variation was found even among these experienced examiners.[15] Their
study suggests that the recording of conduction time or latency may be based

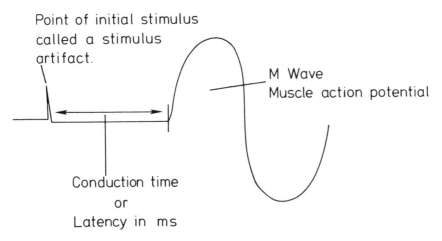

Point of initial stimulus
called a stimulus
artifact.

M Wave
Muscle action potential

Conduction time
or
Latency in ms

Fig. 10-1. A muscle action potential obtained from stimulating over the course of the nerve and recording from the muscle.

on the examiner's perception of where the muscle action potential leaves the baseline. This can vary greatly with examiners. Even in normal or near-normal subjects for whom there is a very clear action potential on the oscilloscope and a relatively straight baseline, there can be differences of opinion as to where the action potential leaves the baseline; causing possible errors of several milliseconds.[10] In my experience, this problem is most notable in those who are just learning to perform the test. Once this problem is discussed with the inexperienced clinician, there is improvement, especially if an example based on the individual clinician's testing can be used to show the importance of the problem. This source of error can be decreased if examiners always use the largest possible amplification of the wave form on the oscilloscope when determining the onset of the potential. Once the wave form is stored on the oscilloscope, calibration of the amplitude measurement is increased so that the point where the wave form leaves the baseline is clearly indicated. An alternative method, if instrumentation does not permit the suggested technique, is the recording of the 10 amplitudes of the stored potential, followed by stimulation and storage of a second potential with the sensitivity set so as to make the potential appear as large as possible on the oscilloscope. If the ulnar nerve is examined and then stimulated at the wrist and elbow, the latency obtained is 3 ms at the wrist and 7 ms at the elbow. Subtracting 3 from 7 leaves a conduction time of 4 ms. The 20-cm distance between sites of stimulation is then divided by the 4-ms factor and velocity is 50 m/sec, or normal. If the latency at the wrist is "under-read" as 2 ms, the latency at elbow was read as 7 ms, the conduction time would be 1 ms longer and would become 5 ms. The resulting velocity would then be 40 m/sec. This might be considered slow and representative of an abnormality. From this example, the importance of obtaining an accurate estimation of the point at which the muscle action potential begins can be appreciated.

MEASUREMENT BETWEEN POINTS OF STIMULATION

When measuring the distance between points of stimulation, one should always use the best possible method of measurement for the specific area of the body that is being examined.[16,17] For example, consider the measurement of distances from a point of stimulation on the radial nerve above the clavicle to a point of stimulation in the axilla.[17] This distance cannot be reliably measured with a tape measure since the length of the tape laid over the external contours of the body will not reflect the length of the radial nerve. Various authors have suggested that most linear measurements can best be obtained by a caliper.[16–18] However, in some areas such as the forearm distances between points of stimulation of the median nerve, tape measurements are probably as valid as those obtained by a caliper. The advantage of measuring by caliper is that body surface contours are eliminated; this does not imply that caliper measurements actually represent the exact distance over which the nerve impulses travel. However, the caliper method will yield more valid results.[17,18]

Many clinicians mark the sites of stimulation on skin with a marking pen. When a large pen is used for marking points of stimulation, care must be taken to measure from midmark to midmark for consistency. Using the previous example of the ulnar nerve and the same latency figures, but distorting the distance between sites of stimulation caused by errors in marking, and using the latencies of 3 ms at the wrist and 7 ms at the elbow, but now recording a measurement of 18 cm instead of 20 cm results in a conduction velocity of 45 m/sec as compared with our previous calculation of 50 m/sec, resulting in a change of 5 m/sec over a fairly long segment. Errors of the same magnitude over shorter segments make even more dramatic changes in computed velocities.

POSITIONING OF LIMBS FOR MEASUREMENT

Measurement between sites of stimulation should be taken with patients positioned exactly as they were when they were stimulated. For example, if a patient was abducted 30° at the shoulder when stimulated, the distance measurement should be made with the arm abducted to 30°. Ulnar nerve studies are often conducted with a patient's elbow flexed to 90°; the same position should then be used for measurement. The position of the extremity effects the length of the nerve. This is probably most evident at the elbow for the ulnar nerve.[19,20] In general, the effects of positioning on nerve conduction velocities have not been investigated.

MEASUREMENT OF THE ACTION POTENTIAL

Stimulation of a motor nerve produces a muscle action potential (MAP). This wave is initially negative and then reverses, becoming positive returning to the baseline and crossing it. The wave then continues in a positive direction before returning finally to the baseline (Fig. 10-1). The amplitude of the action potential in motor nerve conduction testing is usually measured from the baseline to the peak of the negative wave and not from peak to peak.[2,3,10] For MAP testing, a maximum amplitude of response is necessary. To determine if this has been obtained from a supramaximal stimulus, it should be determined that the amplitude of the *negative wave* will not increase with increased intensity of stimulation. Some investigators suggest that the slope of the initial wave form or the duration of the negative wave may have some significance in determining whether there is pathology, but a definitive study of this has not been made. The fastest conducting fibers are thought to make up the first part of the wave form and the average and slower conducting fibers are thought to contribute to the rest of the wave. Therefore, a change in the duration of rise to peak could be indicative of a change in the speed of conduction in some fibers.[2,3]

POSITION OF STIMULATING ELECTRODES AND RELATED PROBLEMS

For proper interpretation of MNCV, stimulation must occur directly over the nerve, and the electrodes must be applied in the proper direction, (i.e., cathode should be distal to the anode.) Braddon and Schuchmann reported latency errors of 0.5 ms in motor conduction studies resulting from reversal of the stimulating cathode and anode.[10] This reversal leads to an erroneously prolonged latency recording.

Meaningful results require that a supramaximal stimulus be delivered to the nerve under study. If a stimulus that is less than supramaximal is used, the fastest conducting fibers may not be stimulated and greater latency values will be recorded. Examiners can often minimize stimulation errors by carefully observing the amplitude of the obtained response and by taking care to assure that they obtain the largest possible response upon stimulation of the nerve.

Volume conduction caused by using a greater than supramaximal stimulation can also cause problems, especially in the upper arm area where the stimulus can spread to an adjacent nerve (as can be the case with the ulnar and median nerves). Most investigators use a standard stimulus duration and a standard rate of stimulation. Stimulation duration is usually 0.05 or 0.1 ms.[2,3] When it is difficult to obtain a response from a nerve, examiners will often use a duration of 0.2 ms. Because it is not clear what the effect the increased duration will have on the amplitude and other measured characteristics of the wave, it may be a mistake to increase duration to 0.2 ms. It is certainly questionable to go above this. For purposes of standardization, I prefer that investigators almost always use the stimulus duration of 0.1 ms for motor conduction velocities. I use a 0.2 ms duration only when no acceptable response can be obtained with the 0.1 ms duration. I then reduce the duration to 0.1 ms after having found the sites for stimulation with the 0.2 ms duration, so that all recordings are with a 0.1 ms duration. Some examiners use the longer duration because this makes it easier to find and to stimulate nerves. However, because the effect of stimulus duration on the measured potential is not fully known, variations in durations may lead to differing clinical interpretations by different examiners. Volume conduction errors can be compounded by increasing the duration of the stimulus.

CALCULATION OF CONDUCTION VELOCITY

The accuracy of calculations of conduction velocities may be different for long and short segments of nerves.[21,22] Calculations are most accurate over the longest nerve segment; however, it is often important to calculate segmental conduction velocities, especially when the clinician is looking for entrapment syndromes.[23] Short nerve segment calculations tend to compound all of the measurement errors noted previously, especially those related to distance measurements and those involved in determining latencies.[21] Examples are the short segments that are calculated for conduction of: the ulnar nerve across the elbow, the peroneal nerve between the popliteal space and the fibular head and the short radial nerve segment between the area above the clavical and the axilla. All of these are subject to increased error because of the shortness of the segment. Errors can be minimized when care is taken in the measurements and when the segments are kept as long as possible. A method has been suggested to minimize error by measuring all nerve conduction velocities over the longest segment possible,[20,21] that is, by examining the ulnar nerve using the segments from the upper arm to the wrist and from the elbow to the wrist and below the elbow to the wrist, rather than measuring the shorter segments from upper arm to above elbow, above elbow to below elbow, and below elbow to wrist. If there is slowing in any one of these longer segments, it should still be apparent even though the measurement is made over a longer segment. However, the long segmental method of computing conduction velocities gives clear evidence of slowing in a particular segment. The longer segment lengths of the second method may "average" the slowing out and borderline abnormalities may be missed. Velocities can be always calculated both ways when problems occur and the examiner can use the best information available. Maynard and Stolov found that competent examiners measuring even on a flat surface still made errors of 3.6 mm on the average; this demonstrates the increased potential for error when measurements are made over body contours.[15]

TEMPERATURE OF BODY PARTS AND ENVIRONMENTS

The temperature of the nerve is a known source of variability in nerve conduction velocity measurements.[24] Recently, some investigators have recommended that a correction formula be used for subjects whose extremities are very cool.[25,26] The method involves determining temperatures of the extremity with a skin thermometer at standard sites. The obtained conduction velocities can then be corrected for the effects of temperatures. Halar et al.[26] suggest the following formula for correction of latency values for computation of conduction velocities:

$$\text{Corrected latency} = \frac{1}{(0.012)(32) - \text{skin temperature (°C)} + 1/\text{latency (ms)}}$$

Patients with peripheral neuropathies are the subjects most likely to have incorrect conduction velocity measurements because of temperature effects. Peripheral neuropathy causes a decrease in limb temperature because of loss of innervation to the vascular and muscular systems. This tends to decrease vascular flow, which in turn causes decreased temperatures in distal regions, especially in the lower extremities. Therefore, a neuropathy may be judged to be more severe than it really is, because decreased limb temperature can lead to reduced conduction velocities.

Controlling room temperature has been suggested as a means of eliminating variability resulting from limb temperature. Some authors suggest making sure that the testing room is always kept at the same temperature and that it is within a comfortable range for patients.[24] Others suggest warming the extremities for 15 to 20 minutes prior to nerve conduction testing.[23] It is probably easier to use a correction formula. It is still important, however, to keep testing room temperatures within a reasonable and narrow range.[25]

SENSORY NERVE CONDUCTION TESTING

Many of the previously described concerns regarding potential sources of error in testing motor nerve conduction velocities, such as distance between electrodes, measurements between points of stimulation, effects of temperature and positioning, may be considered equally important when sensory conduction velocity measurements are made. In addition, there are several unique problems related specifically to sensory nerves: the type of electrode used; the firmness with which it is attached to the skin; measurements of latency; method of stimulation; and measurement distances.

Types of Electrodes

Conduction velocity measurements on upper extremity digital nerves (the ulnar and median nerves) are most commonly made with ring electrodes. Ring electrodes are constructed from a variety of materials, from pipe cleaners to tightly coiled springs.[3] Some manufacturers also provide solid ring electrodes.[27] The question is whether the amplitudes recorded with one type of electrode are the same as those recorded with other types of electrodes.

Most nerve conduction texts published in this country recommend the use of pairs of surface electrodes.[2,3] However, many European authors recommend the use of a monopolar needle electrode technique;[30,31] they believe that very small potentials and the initial positive phase of the potential are missed with surface electrodes. This can affect both latency and amplitude measurements, which are especially important in sensory nerve conduction velocity testing, because the size of the potentials is often the critical element evaluated. Therefore, if some electrodes are more sensitive than others in recording amplitudes, the type of electrode can affect conclusions.

Disk electrodes have been used routinely when recordings are made from the superficial radial nerve, sural nerve, and other sensory nerves where ring electrodes are clearly inappropriate. Variations on the traditional 1-cm disk electrodes had been tried for both the sural and radial nerve.[17,28,29] These have been rectangular electrodes that increase the recording area and therefore increase the number of peripheral branches from which the recording can be taken. The effect of varying the distance between the recording and reference electrodes in the electrode pairs for sensory nerve conduction velocity testing has not been critically examined.

Firmness of Attachment of Electrodes

The firmness with which electrodes are attached to the skin can also be a critical factor in recording sensory potentials. The issue of placement of the ground electrode is the same as in motor conduction velocity testing, except that in sensory testing the amplitudes of recorded potentials are much smaller, making grounding even more critical than in motor nerve testing.

Measurement Techniques

When sensory nerve testing was first used clinically, equipment was not nearly as sophisticated as it is today.[30] With the ability to average a number of responses and with solid-state electronics, sensory potentials can be recorded and displayed much more clearly, in marked contrast to sensory potential recording of 15 or 20 years ago in which there was a great amount of baseline disturbances. Many stimuli were superimposed on one another and permanently displayed, and a photographic technique was needed to show a small change in the baseline configuration (Fig. 10-2). This method resulted in measurements of latencies being taken from beginning of stimulus to peak of the superimposed potentials. Since those early days, sensory potentials have been measured to the peak of the action potential. As a result, there are two different methods for measuring nerve potentials, depending on whether they are from motor or sensory nerves. Even today, with sensory potentials that are easily examined, this difference in measurement technique often persists. With most sensory potentials recorded today, the latency should be measured up to the initiation of the action potential, as it is with motor nerve, rather than to the peak of the action potential (Fig. 10-2).

Investigators who measure to the initiation of the sensory action potential obviously report shorter latencies because of the decreased time to the initiation

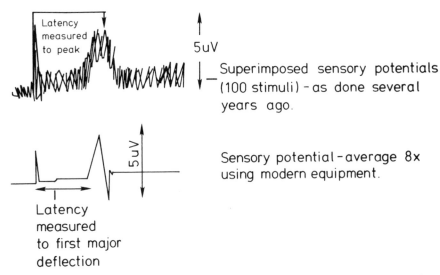

Latency measured to peak

5uV

Superimposed sensory potentials (100 stimuli) - as done several years ago.

5uV

Sensory potential-average 8x using modern equipment.

Latency measured to first major deflection

Fig. 10-2 Sensory potentials—comparing modern averaging with earlier techniques.

of the potential rather than to the peak of the potential; confusion has resulted as to what are the normal latencies of sensory potentials. Investigators also disagree on the proper way of measuring amplitudes of sensory potentials. Some investigators report peak-to-peak measurements as the amplitude for the sensory potentials, whereas other investigators measure sensory potentials from baseline to the peak of the negative wave.[30-32] Problems arise when comparison of results from one examiner is made with those of another, since most examiners are at least internally consistent.

The differences between orthodromic and antidromic stimulation is also controversial. In measuring the ulnar nerve orthodromically stimulation is done through the digital nerves of the fifth finger and recorded over the trunk of the ulnar nerve at the wrist and elbow. If the same nerve were examined antidromically, recording would be made through electrodes over the digital nerves while stimulation was done over the mixed ulnar nerve at the wrist and elbow.

The proponents of antidromic testing state that the technique is easier since the sites for motor stimulation of the nerve are easily found and probably have been marked earlier by the examiner. In routine testing, motor studies are usually done prior to the sensory studies. The amplitude of the sensory potential is greater, and thus justifies use of an antidromic technique. Those in favor of orthodromic technique state that it is possible that the sensory potential can be lost in the motor artifact if there is some slowing or disturbance of the sensory fibers.[23] A slight difference in latency is obtained by use of the orthodromic as opposed to antidromic technique for the same nerve segment; however, in comparing the antidromic with the orthodromic technique, studies have shown that the difference in latencies is not statistically significant.[33] The difference in amplitude of response is statistically significant however, and is a factor in making it easier to obtain sensory potentials on some persons with an antidromic technique.[34] The person who performs nerve conduction testing should be able to use either technique depending on the patient. I recommend use of the antidromic technique first, because it is easier and because it is the only method in common use for some nerves. If for some reason difficulties or problems are suspected that could be better defined by orthodromic technique, I suggest use of the orthodromic method. This approach is based on Ludin's work.[31]

Distances Measurement

One of the problems in sensory nerve conduction testing is that the greater the distance between the site of stimulation and the recording electrodes, the smaller the recorded potentials. This sometimes makes it difficult to compute velocities for sensory nerves over all the segments that are available for computing motor nerve velocities. Because of this, examiners tend to look at only the most distal portion of the sensory nerve.

Other Factors

Some of the factors already mentioned for motor nerves are also importance in trying to control error in sensory conduction testing. Stimulus duration is as important in sensory nerve testing as it is in motor testing. Stimulus duration of >0.1 ms is rarely justified in sensory testing.[30,31] For reasons of patient comfort, the interval between pulses is probably as important in sensory testing as in motor testing. One stimulus interval per second is a comfortable and usable duration for conduction testing. The proper placement of the stimulating electrode over the nerve is probably more important for sensory nerves than for motor nerves because of the smallness of the potentials being recorded. To improve accuracy in sensory conduction testing, one should be very careful about the points of stimulation and the placement of recording electrodes.[15] The effect of temperature is especially important on sensory nerves, since in many peripheral neuropathies sensory changes occur before motor changes.[35]

The effects of positioning have not been studied extensively with regard to sensory nerves. We need to study the effect of wrist position on median nerve sensory potentials because of the common testing for carpal tunnel syndrome. In addition, we need to consider the effect of foot and ankle position when testing the sural nerve and the sensory portions of the lateral and medial plantar nerves.

We must also consider some of the difficulties in testing for second wave forms such as F wave and H reflex.[36] In F wave testing, error may be caused by failure of the examiner to understand the significance of the F wave. F wave testing cannot be averaged because the F wave latency varies for every stimulus; and an F wave does not occur with each stimulus. In 1979, Yates and Brown stated that the then current understanding of the F wave was so poor that using it for evaluation purposes was much too uncertain.[37] Use of the F wave has since increased, but only in limited ways. Our understanding of it has not changed.

In the upper extremity, distance measurements on subjects for F wave studies must be precise in order to duplicate the procedures used to generate the "normograms" used for comparisons,[38,39] as when arm length is measured from the ulnar styloid process to the C_7 cervical vertebra for estimation of arm length for F wave determinations of the upper extremity. The "normograms," which are based on arm length or on height, may not have been based on sufficient numbers of subjects to generate representative values for all members of the population.[38,39] However, because the shortest latency of a series of stimuli is the most important variable measured, many laboratories do not routinely concern themselves with the amplitude of the F wave. The amplitude of this wave often varies with every stimulus, making comparisons between sessions difficult. In most normal subjects, F responses can be readily obtained from the intrinsic muscles of the hands and feet.

There are many problems associated with use of the H reflex. It has been shown to be consistently valuable only for testing of the tibial nerve for either S_1 root lesions or neuropathies.[40–42] The H reflex can be obtained from nearly all nerves in infants and young children, but in adults it can be easily obtained only from the tibial nerve. In adults with central nervous system lesions, H waves can be obtained in nerves other than the tibial nerve, but this cannot be considered diagnostic of "upper motor neuron" lesions. Occasionally, H waves can also be found in the upper extremities of individuals who appear to have chronic peripheral neuropathies; again, this finding is not consistent enough to permit its use for diagnostic purposes.[40]

Those who plan to do testing of F and H waves should practice on a sufficient number of normal subjects until they can obtain the expected results 95 percent of the time. Unless the examiner has gone through this process, the question of whether the expected results can or cannot be obtained may relate more to the difficulty the examiner has in performing the examination than to any pathology present in the patient. To examine the methodological problems in this area, the reader should consult those references already cited.

CLINICAL ELECTROMYOGRAPHY

For the details on performing an EMG examination, any number of standard texts will provide some guidance. Some of the issues discussed in this section will also be found in these sources.[2,32,43,44,48,55]

In discussing measurement issues in clinical electromyography, there are three major problems. First, clinical electromyography remains highly subjective in many ways. The examination consists in large part of what the examiner sees on the oscilloscope and what he hears from the audio system at the time of the examination. Examiners often find it difficult to duplicate the events of the testing situation and to obtain identical results.

Second, there is lack of agreement among electromyographers about the characteristics of the various potentials. This is discussed in more detail below. Characteristics of various EMG potentials and results are interpreted differently in the literature.

Last, errors in reporting and interpretation occur. As with conduction velocity testing, a number of errors may be associated with technique and equipment. Examiners may mistakenly think that an electrode is placed in a muscle or that they see potentials where none are actually present, or they may over- or underinterpret findings.

Evidence of Subjectivity in EMG Examination

As with conduction velocity testing, a number of errors may be associated with technique and equipment. In this section, each of these possibilities will be briefly discussed.

During an EMG examination an examiner first looks for "insertional activity" (noise). Insertional activity has been defined as the EMG activity that occurs while the needle is advancing through muscle tissue.[2,32] Insertional activity can be abnormal if it is either decreased or increased. Decreased insertional activity can represent one of two things: either the muscle tissue is decreased (i.e., atrophied or not present), or the electrode is not in muscle tissue. If the needle is not in muscle tissue, reduced insertional noise is of no significance. However, if the needle is in muscle tissue and there is decreased insertional noise resulting from the decrease of tissue, the decrease of noise is an important clinical finding.

The other possibility is increased insertional activity. Increased insertional activity has been commonly accepted as the continuation of potentials firing for a brief period of time (2 to 3 seconds) after the needle has come to rest.[2,32,44] This is presumably caused by hyperirritability of muscle membranes and is considered normal. Finding specific information about insertional activity in standard texts is difficult.[2,32,44] Judgment of when insertional noise is increased or decreased remains highly subjective. The examiner is making an estimate of the situation. Subjectivity is present throughout the EMG examination.

Some examples of subjectivity may demonstrate the problem. when the needle has come to rest after insertion and the patient is relaxed, no electrical activity should be recorded from a normal subject. Activity seen when the person is presumably at rest is a spontaneous potential. There are several possible explanations. Abnormal potentials may be generated by muscle tissue. Denervation is a the most common abnormality of muscle tissue that causes potentials at rest.[2,32,43,44] However, it is possible to observe small potentials from patients who are not actually relaxed and who are therefore voluntarily firing motor units.[2,32,43,44] An experienced electromyographer can usually distinguish the differences between true spontaneous potentials and volitional activity, but it is a possible source of error based on individual interpretation.

Interpretation-based error is also evident in determinations of the percentage of polyphasic potentials seen on contraction. Polyphasic potentials are motor unit potentials that represent abnormal motor unit function.[2]

Small numbers of polyphasic potentials occur in normal individuals; however, when some "critical" level is exceeded, an abnormality or a pathology is thought to be present.[2] This "critical level" is a subjective determination by the electromyographer. The examiner must consider the number of polyphasic potentials that have been encountered in other muscles. The age of the subject may affect the number of polyphasic potentials that are being displayed.[45] We must then decide what number of polyphasic potentials are no longer considered normal. Levels for polyphasic potentials of 3 percent to 15 percent have been accepted as normal.[2,45,56]

Error also results from volume conduction from normal muscle that is recorded through a needle electrode placed in denervated muscle. Activity is recorded when the surrounding normal muscle contracts.[2,43] These potentials are usually distant and indistinct in display.[2] Some electromyographers occasionally interpret these potentials as activity from the muscle where the needle is located. The experienced electromyographer can prevent this type of error.

Characteristics of EMG Potentials as a Potential Source of Error

Problems are also caused because electromyographers differ as to what they accept as normal characteristics of a person's potentials. Five characteristics of an EMG potential can be examined: (1) duration of the potential, (2) frequency of occurrence of the potential; (3) size or the amplitude of the potential; (4) characteristics of the wave form (number of phases and configuration of the potential); and (5) sound that is generated by the potential.[47]

Four or five of the standard EMG textbooks show numerous variations and omissions in the description of some of the wave forms, such as differences in description of the normal motor unit. The following discrepancies can be found: normal motor unit durations are cited as being 2 to 10 ms or 4 to 17 ms in duration.[2,47] A 17-ms duration is 7 ms longer than the first upper limit: this is a large difference.

The frequency of firing for the normal motor unit has been described as varying from 20 to 50 Hz by some authors, whereas others have reported that a single motor unit can fire up to 60 Hz.[2,47] It must be understood that the frequency of firing of a motor unit is under voluntary control. When a person is asked to perform muscular activity at higher and higher levels of demand, he or she then recruits more motor units, and/or the motor units are fired at higher frequencies.

In clinical EMG, it is difficult to determine firing rates of motor units beyond a certain level of muscular effort unless there is a decreased number of motor units that are active. With increased activity, the counting of the firing rates of individual motor units becomes increasingly difficult. When there is a decrease in the number of available motor units, as in partially innervated muscle, it is easier to count frequencies of motor units because the response to increased demand is increased frequencies.

The amplitude of the normal motor unit potential is another variable that lacks a standard description for "normal." Many investigators state that motor units that are larger than 2 mV are abnormal.[44,47] However, other electromyographers state that 5 mV potentials are common and should not be considered pathological.[2] EMG potentials are generally measured from peak to peak of the wave.[48] In some of the standard texts, it is not clear what is being measured.[2,47]

Descriptions of fibrillation potentials also vary. This potential is of such fundamental importance in electromyography that there should be fairly high levels of agreement about its characteristics. The duration of fibrillation potentials is reported by some authors as of a very short duration of (2 ms or less).[47] Others have reported durations of fibrillation potentials as long as 5 ms.[49] There is also inconsistency in descriptions of frequency of firing in fibrillation potentials. Frequencies of 10 to 15 Hz and of frequencies up to 60 Hz have been reported.[2,47-49] Examiners should report what is most commonly seen during an examination. Fibrillation potentials often have a frequency of 10 to 15 Hz. Occasionally, higher frequencies may be seen; lower firing rates are commonly seen.

There is also disagreement about the amplitude of fibrillation potentials, with amplitudes of 600 to 800 μV or higher being reported.[2,47-49] Fibrillation potentials are commonly between 50 and 150 μV. Even descriptions of fibrillation forms are a subject of controversy. Most investigators report that the wave form is biphasic and that the initial wave is always positive, but some authors have reported that the initial wave can be negative and that sometimes a complex wave form for some fibrillation potentials is seen. These discrepancies make it extremely difficult for the electromyographer to know what to expect. There is no universal definition even for something as simple as a fibrillation potential. I keep life as simple as possible and draw arbitrary limits on the definition of a fibrillation potential by assuming that it should be biphasic with an initial positive phase and should have a short duration (3 ms or less).

In future studies, all of the different EMG potentials that have been described should be discussed and differences described by various authors on the characteristics of each of these potentials should be sorted out.[2,32,43-45,47,48] It is important to realize that these differences exist, because many measurement issues in clinical electromyography must be resolved.

This very important measurement principle must be considered when sophisticated equipment is used. Clinical electromyographic equipment has become more and more sophisticated, making possible better and easier displays of the electrical activity recorded from a muscle. This has included improvements such as digital storage and the ability to store larger amounts of EMG activity for review. The equipment, however, does not make decisions about what the electromyographer sees on the oscilloscope. The improvement in electromyographic equipment probably has decreased errors because of the subjectivity of electromyographers. If a potential can be stored its amplitude, its duration, its frequency, and the wave form certainly can be measured more easily than it is when storage is not available. However, differences in interpretation still exist.

There is a tendency at times to make judgments based on the use of sophisticated equipment rather than on sound clinical observations. In electromyography it is possible (and dangerous) to substitute sophisticated testing for clinical judgment. Some physicians routinely refer patients for EMG examinations for such problems as low back pain. A patient may have no signs or symptoms of nerve root pathology, but finds himself being examined by an electromyographer because the primary practitioner doubts his own clinical judgment that the patient has no nerve root problem related to low back pain.

Literature describing electromyography is voluminous, making it difficult for any one electromyographer to be aware of all the nuances therein. A good example is shown in the discussion of the descriptions and names used for wave forms. We have described some of the characteristics of a normal motor unit and some of the problems in defining those characteristics precisely. Several years ago, Taverner described a group of motor units (that he called, for lack of a better name, abnormal motor units)[50] that were either shorter in duration or longer in duration than normal motor units, but that otherwise had all the characteristics of normal motor units. He felt that these disturbances probably represented a neuropathic abnormality. Very few other electromyographers have discussed this particular group of motor unit potentials.

Smorto and Basmajian used the term "skewed potentials" to describe a group of potentials that he felt were connected primarily with chronic neuropathic problems.[43] The wave forms were usually in the positive direction and of longer duration and larger amplitude than is normal. They also stated that they frequently found these potentials to be the primary manifestation of old neuropathic problems. To my knowledge, they are the only authors who have referred to these potentials; this presents a problem. If I see these kinds of potentials and have read Smorto and Basmajian's description of them, I also refer to them as "skewed potentials" and interpret the potentials as they did.[9] One has to ask if these potentials have only recently come into being or if there is a tendency among clinical electromyographers to ignore things that they see on the oscilloscope or hear on the loudspeaker and do not understand or for which they have no categories. To attempt to solve this problem, terms should be more precisely and universally defined.[51]

Techniques and Equipment as Sources of Error

The effect of electrode type on potentials has not received full discussion in the literature.[2,32,44,52-54] Two kinds of needle electrodes are commonly used clinically. The coaxial needle electrode has an active or recording electrode, which is a platinum wire embedded in a hypodermic needle. Insulation is inserted between the active electrode and the surrounding needle. The surrounding needle becomes the reference electrode, and the recording area is the bare tip of the active electrode exposed at the end of the needle. With this electrode arrangement, the interelectrode distance remains the same at all times. The second commonly used electrode is the monopolar needle, usually a needle covered with teflon except for the bare tip used for recording. Monopolar electrodes are used with small disk electrodes placed on the surface of the skin near the needle. The disk serves as the reference electrode. Occcasionally an electromyographer uses two needle electrodes, one a surface needle electrode that is inserted into the skin as a reference electrode.

Clinical electromyographers tend to use the type of needle electrode that was suggested to them by the person who taught them electromyographic technique, rather than choosing an electrode based on the advantages of one type over another. Each electrode has advantages. The coaxial electrode is easier to move from one site to another since there is no reference electrode that has to be moved. This allows the electromyographer to move quickly and easily from one muscle site to the next. The coaxial needle electrode has a disadvantage in that it has a slightly larger bore than a monopolar needle and therefore causes more patient discomfort. With the coaxial needlle, the interelectrode distance does not change and the recording area is smaller than it is with a monopolar electrode.

Those who favor the monopolar needle cite its comfort for the patient. It has a narrower bore and a teflon coating that permits it to slide through the tissues more easily than does the noncoated coaxial needle. A major difference between coaxial and monopolar electrodes is the size of the recording area. The area is much larger with monopolar electrodes as is the inter-electrode distance. The distance actually varies with each needle insertion since the reference electrode remains in one place. One of the problems with the use of monopolar needles is that some examiners do not maintain a rigid clinical technique of keeping the reference electrode close to the monopolar needle. I have seen electromyographers use monopolar electrodes 6 or more inches away from their reference electrode. One can appreciate the differences in inter-electrode distances that occur when a monopolar needle that is approximately 2 inches in length is fully inserted into a muscle as compared with the difference when the needle has been withdrawn to more and more superficial areas. The inter-electrode distance can vary from $2\frac{1}{2}$ inches at the deepest location to only $\frac{1}{2}$ inch at the most superficial location. This factor is magnified when the monopolar needle is approximately 5 or 6 inches away from the reference electrode.

There are differences in reported amplitudes, complexity of wave forms, and even the possibility of more frequently reported positive sharp waves by those who use monopolar needles as opposed to those who use coaxial needles.[52–54] The difference between the two needle types may be of clinical significance, and since it is a possible source of variability in findings, it is a continuing issue in measurement.

Reporting and Interpretation Errors

In clinical electromyography, error often occurs in reporting of results. Johnson states that electromyographers must know which muscle they are recording information from because they may have made an anatomical error.[55] This could certainly be of significance in determining a patient's problem, and can result from a failure to understand the cross-sectional anatomy of the area in which the needle electrode is inserted. The needle is sometimes inserted all the way through the muscle that is being examined and as a result records from deeper muscles. The needle electrode sometimes passes in a lateral direction into an adjacent muscle.

Errors in reporting the amount of interference activity obtained on full resisted muscle activity may occur. Electromyographers may misinterpret the amount of activity present because they misjudge the patient's effort; therefore, examiners may state there is a decreased interference pattern. Pain may inhibit muscle activity and lead to a decreased interference pattern that may have nothing to do with the number of active motor units available.

Error also results from anomalous innervation. The literature contains many reports of common variations in the innervation of muscles,[56,57] such as the Martin-Gruber anastomosis between the ulnar and median nerves described in nearly every anatomy textbook and Spinner's work on the upper extremity. Great variations in innervation can exist at both peripheral nerve and nerve root levels. Therefore, errors can occur because of a failure to appreciate the patient's anomalous innervation.[56] Electromyographers must be aware of the most common anomalous innervations in the extremities that they are testing.

It is important to realize that both nerve conduction velocity and EMG testing are commonly performed together. Because nerve conduction velocity and electromyographic testing often accompany each other, they can be used together to detect anomalous innervations that could not be detected with a single technique.

Johnson reports other common faults in reporting, one of the most common being a failure to perform an adequate examination.[55] Electromyographers probably should err on the side of doing too much examination rather than too little. Reports of electromyographers who have based conclusions on very limited muscle sampling have often astonished me. Often, errors in the EMG examination technique cause error in interpretation. An electromyographer often examines a preselected set of muscles and nerves rather than basing his or her study on the clinical problem of the patient, as when six preselected muscles in the lower extremity are examined for suspected nerve root pathology of the lumbar area.

Another problem is the over-interpretation of EMG findings. A few abnormal potentials are not indicative of pathology in most persons.[55] Problems inn electromyographic interpretation are similar to those that occur in interpretation of a research project; there is a danger that some may over-interpret the results of an examination; the other danger is lies in under-interpretation. Important information is sometimes not properly or adequately interpreted; therefore, its significance is missed.

EMG AS A KINESIOLOGICAL RESEARCH TOOL

The use of electromyography as a kinesiological research tool is certainly not new; the book *Muscles Alive*, authored by Basmajian, now in its 4th edition, is evidence of this.[52] Use of kinesiological EMG has been a very important tool for the analysis and understanding of muscle function. Major issues in Kinesiological EMG will be briefly considered here.

There has been a continuing controversy about both electrode placement and the electrode types used in kinesiological EMG. Exhaustive discussions of these topics, are presented in several standard reference texts.[52,58] There is controversy about the type and quality of data that can be recorded with surface, fine wire, or needle electrodes. The choice of electrode depends on the kind of information the investigator is seeking. Surface electrodes are appropriate for recording EMG activity when one is concerned with whether the muscle under the electrode is active during certain movements. The electrodes in this instance are placed over relatively large muscle masses. Needle or wire electrodes are obviously needed if the same question is asked about muscles that are not superficial. One of the difficulties with wire or needle electrodes is that the recording area is very small, much smaller than that of a surface electrode. With wire or needle electrodes, the information obtained can be related specifically to the muscle in which the electrode is embedded.[52]

A major concern of the kinesiologist deals with the relationship of the electrical activity measured with the muscle force being produced. Most investigators believe that there can only be a rough approximation between the amount of EMG activity recorded and muscle force measures.[30,58] The more EMG activity recorded, the more active the contraction; therefore, more motor units fire or they fire more frequently. But there is not always a linear relationship for measures between EMG and muscle activity.[30,58] One reason for this may be the volume conduction that is recorded when surface electrodes are used, particularly if the surface electrodes are not placed directly over the muscle belly. When one uses needle or wire electrodes and is trying to make an approximation between muscle activity and muscle efforts, the small size of the recording field may have an effect on the information recorded.[52,54]

Kinesiological EMG measurements are often normalized. Normalization means to "make normal or according to the standard."[31,60] In electromyography, one of the questions often asked is whether one activity involves more electrical activity from the muscle than another exercise or functional activity. Researchers will often use a standard contraction that everyone will understand as the standard for comparison with the other activities, as when they want to know how much activity was recorded from the tibialis anterior during a particular functional activity or exercise. One might perform a manual muscle test for the tibialis anterior and record the EMG activity. This value could then be used as the standard against which the other activities will be measured. In other words, all other EMG values would be expressed as a percentage of the EMG measured during the maximal contraction. This is one form of normalization. The purpose of normalization is to assist the researcher in interpreting the data obtained from an experiment. This is achieved by making the normalized activity for each subject the measurement that is used for all comparisons of activity that are of interest to the researcher. This eliminates the need to control for the variability that occurs across subjects (because of anatomical differences) and the variability seen in data collected on different days when electrodes must be reapplied to the same subject.

The International Society of Electrophysiological Kinesiology (ISEK) has published a paper that describes the terminology and standards used in EMG research.[59] This document discusses the important measurement issues in kinesiological EMG and describes the importance of reporting how the research was conducted, particularly the type of electrode used, inter-electrode distance, manner of skin preparation used for surface electrodes, the type of electrode paste used, etc. Also discussed are the issues surrounding use of terminology such as "integrated EMG" and "averaged EMG". The term, integrated EMG, has not always been used in the same way by all investigators. The recording equipment used has a great influence on whether the EMG is truly integrated or whether it is merely an average of the electrical activity seen by the electrodes. The ISEK report also has sections of definitions for contraction types and some biomechanical terms. Use of the ISEK paper would assist EMG investigators and improve communications about EMG research.

This brief discussion of some of the measurement issues in kinesiological EMG is far from exhaustive, it is hoped that the reader who contemplates using EMG will consult some of the literature in this area and be aware of potential sources of measurement error.

SUMMARY

This chapter has discussed some of the difficulties in the clinical uses of nerve conduction testing and electromyography. There has been tremendous growth in the interest in this type of testing. The sophistication of the equipment used to perform clinical testing has improved. Use of both nerve conduction studies and EMG have made contributions to the understanding of musculoskeletal and neuromuscular problems and to the clinical management of many of these problems. In the hands of an experienced and careful examiner, these studies can provide the clinician with reliable and valid information. In this chapter, some of the difficulties in interpreting some of these studies have been discussed in order to bring this information to the attention of clinicians. This does not in any way minimize the importance of EMG and nerve conduction studies; it just means that intelligent examiners should be aware of the problems associated with this important clinical technique.

REFERENCES

1. Hodes R, Larabee MG, German W: The human electromyogram in response to nerve stimulation and the conduction velocity of motor axons. Studies on normal and on injured peripheral nerves, Arch Neurol Psychiatry 60:340, 1984
2. Goodgold J, Eberstein A: Electrodiagnosis of Neuromuscular Disease, 2nd Ed., Williams & Wilkins, Baltimore, 1978

3. Smorto MR, Basmajian JV: Clinical Electroneuromyography, 2nd Ed., Williams & Wilkins, Baltimore, 1979

4. Dawson GD, Scott JW: The recording of nerve action potentials through the skin in man. Neurol Neurosurg Psychiatry 12:259, 1949

5. Currier DP: Value of the magnitude of the muscle action potential. Phys Ther 51:1000, 1971

6. Currier DP: Placement of recording electrode in median and peroneal nerve conduction studies. Phys Ther 55:356, 1975

7. Burke J: Electrode placement and muscle action potential amplitudes. Phys ther 53:127, 1973

8. Pinelli P: Physical, anatomical and physiological factors in the latency measurement of the M response. Electroenceph Clin Neurophys 17:86, 1964

9. Klein B, Echternach J, Levy F: Inter- and intra-tester reliability in the performance of nerve conduction testing. Proceedings of APTA Annual Conference, June 1981

10. Braddon RH, Schuchmann J: In Johnson EW (ed): Motor Conduction in Practical Electromyography, Williams & Wilkins Baltimore, 1980

11. Buchtal F, Rosenfalk A, Torjaborg W: Electrophysiological findings in entrapment of the median nerve at the wrist and elbow. J Neurol Neurosurg Psychiatry 37:340, 1974

12. Melvin JL, Harris DH, Johnson GW: Sensory and motor conduction velocity in ulnar and median nerves. Arch Phys Med Rehab 42:57, 1966

13. Jebsen RH: Motor conduction in the median and ulnar nerves. Arch Phys Med Rehab 48:185, 1976

14. Johnson EW, Ortiz PR: Electrodiagnosis of tarsal tunnel syndrome. Arch Phys Med Rehabil 47:776, 1966

15. Maynard FM, Stolov WC: Experimental error in determination of nerve conduction velocity. Arch Phys Med Rehab 43:362, 1972

16. Checkles NS, Barley JA, Johnson EW: Tape and caliper surface measurements in determination of peroneal nerve conduction study. Arch Phys Med Rehab 50:214, 1969

17. Echternach JL, Levy F: Motor conduction velocities of the radial nerve: an analysis of measurement errors. Proceedings of USPHS Professional Association, Crystal City, VA, 1980

18. Gassel MM: Sources of error in motor nerve conduction studies. Neurology 14:825, 1964

19. Checkles NS, Russakov AD, Piero DL: Ulnar nerve conduction velocity: effect of elbow position on measurement. Arch Phys Med Rehab 52:362, 1971

20. Nelson RM: Effects of elbow position in motor conduction velocity of the ulnar nerve. Phys Ther 60:780, 1980

21. Schubert HA: Conduction velocities along the course of the ulnar nerve. J Appl Physiol 19:423, 1964.

22. Jebsen RH: Motor conduction velocity in the median and ulnar nerves. Arch Phys Med Rehab 48:185, 1967

23. Oh SJ: Clinical electromyography: Nerve conduction studies. pp. 47–64. In Nerve Conduction Techniques. University Park Press, Baltimore, 1984

24. Hendriksen J: Conduction velocity of motor nerves in normal subjects and patients with neuromuscular disorders. Master's thesis, University of Minnesota, 1956

25. Halar EM, DeLisa JA, Brozovich FV: Peroneal nerve conduction velocity: the importance of temperature correction. Arch Phys Med Rehab 62:439, 1981

26. Halar EM, DeLisa JA, Brozovich FV: Nerve conduction velocity: relationship of skin subcutaneous and intramuscular temperature. Arch Phys Med Rehab 61:199, 1980

27. Goldberg NJ, Rogoff JB, Levine B: A spring-loaded electrode for sensory nerve conduction. Arch Phys Med Rehab 49:665, 1968

28. Shahani B, Goodgold J, Spielholz N: Sensory nerve action potentials in the radial nerve. Arch Phys Med Rehab 48:602, 1969

29. DiBenedetto M: Sensory nerve conduction in the lower extremities. Arch Phys Med Rehab 51:253, 1970

30. Buchthal F, Rosenfalk A: Evoked action potentials and conduction velocity in human sensory nerves. Brain Res 3:1, 1966

31. Lundin H, Tackmann W: Sensory Neurography, Thieme-Stratton, New York, 1981

32. Aminoff MJ: Electromyography in Clinical Practice. Addison-Wesley, Menlo Park, New Jersey, 1978

33. Liberson Gratzer M, Zales A, et al: Comparison of conduction velocities of motor and sensory fibers determined by different methods. Arch Phys Med Rehab 47:17, 1966

34. Ruskin P, Rogoff JB: Simultaneous sensory and motor conduction latency noting effect of topical anesthasia. Arch Phys Med Rehab 45:597, 1964

35. Ludin HP, Beyeler F: Temperature dependency of normal sensory nerve action potentials. J Neurol 216:173, 1977

36. Magladery JW, McDougal DB: Electrophysiological studies of nerve and reflex activity in normal man. The identification of certain reflexes in the electromyogram and the conduction velocity of peripheral nerve fibers. Bull Johns Hopkins Hosp 86:265, 1950

37. Yates SK, Brown WF: Characteristics of the F response: a single motor unit study. J Neurol, Neurosurg Psych 42:161, 1979

38. Weber RJ, Piero DL: F wave evaluation of thoracic outlet syndrome: a multiple regression derived F wave latency predicting technique. Arch Phys Med Rehab 59:464, 1978

39. Eisen A, Schomer D, Melmed C: The application of F wave measurements in the differentiation of proximal and distal upper limb segments. Neurology 27:662, 1977

40. Lachman T, Shahani BT, Young RR: Late responses as aides to diagnosis in peripheral neuropathy. J Neurol Neurosurg Psych 43:156, 1980

41. Braddon RI, Johnson EW: Standardization of H reflex and diagnostic use in S1 radiculopathy. Arch Phys Med Rehab 55:161, 1974

42. Wager EW, Buerger, AA: H-reflex latency and sensory conduction velocity in normal and diabetic subjects. Arch Phys Med Rehab 55:126, 1974

43. Smorto MR, Basmajian JV: Electrodiagnosis, A Handbook for Neurologists. Harper and Row, Hagerstown, Maryland, 1977

44. Aminoff MJ: Electrodiagnosis in Clinical Neurology. Churchhill Livingstone, New York 1980

45. Marinacci AA: Applied Electromyography. Lea & Febiger, Philadelphia 1968

46. Hoover BB, Caldwell JW, Krusen EM, et al: Value of polyphasic potentials in diagnosis of lumbar root lesions. Arch Phys Med Rehab 51:546, 1970

47. Rodriquez AA, Oester YT: Fundamentals of Electromyography. p. 297. In Licht S (Ed): Electrodiagnosis and Electromyography, E. Licht, New Haven, 1971

48. Johnson EW, Parker WD: Electromyographic examination. p. 1. In Johnson EW (ed): Practical Electromyography, Williams & Wilkins, Baltimore, 1980

49. Buchthal F, Rosenfalck P: Spontaneous electrical activity of human muscle. Electroenceph Clin neurophys 20:321, 1966

50. Taverner D: Clinical Applications of Electromyography, p. 342. In Licht S (ed): Electrodiagnosis and Electromyography, 2nd Ed. E. Licht, New Haven, 1965
51. Glossary of Terms Used in Clinical Electromyography. Compiled by The Nomenclature Committee of the American Association of Electromyography and Electrodiagnosis, Rochester, Minesota, 1980
52. Basmajian JV: Muscles Alive: Their Functions Revealed by Electromyography, 4th Ed., Williams & Wilkins, Baltimore, 1978
53. Reiner S, Rogoff JB: Instrumentation, p. 349. In Johnson EW (ed): Practical Electromyography. Williams & Wilkins, Baltimore, 1980
54. Geddes LA: Electrodes and the Measurement of Bioelectric Events. Wiley, New York, 1972
55. Johnson EW, Parker WD: Interpreting and Reporting, p. 308. In Johnson EW (ed): Practical Electromyography. Williams & Wilkins, Baltimore, 1980
56. Spinner M: Injuries to the Major Branches of Peripheral Nerves WB Saunders, Philadelphia, 1972
57. Guttmann L: Important anomalous innervations of the extremities. Minimonograph No. 2, American Association of electromyography and Electrodiagnosis, Rochester, Minnesota, 1981
58. DeLuca CJ: Towards understanding the EMG signal, p. xxx. In Basmajian JV (ed): Muscles Alive, 4th Ed. Williams & Wilkins, Baltimore, 1978
59. Report by the Ad Hoc Committee of the International Society of Electrophysiological Kinesiology: Units, Terms and Standards in Reporting of EMG Research, August, 1980
60. Stedman's Medical Dictionary, 23rd Ed., Williams & Wilkins, Baltimore, 1976

Index